RADIOLOGY

CASE REVIEW SERIES | Breast Imaging

RADIOLOGY

CASE REVIEW SERIES | Breast Imaging

Chris I. Flowers, MD, FRCR, FSBI

Director of Breast Imaging and Research
Department of Diagnostic Imaging
H. Lee Moffitt Cancer Center & Research Institute

Associate Professor of Radiology
Department of Oncological Sciences
College of Medicine
University of South Florida
Tampa, Florida

Markus K. Holzhauer, MD

Windsong Radiology Group
Williamsville, New York

SERIES EDITOR

Roland Talanow, MD, PhD

President
Department of Radiology Education
Radiolopolis, a subdivision of InnoMed, LLC
Stateline, Nevada

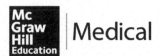

New York   Chicago   San Francisco   Athens   London
Madrid   Mexico City   Milan   New Delhi   Singapore
Sydney   Toronto

Radiology Case Review Series: Breast Imaging

Copyright © 2014 by McGraw-Hill Education. All rights reserved. Printed in the United States of America. Except as permitted under the United States Copyright Act of 1976, no part of this publication may be reproduced or distributed in any form or by any means, or stored in a data base or retrieval system, without the prior written permission of the publisher.

9 LKV 24

ISBN 978-0-07-178719-2
MHID 0-07-178719-4

This book was set in Times LT Std. by Thomson Digital.
The editors were Michael Weitz and Robert Pancotti.
The production supervisor was Catherine H. Saggese.
Project management was provided by Ritu Joon, Thomson Digital.
The text designer was Elise Lansdon; the cover designer was Anthony Landi.
LSC Communications was the printer and binder.

This book is printed on acid-free paper.

Library of Congress Cataloging-in-Publication Data

Flowers, Chris, author.
  Breast imaging / Chris I. Flowers, Markus K. Holzhauer.—Edition 1.
    p. ; cm.—(Radiology case review series)
  Includes bibliographical references and index.
  ISBN-13: 978-0-07-178719-2 (softcover : alk. paper)
  ISBN-10: 0-07-178719-4
  I. Holzhauer, Markus K., author. II. Title. III. Series: Radiology case review series.
  [DNLM: 1. Mammography—methods—Case Reports. 2. Mammography—methods—Problems and Exercises. 3. Breast Diseases—radiography—Case Reports. 4. Breast Diseases—radiography—Problems and Exercises. WP 815]
  RG493.5.R33
  618.1'907572—dc23
                                                                                    2013028633

McGraw-Hill Education books are available at special quantity discounts to use as premiums and sales promotions or for use in corporate training programs. To contact a representative, please visit the Contact Us pages at www.mhprofessional.com.

To our wives and families who have had to put up
with endless hours of poring over cases and our computers,
when we could have been taking the family to the Mall or
off on road trips. Thank you for your patience,
and here is the reward.

Contents

Series Preface

Maybe I have an obsession for cases, but when I was a radiology resident I loved to learn especially from cases, not only because they are short, exciting, and fun—similar to a detective story in which the aim is to get to "the bottom" of the case—but also because, in the end, that's what radiologists are faced with during their daily work. Since medical school, I have been fascinated with learning, not only for my own benefit but also for the sake of teaching others, and I have enjoyed combining my IT skills with my growing knowledge to develop programs that help others in their learning process. Later, during my radiology residency, my passion for case-based learning grew to a level where the idea was born to create a case-based journal: integrating new concepts and technologies that aid in the traditional learning process. Only a few years later, the *Journal of Radiology Case Reports* became an internationally popular and PubMed indexed radiology journal—popular not only because of the interactive features but also because of the case-based approach. This led me to the next step: why not tackle something that I especially admired during my residency but that could be improved—creating a new interactive case-based review series. I imagined a book series that would take into account new developments in teaching and technology and changes in the examination process.

As did most other radiology residents, I loved the traditional case review books, especially for preparation for the boards. These books are quick and fun to read and focus in a condensed way on material that will be examined in the final boards. However, nothing is perfect and these traditional case review books had their own intrinsic flaws. The authors and I have tried to learn from our experience by putting the good things into this new book series but omitting the bad parts and exchanging them with innovative features.

What are the features that distinguish this series from traditional series of review books?

To save space, traditional review books provide two cases on one page. This requires the reader to turn the page to read the answer for the first case but could lead to unintentional "cheating" by seeing also the answer of the second case. Doesn't this defeat the purpose of a review book? From my own authoring experience on the *USMLE Help* book series, it was well appreciated that we avoided such accidental cheating by separating one case from the other. Taking the positive experience from that book series, we decided that each case in this series should consist of two pages: page 1 with images and questions and page 2 with the answers and explanations. This approach avoids unintentional peeking at the answers before deciding on the correct answers yourself. We keep it strict: one case per page! This way it remains up to your own knowledge to figure out the right answer.

Another example that residents (including me) did miss in traditional case review books is that these books did not highlight the pertinent findings on the images: sometimes, even looking at the images as a group of residents, we could not find the abnormality. This is not only frustrating but also time consuming. When you prepare for the boards, you want to use your time as efficiently as possible. Why not show annotated images? We tackled that challenge by providing, on the second page of each case, the same images with annotations or additional images that highlight the findings.

When you are preparing for the boards and managing your clinical duties, time is a luxury that becomes even more precious. Does the resident preparing for the boards truly need lengthy discussions as in a typical textbook? Or does the resident rather want a "rapid fire" mode in which he or she can "fly" through as many cases as possible in the shortest possible time? This is the reality when you start your work after the boards! Part of our concept with the new series is providing short "pearls" instead of lengthy discussions. The reader can easily read and memorize these "pearls."

Another challenge in traditional books is that questions are asked on the first page and no direct answer is provided, only a lengthy block of discussion. Again, this might become time consuming to find the right spot where the answer is located if you have doubts about one of several answer choices. Remember: time is money—and life! Therefore, we decided to provide explanations to *each* individual question, so that the reader knows exactly where to find the right answer to the right question. Questions are phrased in an intuitive way so that they fit not only the print version but also the multiple-choice questions for that particular case in our online version. This system enables you to move back and forth between the print version and the online version.

In addition, we have provided up to 3 references for each case. This case review is not intended to replace traditional textbooks. Instead, it is intended to reiterate and strengthen your already existing knowledge (from your training) and to fill potential gaps in your knowledge.

However, in a collaborative effort with the *Journal of Radiology Case Reports* and the international radiology community Radiolopolis, we have developed an online repository with more comprehensive information for each case, such as demographics, discussions, more image examples, interactive image stacks with scroll, a window/level feature, and other interactive features that almost resemble a workstation. In addition, we are planning ahead toward the new Radiology Boards format and are providing rapid fire online sessions and mock examinations that use the cases in the print version. Each case in the print version is crosslinked to the online version using a case ID. The case ID number appears to the right of the diagnosis heading at the top of the second page of each case. Each case can be accessed using the case ID number at the following web site: www.radiologycasereviews.com/case/ID, in which "ID" represents the case ID number. If you have any questions regarding this web site, please e-mail the series editor directly at roland@talanow.info.

I am particularly proud of such a symbiotic endeavor of print and interactive online education and I am grateful to McGraw-Hill for giving me and the authors the opportunity to provide such a unique and innovative method of radiology education, which, in my opinion, may be a trendsetter.

The primary audience of this book series is the radiology resident, particularly the resident in the final year who is preparing for the radiology boards. However, each book in this series is structured on difficulty levels so that the series also becomes useful to an audience with limited experience in radiology (nonradiologist physicians or medical students) up to subspecialty-trained radiologists who are preparing for their CAQs or who just want to refresh their knowledge and use this series as a reference.

I am delighted to have such an excellent team of US and international educators as authors on this innovative book series. These authors have been thoroughly evaluated and selected based on their excellent contributions to the *Journal of Radiology Case Reports*, the Radiolopolis community, and other academic and scientific accomplishments.

It brings especially personal satisfaction to me that this project has enabled each author to be involved in the overall decision-making process and improvements regarding the print and online content. This makes each participant not only an author but also part of a great radiology product that will appeal to many readers.

Finally, I hope you will experience this case review book as it is intended to be: a quick, pertinent, "get to the point" radiology case review that provides essential information for the radiology boards in the shortest time available, which, in the end, is crucial for preparation for the boards.

Roland Talanow, MD, PhD

Preface

For physicians working in the breast imaging field, there have been more challenges than in most disciplines in radiology. Breast cancer diagnosis and treatment have changed significantly over the last decade or two, along with the technologies that have been used and the planes in which we have visualized the breast. Along with the changes in techniques and advances in knowledge have come the requirements of regulatory and quality control, in both the United States and Europe. In the United States, the US Food and Drug Administration regulates the field according to the Mammography Standards Quality Act (MSQA), with minimum requirements for physicians practicing in this field. At the same time, the US board examinations have changed to include a high standard of knowledge in a few subjects in the final examination.

With this background, the authors, who both are of European origin and work in the United States, one in academic practice and one in community (private) practice, have produced a case review book that consists of images, test questions, and easy-to-read answers. For those readers preparing to take their final board examinations, the cases, discussions, and pearls should cover most of the topics that may appear on the examination. For those who seek more extensive learning, the book is supplemented with an interactive online component that includes high-resolution images and extra teaching points. We hope that you enjoy reading through this textbook and that you benefit greatly from using it.

Any abnormality in the left breast?

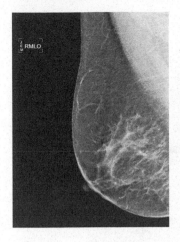 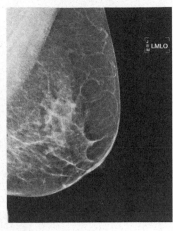 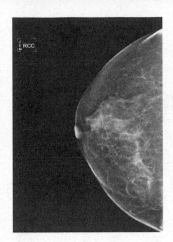 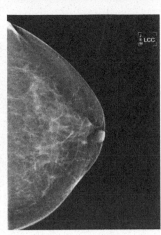

1. If there is a one-view-only asymmetry, what could be the next step?

2. If a patient was in the office at the time of the exam, what could be the next step?

3. What is a technical repeat in general?

4. What is the most likely malignancy explaining a one-view-only asymmetry?

5. What are the factors that make the judgment difficult, if this is a real finding?

Case ranking/difficulty: 🍁

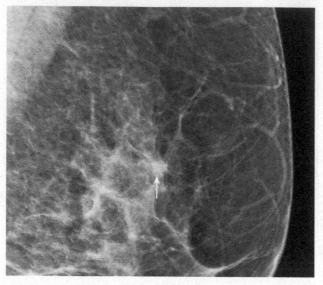

Electronically magnified image of the left MLO screening view.

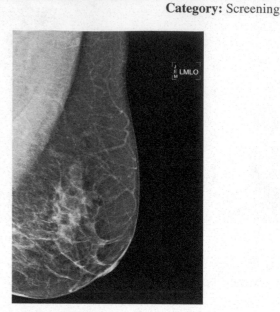

Repeat left MLO view with different angle demonstrating resolution of the questionable asymmetry.

Answers

1. If there is an asymmetric density seen in one view only, decision has to be made first whether this is real or it is a result of projection and overlying tissue. If the finding is believed to be real, the patient has to be recalled, and if the finding is believed to be the result of projection, then the patient can be classified as BI-RADS 1 negative.

2. If the patient is still in office, a repeat MLO view with different angle could be done and the patient could still be handled as a screening patient. This is not a common environment, since batch reading is performed in the vast majority of places in the United States. If a spot compression view is performed, the patient had to be handled as "recall" and the exam should be labeled as diagnostic mammogram.

3. If there is an indeterminate finding that needs workup, it is called a diagnostic mammogram. If there is limited exam because of motion, incomplete inclusion of tissue, or bad compression, repeat standard views or XCCL view can be added as a "technical repeat."

    If this mammogram is obtained with the patient still available in the office, an additional image can be added with a different angle and the exam could still be classified as a screening exam. However, this scenario is not common, since most screening exams are read without the patient being present (batch reading).

4. Lobular invasive carcinoma is most likely the type of malignancy that can manifest in the form of an asymmetry seen on one view only.

5. One way to eliminate the call back of "one-view-only findings" is to correlate the images with prior studies. Also helpful is if the breast is not very dense which makes correlation with the other plane easier. In case of nipple discharge or palpable abnormality, the patient should be diagnosed in the first place.

Pearls

- The overwhelming numbers of one-view-only densities are the result of superimposed breast tissue.
- According to the study of Sickles, 82.7% of these cases could be classified as superimposed tissue based on the standard views or through additional workup.
- Of the remainder of the cases, only a very small fraction turned out to be malignant (less than 2%). Of these cases, most were lobular invasive carcinomas.

Suggested Readings

Pearson KL, Sickles EA, Frankel SD, Leung JW. Efficacy of step-oblique mammography for confirmation and localization of densities seen on only one standard mammographic view. *AJR Am J Roentgenol.* 2000;174(3):745-752.

Sickles EA. Findings at mammographic screening on only one standard projection: outcomes analysis. *Radiology.* 1998;208(2):471-475.

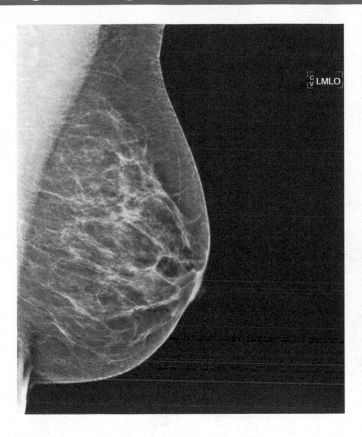
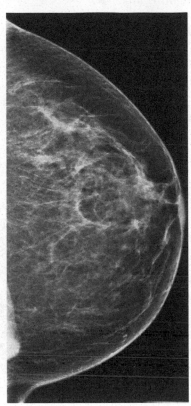

1. If you see this density on the CC view on screening mammogram, what is the next step?

2. What other options might help if there is clinical concern?

3. How frequent is that finding?

4. What else could be helpful to determine if density in the medial posterior breast is benign?

5. If this was a new suspicious finding, where could it likely hide on the MLO view?

Case ranking/difficulty:

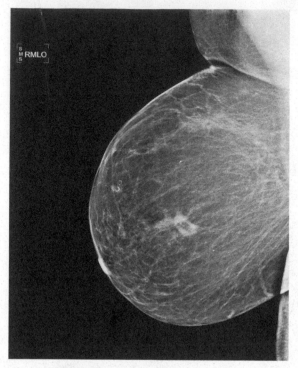

Screening mammogram, right MLO view.

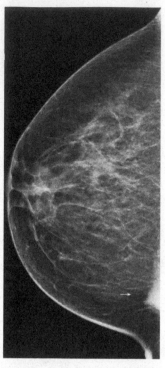

Screening mammogram, right CC view.

Answers

1. This is a typical appearance of a sternalis muscle; in this particular case, bilaterally—it is considered a congenital variant—patient can return after 1 year for screening.

2. If clinical concern, further workup with modified CC views and possible ultrasound might be considered. If this is a sternalis muscle, ultrasound will be normal. As an alternative, correlation with old chest CT could be helpful.

3. It is present in about 8% of the population based on cadaver studies—in about 30% of these, it would show up on the mammogram.

4. If seen bilaterally and if it is stable since prior studies, there is no doubt this is a presentation of sternalis muscle and benign. If it is seen on one view only, and does not show the typical form and location for the presence of sternalis muscle, it is more of a concern—it might not be covered on the MLO view and workup might be necessary.

5. Finding such as seen above in the right CC view of the screening mammogram could hide in the inframammary fold. However, in this case, it is benign finding, consistent with sternalis muscle, given the typical shape, form, and location.

Pearls

- The sternalis muscle is an uncommon anatomic variant of the chest wall musculature, which is present in about 8% of both males and females, based on cadaver studies.
- The sternalis muscle is more frequently unilateral than bilateral; it is longitudinal in extent and parasternal in location and it is more superficial than the rectus abdominis muscle.
- The correct diagnosis on a mammogram can be achieved by recognizing the typical location and configuration.
- If there is remaining concern, correlation with old CT of the chest or further evaluation with chest CT could be helpful.

Suggested Reading

Bradley FM, Hoover HC, Hulka CA, et al. The sternalis muscle: an unusual normal finding seen on mammography. *AJR Am J Roentgenol.* 1996;166(1):33-36.

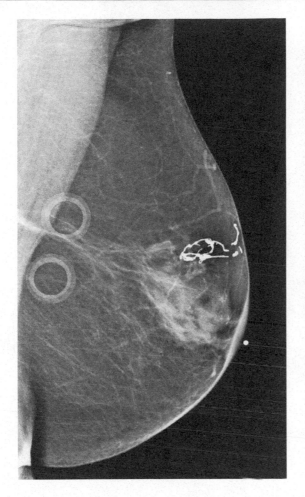
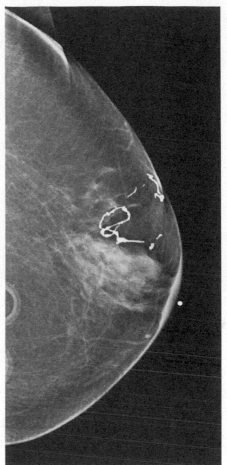

1. What BI-RADS classification is used for this entity?

2. What is the one most likely cause for these findings?

3. What is the next best imaging test?

4. What type of biopsy should be performed as one of these is palpable?

5. What type of surgical suture is more prone to calcify on mammograms?

Case ranking/difficulty:

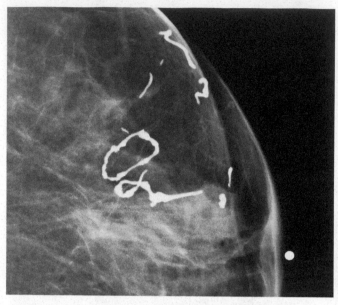

Close-up image shows one of the sutures has a tie.

4. The most prudent thing would be to leave them alone. Catgut sutures are supposed to be reabsorbed over time, but they now have fat necrosis around them. Sometimes, the patient would prefer to see a surgeon to discuss removal. Removal of foreign bodies (eg, biopsy clips) can be done using vacuum-assisted biopsy, so in theory, it could be used here.

5. Catgut usually gets reabsorbed over a period of months or years. However, the sutures can potentially give rise to a severe form of fat necrosis due to the foreign proteins in the catgut. For this reason, many man-made sutures have been used over the years, some of which are still broken down by the human body, and others that have more permanent properties.

Pearls

• Common in older patients, as this was more commonly found with older catgut suture. A variant of fat necrosis with calcifications around the body of the suture, which then does not get resorbed.

Answers

1. If you do not describe the abnormality, and as there is nothing else in the breast, you could use BI-RADS 1. However, it is difficult to get away without describing the findings here, and so a more appropriate impression would be BI-RADS 2: benign.

2. Postradiation changes may cause calcifications in vessels and coarse ductal calcification as part of induced apoptosis. Calcifications postimplant removal are more typically at the posterior aspect of the breast disc, and there may be associated silicone granulomas. Calcified guinea worm is sometimes found in women from an area where the worm is prevalent. Ruptured oil cysts show discontinuous calcifications.

3. No further imaging tests are required for this calcified foreign body. The imaging features are diagnostic of calcified sutures.

Suggested Readings

Libshitz HI, Montague ED, Paulus DD. Calcifications and the therapeutically irradiated breast. *AJR Am J Roentgenol*. 1977;128(6):1021-1025.

Stacey-Clear A, McCarthy KA, Hall DA, et al. Calcified suture material in the breast after radiation therapy. *Radiology*. 1992;183(1):207-208.

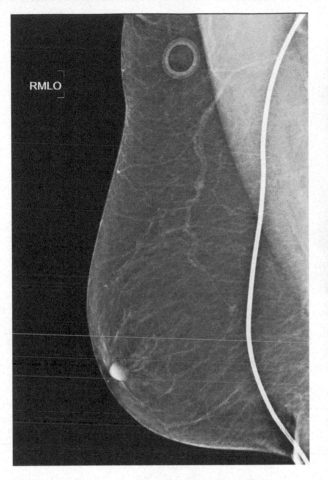
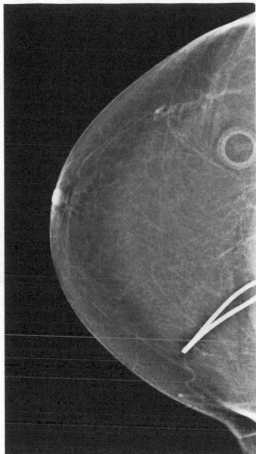

1. What BI-RADS classification should be used here?

2. What is the one most likely cause for these findings?

3. What produce calcified lesions that can be identified on mammography?

4. What is the best view to identify the track of a VP shunt?

5. What is the risk of malignant transformation around a VP shunt?

Case ranking/difficulty: 🦴

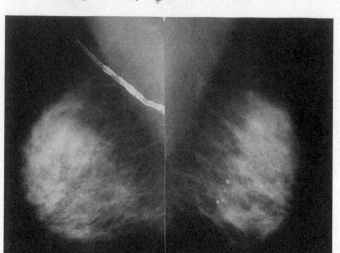

Bilateral MLO exam showing another case of a calcified ventricle-peritoneal shunt that had been in situ for the life of the patient.

4. In general, the MLO view shows the tube entering from the superior breast and exiting through the inferior part. There are variable appearances on the CC, depending on its track. XCCL, cleavage views, and laterals sometimes help if you cannot see the tube adequately, but they are not usually required for diagnosis.

5. There is a published case report of a multifocal tumor around a VP shunt, but this is likely to be a very rare finding.

Pearls

- It is a calcified artificial structure, so what kind of tube is it?
- What is the direction (from/to)?
- The answers you come up with will lead you to the correct finding.

Answers

1. In general, if you describe a finding, then BI-RADS 2 should be used. However, a BI-RADS 1 could equally be used as the finding is not within the breast itself.

2. This is typical of a ventriculoperitoneal shunt, as treatment for hydrocephalus.

3. Dracunculiasis is a guinea worm. When the parasite dies, it calcifies and appears as a loosely coiled tubular structure. Sutures may calcify, particularly if the patient has had radiation treatment. Surgical clips are inert and do not typically calcify. Pacemaker wires have occasionally been reported as calcified in the subdermal portion of its track. VP shunts calcify in the two examples shown here, as they are in the body for a very long time.

Suggested Readings

Ioannis K, Ioannis K, Angelos L. Routine mammographic imaging: it was only a needle. *Breast J.* 2006;12(5):493.

Lee D, Cutler B, Roberts S, Manghisi S, Ma AM. Multi-centric breast cancer involving a ventriculoperitoneal shunt. *Breast J.* 2010;16(6):653-655.

Vimalachandran D, Martin L, Lafi M, Ap-Thomas A. Cerebrospinal fluid pseudocyst of the breast. *Breast.* 2003;12(3):215-216.

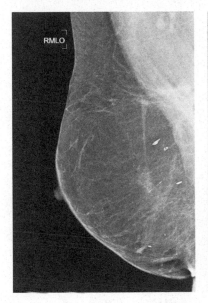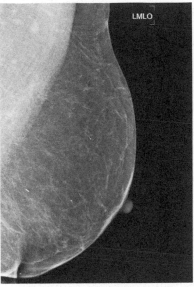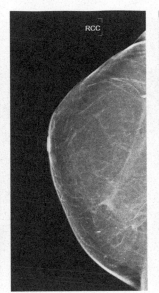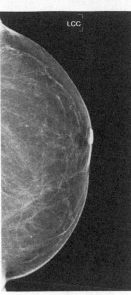

1. What BI-RADS classification should be used here?

2. What should be the next diagnostic imaging exam?

3. What type of surgery may this patient have had?

4. What type of biopsy should be performed?

5. What type of follow-up surveillance would you recommend?

Case ranking/difficulty: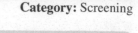

Category: Screening

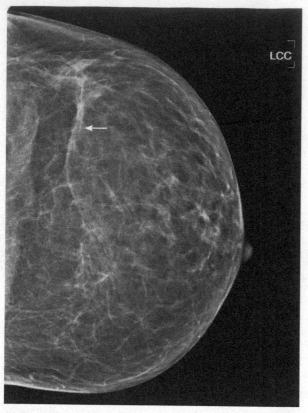

LCC

Pearls

• Common, benign appearance. Watch for swirling lines that do not correspond to normal anatomy, particularly in the lower half of the breast.

Suggested Readings

Beer GM, Kompatscher P, Hergan K. Diagnosis of breast tumors after breast reduction. *Aesthetic Plast Surg.* 1997;20(5):391-397.

Muir TM, Tresham J, Fritschi L, Wylie E. Screening for breast cancer post reduction mammoplasty. *Clin Radiol.* 2010;65(3):198-205.

Rubin JP, Coon D, Zuley M, et al. Mammographic changes after fat transfer to the breast compared with changes after breast reduction: a blinded study. *Plast Reconstr Surg.* 2012;129(5):1029-1038.

Another case of breast reduction showing a transverse line across the posterior part of the breast disc. Lines occurring that are not expected.

Answers

1. The findings of the scars are characteristic. You can ignore the scars and give a negative for malignancy BI-RADS 1 assessment, or describe the finding and give it a BI-RADS 2, benign.

2. No further workup is required, as the finding is normal postsurgical appearances.

3. These are the scars from a mastopexy (otherwise known as a breast reduction). TRAM reconstruction has its own characteristic imaging findings. Bilateral lumpectomy scars or multiple benign surgical biopsies could in theory give these appearances.

4. No biopsy is required as this is an "Aunt Minnie" appearance of postreduction scars. Biopsy may be required of palpable areas of fat necrosis occurring following this type of surgery.

5. The patient can be followed with routine screening, unless the operation was relatively recent, in which case annual diagnostic mammography is recommended.

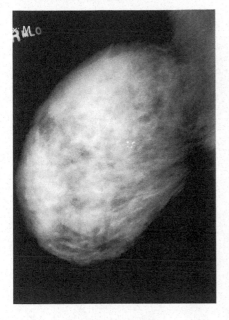
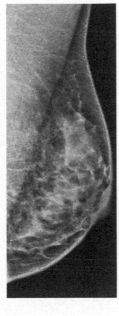
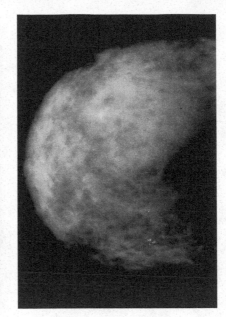
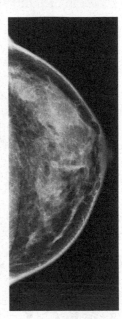

1. What are the different choices in BI-RADS lexicon for relatively dense breasts?

2. What are the two choices in BI-RADS lexicon for relatively less dense breasts?

3. What is the consequence of very dense fibroglandular tissue?

4. Why is mammography not worthless in very dense patients?

5. What other breast screening exams exist in the United States?

Case ranking/difficulty:

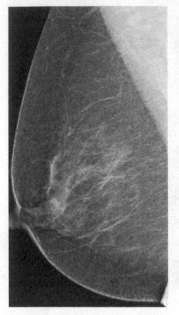 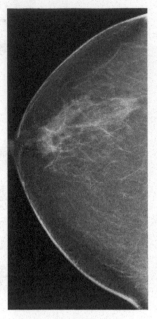 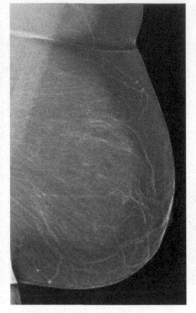 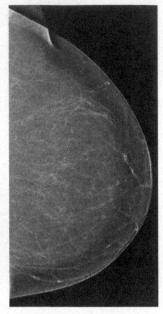

Screening mammogram, right MLO view demonstrating "scattered fibroglandular tissue."

Screening mammogram, right CC view demonstrating "scattered fibroglandular tissue."

Screening mammogram, left MLO view demonstrating "almost entirely fatty replaced" tissue.

Screening mammogram, left CC view demonstrating "almost entirely fatty replaced" tissue.

Answers

1. There are four categories to describe the composition of the breast: The two categories describing denser breasts are (1) "extremely dense" (>75% glandular tissue) and (2) "heterogeneously dense" (51–75% glandular tissue).

2. There are two categories describing less dense breast compositions: (1) "scattered fibroglandular tissue" (25–50% glandular tissue) and (2) "almost entirely fatty replaced" (<25% glandular tissue).

3. The sensitivity of mammography is significantly reduced and this results in less value of the mammogram. However, it is still valuable and does not eliminate the need for screening. To obtain old images is even more important. Additional exams, such as MRI and ultrasound, might be helpful. In the United States, only screening MRI is officially accepted as additional screening exam. Ultrasound is more controversial.

4. Mammography is still very helpful. It can still show calcifications, and might be able to show distortion or masses. Mammography will be limited in value because of its reduced ability to detect developing densities.

5. Only MRI is accepted by insurance companies for screening, but only in high-risk patients (lifetime risk of more than 20–25%). Ultrasound is not accepted as a screening exam but sometimes ordered by referring physicians (gray zone) with the indication such as "fibrocystic changes."

Pearls

- The amount of fibroglandular tissue in general is more prominent in younger patients in the reproductive age and decreases over time.
- The amount of fibroglandular tissue also depends on the hormonal status, including intake of estrogens, and it is related to congenital differences.
- Dense fibroglandular tissue is considered risk factor for breast cancer in several regards: (1) It does limit the value of mammography and its sensitivity to detect cancer. (2) Because of higher quantity of tissue, the likelihood to develop malignancy is higher. (3) There is correlation to some proliferative forms of aging of the parenchyma that is often times considered as risk factor for malignancy.

Suggested Readings

Boyd NF, Martin LJ, Bronskill M, Yaffe MJ, Duric N, Minkin S. Breast tissue composition and susceptibility to breast cancer. *J Natl Cancer Inst*. 2010;102(16):1224-1237.

Boyd NF, Martin LJ, Yaffe MJ, Minkin S. Mammographic density and breast cancer risk: current understanding and future prospects. *Breast Cancer Res*. 2011;13(6):223.

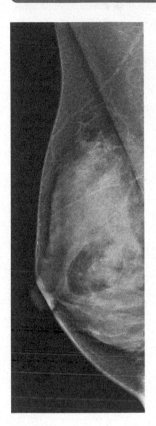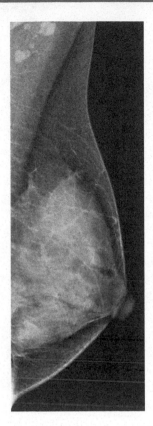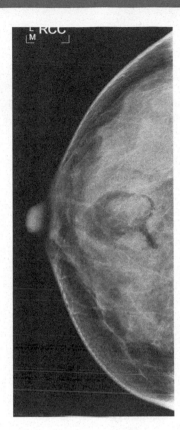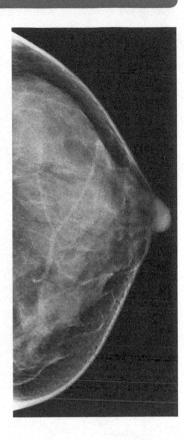

1. What BI-RADS classification should be used here?

2. What type of tissue is this lesion composed?

3. What is the next best imaging test?

4. What type of biopsy would you recommend?

5. What are the likely clinical findings on palpation?

Case ranking/difficulty: 🝔

Answers

1. This lesion is characteristically benign, BI-RADS 2.

2. This lesion is composed of fat (adipose). The lesion would have glandular density and therefore invisible if it were composed of normal fibroglandular elements. Cooper's ligaments are the small curvilinear lines attaching the glandular disc to the skin.

3. This finding is characteristic enough to recommend return to routine screening. It should be visible on prior examinations. Lipomas can be surprisingly hard to demonstrate on ultrasound. Non-fat sat T1 MRI can confirm that the lesion contains fat. Tomosynthesis should be able to demonstrate the findings clearly, compared with conventional 2D mammograms.

4. Clearly, if this lesion is diagnostic of a lipoma, then biopsy is not indicated.

5. The palpation findings of a lipoma are usually either nothing or a soft lump. Sometimes, the margins may not be easily felt, and then described as a vague soft lump. In rare instance that a lipoma gets infected, the findings may be of a hard lump, but there are clearly other signs of infection.

Pearls

- Aunt Minnie type of case.
- Harmless fatty density mass.

Suggested Readings

Kapila K, Pathan SK, Al-Mosawy FA, George SS, Haji BE, Al-Ayadhy B. Fine needle aspiration cytology of breast masses in children and adolescents: experience with 1404 aspirates. *Acta Cytol*. 2009;52(6):681-686.

Kirova YM, Feuilhade F, Le Bourgeois JP. Breast lipoma. *Breast J*. 2002;8(2):117-118.

Lanng C, Eriksen BØ, Hoffmann J. Lipoma of the breast: a diagnostic dilemma. *Breast*. 2004;13(5):408-411.

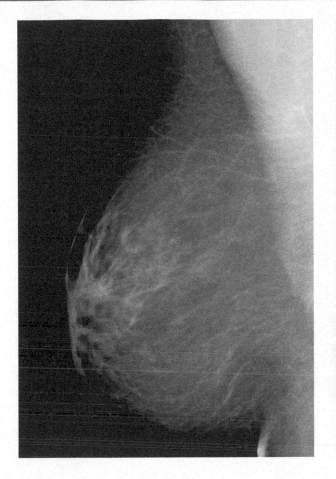
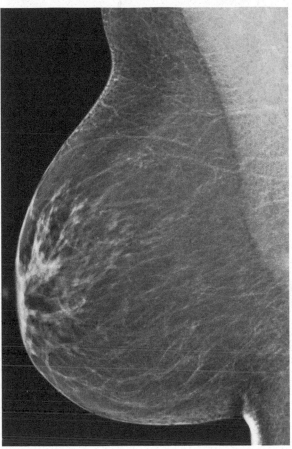

1. Can you see any abnormality on the new screening mammogram?

2. Which of the mammogram is digital?

3. What is the advantage of digital mammogram over film mammography?

4. What is the disadvantage of digital mammography in comparison with film mammography?

5. What are the practical consequences reading digital mammograms?

Case ranking/difficulty:

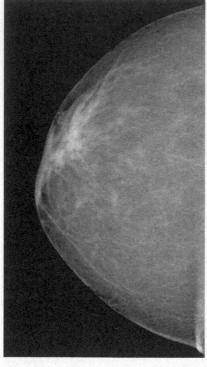

Screening film mammogram, right CC view 2006.

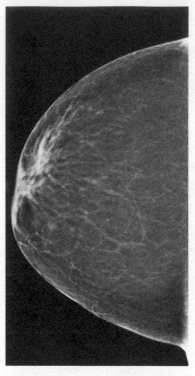

Screening digital mammography, right CC view 2011.

Answers

1. The exam from 2011 does not demonstrate any abnormality in comparison with the exam from 2009.

2. The 2011 exam is digital, whereas the 2009 exam is screen film mammography. The digital study demonstrates better contrast resolution.

3. Digital mammography has the advantage of better contrast resolution, which is helpful to detect developing malignancy in dense breast tissue.

4. Digital mammography has less spatial resolution then film mammography—this was for a long time the limiting factor in establishing digital mammography. The advantage of better contrast resolution, however, has been shown to outweigh the disadvantage of less spatial resolution.

5. Switching from reading screening film mammograms to reading screening digital mammograms requires to adjust the threshold to recall patient for densities as a result of the increased contrast resolution and to adjust the threshold to recall patient for calcifications as well.

Pearls

- Digital mammography has superior contrast resolution, whereas film mammography has an advantage of spatial resolution.
- Digital mammography has better sensitivity to detect developing "asymmetries" in dense breast tissue.
- Digital mammography also has higher sensitivity for detection of calcifications.

Suggested Readings

Karssemeijer N, Bluekens AM, Beijerinck D, et al. Breast cancer screening results 5 years after introduction of digital mammography in a population-based screening program. *Radiology*. 2009;253(2):353-358.

Lewin JM, Hendrick RE, D'Orsi CJ, et al. Comparison of full-field digital mammography with screen-film mammography for cancer detection: results of 4,945 paired examinations. *Radiology*. 2001;218(3):873-880.

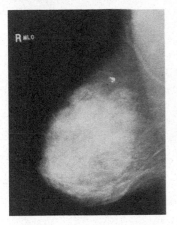 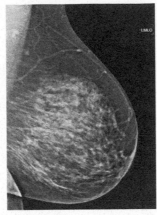 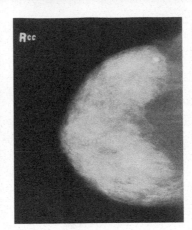 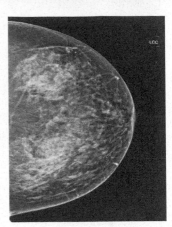

1. What BI-RADS classification should be used here?

2. In which groups of women did the DMIST study show benefit?

3. What is the dose of a digital mammogram relative to analog?

4. Which of the following are some of the benefits of digital versus analog?

5. What of the following findings or structures are better seen with digital mammography?

Answers

1. Normal dense breast tissue, better seen on digital. The appropriate BI-RADS classification is therefore 1: negative for malignancy. The first time a digital mammogram is performed on the woman, there is a higher probability of finding calcifications that you are not sure could be seen on the analog mammogram. In that instance, you need to give a BI-RADS 0 and recall for workup.

2. The DMIST study was performed to answer the question as to whether digital mammography was better than analog mammography, but only really had to show equivalence to gain acceptance. There were three groups of women where some benefit was shown: those with dense breasts, women younger than 50 years, and perimenopausal women. There is some evidence that digital mammography is less effective than screen-film mammography in women with fatty breasts. However, this is being addressed by some manufacturers, changing their anodes to tungsten from molybdenum.

3. It can vary by tissue type, but there has generally been a drop in mean glandular radiation dose during the switch to digital. Further reductions have also occurred using photon counting techniques, where radiation doses are approximately 50% lower than regular mammograms. Tomosynthesis as a new technology started at approximately three times the regular dose of mammography as the FDA required a regular mammogram in addition to the 3D exam. Measures have been taken, which has reduced to approximately 1.6 times, and still within the 2 mGy FDA requirement.

4. The effects on the environment and concerns over the disposal of silver used to be a big concern. There is little difference in radiation dose compared with analog mammography, except for a few systems, for example, Philips MicroDose, which has approximately 50% normal radiation dose. Digital allows you to perceive calcifications much easier. A small digital reimbursement supplement that is likely to disappear now as analog is virtually extinct. CAD has been available for analog systems, but it is more efficient on digital systems.

5. Most of the above are correct, and some may argue that all are correct, as the dynamic range of digital and the contrast resolution of digital mammography makes everything easier to see.

Pearls

- Digital mammograms show normal breast tissue clearly, especially in patients with denser breast tissue.
- Microcalcifications are also much easier to identify and to characterize.

Suggested Readings

Kopans DB, Pisano ED, Acharyya S, et al. DMIST results: technologic or observer variability? *Radiology.* 2008;248(2):703; author reply 703.

Pisano ED, Hendrick RE, Yaffe MJ, et al. Diagnostic accuracy of digital versus film mammography: exploratory analysis of selected population subgroups in DMIST. *Radiology.* 2008;246(2):376-383.

Zuley M. How to transition to digital mammography. *J Am Coll Radiol.* 2007;4(3):178-183.

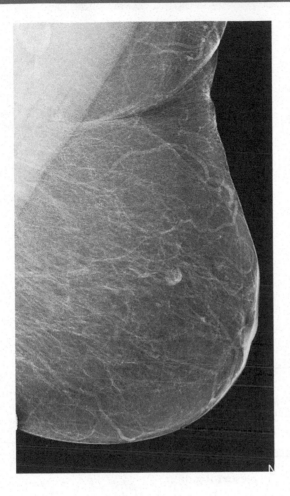
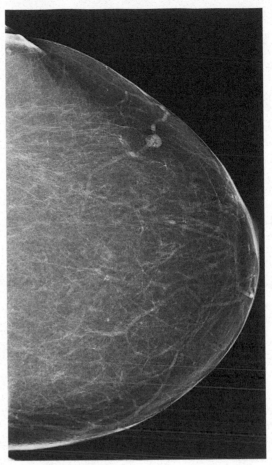

1. What is the workup for "round" mass seen on first mammogram?

2. What is the next step if fat cannot be visualized?

3. What is the characteristic finding of an intramammary lymph node?

4. Where is the location of the mass?

5. What would you do if the mammogram does not show fat but ultrasound demonstrates a large fatty hilum?

Case ranking/difficulty: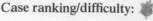

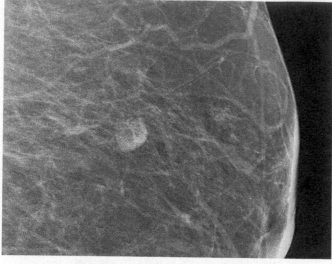

Diagnostic mammogram, left MLO view demonstrates benign-appearing mass with fat.

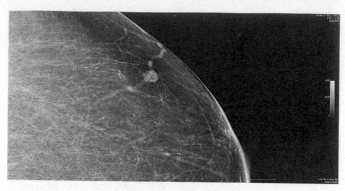

Diagnostic mammogram, left CC view demonstrates benign-appearing mass with fat.

Answers

1. Next step in general is workup with spot compression views.

2. Ultrasound can be used for further characterization. If that does not show any abnormality, the finding is probably benign and 6-month follow-up mammography is recommended. If ultrasound demonstrates the mass, it can be further characterized on ultrasound. If ultrasound demonstrates cysts in internal echoes or thin membranes ("complicated cyst"), cyst aspiration or as an alternative 6-month follow-up and ultrasound surveillance over 2 years is recommended.

3. It is generally located in the upper outer quadrant. If fat is seen on the mammogram, it is diagnostic for lymph node. Lymph nodes are also sometimes located in other parts of the breast. They are in general well circumscribed.

4. It is located slightly superior on MLO and very lateral on CC view.

5. In this case, the ultrasound finding likely does not correlate to the mammogram. Mammogram should show fat as well. The ultrasound finding is benign and does not need follow-up. The mammogram finding does need follow-up if it is not new but seen on first mammogram and does not contain definitely fat. Bottom line: if ultrasound finding does not correlate, 6-month follow-up mammogram is recommended for a well-circumscribed mass seen on first mammogram.

Pearls

- Typical location for intramammary lymph node is the upper outer quadrant; however, they can exist anywhere in the breast.
- If fat can be identified on screening mammogram in a well-circumscribed mass, it is in general consistent with lymph node and mammogram can be classified as BI-RADS 2, benign.

Suggested Reading

Meyer JE, Ferraro FA, Frenna TH, et al. Mammographic appearance of normal intramammary lymph nodes in an atypical location. *AJR Am J Roentgenol.* 1993;161: 779-780.

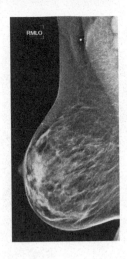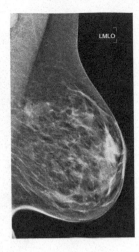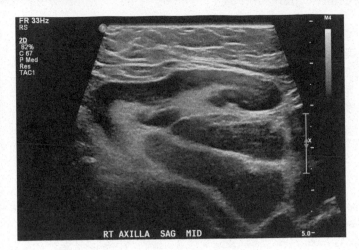

1. What BI-RADS classification should be used here?

2. What is the next best imaging test?

3. Which of the following are known causes of bilateral axillary adenopathy?

4. From which cell line does Non-Hodgkin lymphoma (NHL) arise?

5. How does primary breast lymphoma present?

Case ranking/difficulty:

Category: Diagnostic

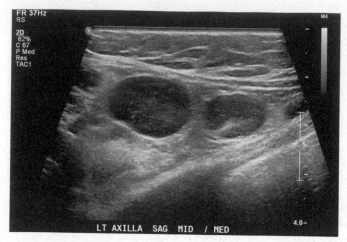

Axilla ultrasound shows one oval solid node with loss of the normal hilum, and a second with diffuse thickening of the cortex and effacement of the hilum.

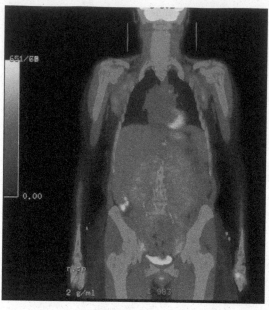

Note multiple enlarged lymph nodes in both axillae.

Answers

1. These lymph nodes are abnormal and do not look like lymphatic spread from a breast cancer. If the patient is with a known lymphoma and under treatment, you could use BI-RADS 2: benign for the breasts, but make a note of the axillary findings. If not known about, then a BI-RADS 0 could be used to get the patient seen, and ultrasound of the axilla performed and possibly biopsied so that they can be passed on to the hematologists.

2. In the setting of likely lymphoma, following a needle biopsy, a PET/CT may give the most staging information before a decision is made.

3. HIV-related lymphadenopathy, systemic inflammatory condition, and lymphoma/chronic lymphocytic leukemias can present with nodes. Inflammatory breast cancer usually presents with unilateral lymphadenopathy. Breast abscesses can also present as unilateral lymphadenopathy. Pelvic abscess does not usually present with axillary nodes.

4. NHL can arise from any of the T or B line white cells, progenitors, or more mature cells; 10% to 35% of patients have extranodal primary lymphoma at the time of presentation.

5. Very uncommon as breast primary, but breast commonly involved when known systemic lymphoma. Painless breast mass usually affecting the right breast; 30% to 40% have ipsilateral axillary adenopathy; average age 55 to 60 years, and right breast more common than left.

Pearls

- Bilateral nodes seen in axilla on mammography are not necessarily benign.
- Systemic disease can manifest itself on mammograms.
- Do not forget lymphatic disorders as a cause of axillary adenopathy on mammograms.

Suggested Readings

Gorkem SB, O'Connell AM. Abnormal axillary lymph nodes on negative mammograms: causes other than breast cancer. *Diagn Interv Radiol.* 2012;18(5):473-479.

Valente SA, Levine MD, Silverstein MD, et al. Accuracy of predicting axillary lymph node positivity by physical examination, mammography, ultrasonography, and magnetic resonance imaging. *Ann Surg Oncol.* 2012;19(6):1825-1830.

Walsh R, Kornguth PJ, Soo MS, Bentley R, DeLong DM. Axillary lymph nodes: mammographic, pathologic, and clinical correlation. *AJR Am J Roentgenol.* 1997;168(1):33-38.

Palpable abnormality

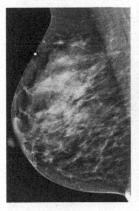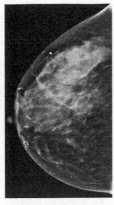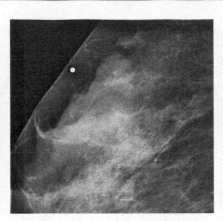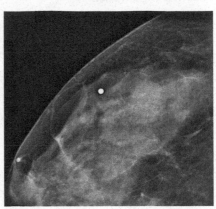

1. What is the finding on the diagnostic mammogram?

2. What is the next step in the workup of the patient?

3. If ultrasound does not show any abnormality, what is the next step?

4. What would be the next step if ultrasound demonstrates hypoechoic nodule with internal echoes?

5. What is the definition of a simple cyst—if that is the ultrasound finding what is the next step?

Case ranking/difficulty: 🍁

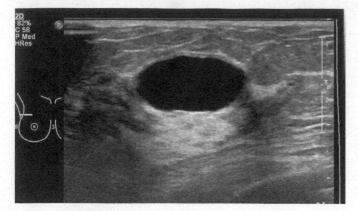

Gray-scale ultrasound demonstrating "anechoic," "well-circumscribed" mass with "posterior acoustic enhancement."

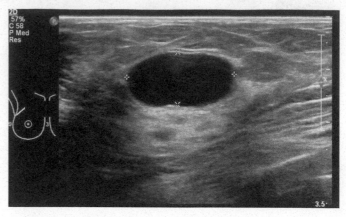

Gray-scale ultrasound demonstrating simple cyst.

Answers

1. Mammogram of right breast, including spot compression views, does not show any definite abnormality.

2. Next step in workup is targeted ultrasound directed to the right upper outer quadrant.

3. If ultrasound does not show abnormality, the final assessment is BI-RADS 1 negative, and a sentence should be added that "further assessment of the palpable abnormality should be based on clinical grounds." If patient is high risk or if the clinical findings are overwhelming and the breast parenchyma is dense and might obscure abnormality, MRI might be an option as problem-solving tool.

4. In case of corresponding hypoechoic mass with internal echoes but without flow on duplex, this is called "complicated cyst" and cyst aspiration should be performed. Since the mass was not seen on mammogram, there is no need to repeat mammogram. Alternative could be to call "complicated cyst" "probably benign" and perform follow-up ultrasound in 6 months, another after 6 months, and then after 1 year.

5. Simple cyst is defined as round and oval "well-circumscribed," "anechoic" mass with "posterior acoustic enhancement." This is the description of the finding seen on this particular patient. Assessment is BI-RADS 2, benign, and patient can return to normal screening exam.

Pearls

- If ultrasound can prove that simple cyst explains lump felt by the patient, the final assessment is "benign"-BI-RADS 2 and patient can return in 1 year for next screening mammogram.
- If there is any doubt that this a simple cyst, as a result of the internal echoes or debris, it should be called "complicated cyst" and cyst aspiration can be performed.
- Alternative management can be to follow "complicated cyst" over 2 years with ultrasound and call it "probably benign," in particular in case of more than one "complicated cysts."
- If there are scattered cysts bilaterally of which some are "complicated," they can be called "benign" and no follow-up is necessary.
- If there are mural nodules at the wall, or if there was thickening of the wall or the presence of thick membrane, finding is called "complex mass" and core biopsy should be performed.

Suggested Readings

Berg WA, Campassi CI, Ioffe OB. Cystic lesions of the breast: sonographic-pathologic correlation. *Radiology*. 2003;227(1):183-191.

Dennis MA, Parker SH, Klaus AJ, Stavros AT, Kaske TI, Clark SB. Breast biopsy avoidance: the value of normal mammograms and normal sonograms in the setting of a palpable lump. *Radiology*. 2001;219(1):186-191.

Rinaldi P, Ierardi C, Costantini M, et al. Cystic breast lesions: sonographic findings and clinical management. *J Ultrasound Med*. 2010;29(11):1617-1626.

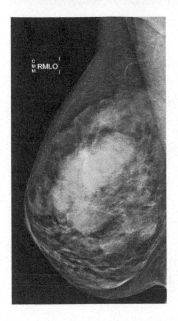 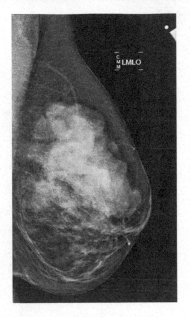 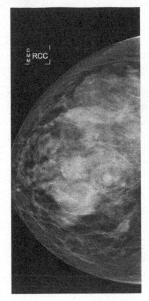 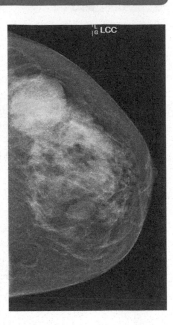

1. What BI-RADS classification should be used here?

2. What are the potential pathologies based on the imaging?

3. What should be the next imaging investigation?

4. How should the lesion be managed if it turns out to be a cystic lesion?

5. If you aspirate a cyst, should you send the fluid for cytology?

Case ranking/difficulty: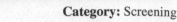

Answers

1. This is a characteristic finding, where using the 'multiple masses' finding note allows you to give this a BI-RADS 2. If you are uncertain about any of the masses, with indistinct margins, or the mass is partially obscured, you should give the patient a BI-RADS 0 and perform a diagnostic workup to include spot views and ultrasound scanning.

2. The most common cause of these findings are cysts and fibroadenomas, sometimes a mix of both. Metastases have circumscribed margins and should be considered in the presence of a known OTHER cancer, which could potentially metastasize to the breast. Rarely a triple negative ductal cancer may present as a circumscribed mass, but does not tend to have the appearances as of this exam.

3. If you have not used the multiple masses, and given a BI-RADS 2, then the next test should be a routine follow-up mammogram (1 year in the United States). If the patient has a palpable lump being worked up, then an ultrasound may be the best first-line investigation, as we need to confirm whether the lump is cystic or solid. For margins, a single tomosynthesis projection is showing promise in the workup of women with masses.

4. Simple cysts can come and go rapidly, changing even day to day. Some cysts remain over a long period, developing thick proteinaceous debris, which may show as a snowstorm appearance on ultrasound. Sometimes, this debris is adherent to a cyst wall, and prompt short-term surveillance or even biopsy. Historically, cysts were sometimes surgically excised.

5. Cyst aspirations are not routinely performed anymore. It may help if the fluid is bloody, but this is usually due to a traumatic tear of a small vessel around the cyst wall, and not related to the cyst at all (a bloody tap—especially at the end of aspiration).

Pearls

- Circumscribed mass in young woman likely to be either a cyst or fibroadenoma.
- PROVISO: triple negative breast cancer can present as circumscribed masses in young women, although rare in everyday practice.
- Ultrasound is the quickest, easiest, and non ionizing test to rule out a solid mass, and confirm a cyst.

Suggested Readings

Lister D, Evans AJ, Burrell HC, et al. The accuracy of breast ultrasound in the evaluation of clinically benign discrete, symptomatic breast lumps. *Clin Radiol*. 1998;53(7): 490-492.

Shetty MK, Shah YP. Sonographic findings in focal fibrocystic changes of the breast. *Ultrasound Q*. 2002;18(1):35-40.

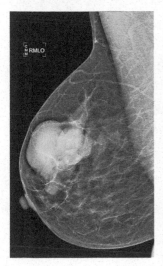
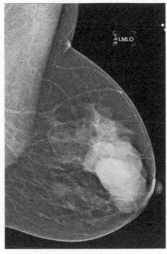
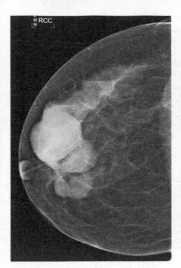
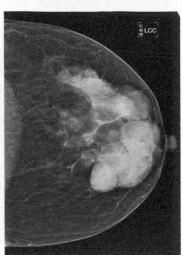

1. What BI-RADS classification should be used here?

2. What is the most likely pathology based on the imaging?

3. What is the next best imaging test?

4. What type of intervention would you recommend?

5. What is the risk of breast cancer in patients with multiple cysts?

Case ranking/difficulty: 🌸

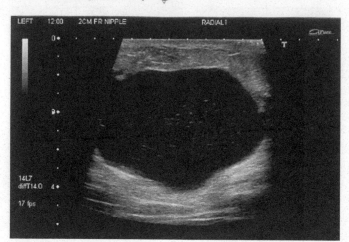

LEFT 12:00 2CM FR NIPPLE RADIAL1

14L7
diffT14.0
17 fps

Multiple simple cysts in both breasts confirmed on ultrasound exam.

Answers

1. The multiple, noncalcified, circumscribed, bilateral masses are likely due to fibroadenomas or cysts. A BI-RADS 2, benign, note is appropriate.

2. The findings are most likely cysts or fibroadenomas, although rarely you can get multiple phyllodes tumors in both breasts; the key here is that those lesions are not stable and tend to be rapidly growing. Metastases to the breast can look identical to this, but is in the setting of a known "other" cancer that has the potential to metastasize to the breast.

3. If you wish to work this up, then ultrasound on its own can distinguish between solid and cystic masses. Some claim that tomosynthesis has a role here, but the data are currently lacking. As this is a benign finding, routine mammograms are indicated.

4. No intervention is required for multiple benign lesions.

5. There was a reported statistical relationship between simple cysts and subsequent breast cancer, likely related to the sensitivity of breast tissue to circulating estrogens, but this has not been validated, and does not reach the risk levels associated with hyperplastic or borderline neoplastic lesions of the breast.

Pearls

- Multiple noncalcified masses in the breast are a benign finding, and are described in the BI-RADS manual as a special case.
- To meet the criteria, the masses have to be circumscribed, not calcified, and to have at least two on one side and one on the contralateral breast.

Suggested Readings

Berg WA, Sechtin AG, Marques H, Zhang Z. Cystic breast masses and the ACRIN 6666 experience. *Radiol Clin North Am.* 2010;48(5):931-987.

Chang YW, Kwon KH, Goo DE, Choi DL, Lee HK, Yang SB. Sonographic differentiation of benign and malignant cystic lesions of the breast. *J Ultrasound Med.* 2007;26(1):47-53.

Heinig J, Witteler R, Schmitz R, Kiesel L, Steinhard J. Accuracy of classification of breast ultrasound findings based on criteria used for BI-RADS. *Ultrasound Obstet Gynecol.* 2008;32(4):573-578.

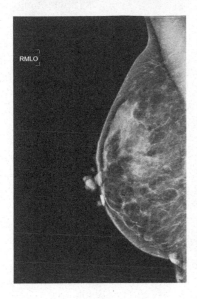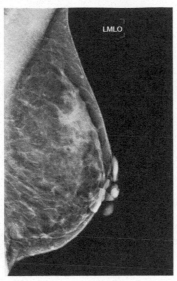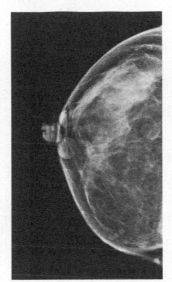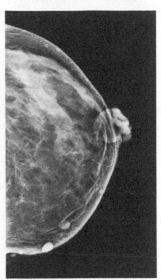

1. What BI-RADS classification should be used here?

2. What is the inheritance pattern of neurofibromatosis?

3. Which chromosome is affected by the NF-1 mutation?

4. What type of breast biopsy should be performed to confirm the diagnosis?

5. What are the other supportive features for the diagnosis of NF-1?

Case ranking/difficulty:

Category: Screening

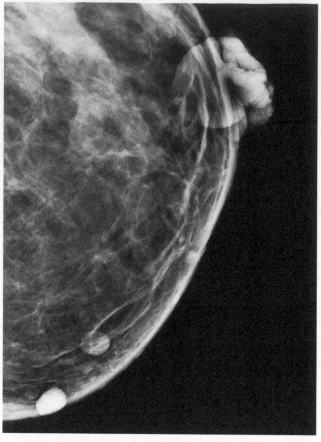

Close-up view of irregular, lobulated, overgrowth of nipple, and two circumscribed superficial masses.

Answers

1. This is a benign finding, and therefore a BI-RADS 2 assessment would be appropriate.

2. The defect on chromosome 17 arises by autosomal dominant genetics, but 50% occur by spontaneous mutation.

3. Chromosome 17 has the locus for the mutated gene affected in NF-1.

4. No biopsy of the breast needs to be performed to confirm the diagnosis. The diagnosis is usually obvious on physical examination. Also, they may be under preexisting care for known neurofibromatosis.

5. The NF-1 gene is on chromosome 17 and affects cell signaling. As a result, there is overgrowth causing benign tumors and also scoliosis (in 20%) or other limb deformities. Epilepsy is observed in approximately 7% of patients. Learning difficulties or other psychological issues are common. The gastrointestinal system is generally not involved with tumors in NF-1. Tumors are more common in the nervous system with plexiform neurofibromas, and schwannomas. Pheochromocytoma is a complication.

Pearls

- Cutaneous masses. Usually, this is obvious when you look at the patient.
- A defect in the NF-1 gene on chromosome 17 (type 1 neurofibromatosis).
- Autosomal dominant pattern of inheritance, but up to 50% of NF-1 cases arise because of spontaneous mutation.
- 1:3500 live births

Suggested Readings

Cao MM, Hoyt AC, Bassett LW. Mammographic signs of systemic disease. *Radiographics*. 2012;31(4):1085-1100.

Goksugur N, Gurel S. Neurofibromatosis of nipple-areola complex. *Breast J*. 2012;17(4):424.

Sherman JE, Smith JW. Neurofibromas of the breast and nipple-areolar area. *Ann Plast Surg*. 1981;7(4):302-307.

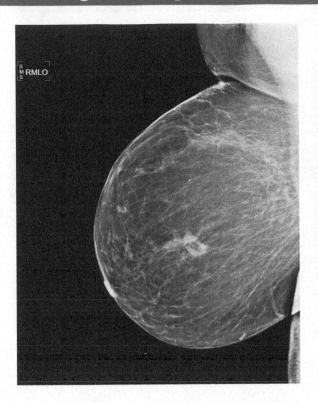
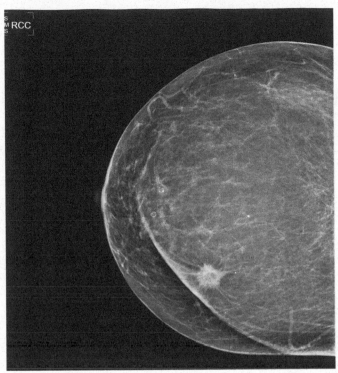

1. What is the significance of the lesion in the right breast?

2. What is the diagnosis?

3. How can fat necrosis appear on mammogram?

4. If there is concern for recurrent malignancy, what would be the next step?

5. If there is remaining concern for recurrent malignancy, what would be the next step?

Case ranking/difficulty: 🌑

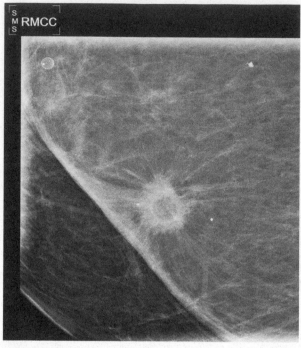

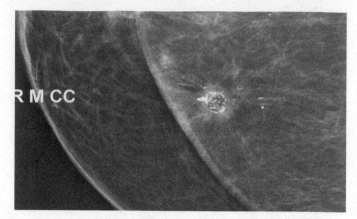

Current mammogram, right spot compression CC view demonstrating retraction of the scar and development of "coarse, heterogenous" calcifications.

Old mammogram, right spot compression CC view demonstrating fat necrosis.

postoperative enhancement due to granulation tissue from enhancement as a result of recurrent tumor.

Answers

1. Focal area does contain fat and is a benign finding. This is a benign lesion BI-RADS 2. Correlate with history—patient had lumpectomy.

2. This is typical appearance of scar after lumpectomy with fat necrosis.

3. Fat necrosis can present a wide variety of morphology, of which some are more pathognomonic and some are more difficult to distinguish from possible malignancy. If there is fat within the focal finding or the abnormality contains "coarse and heterogeneous" calcifications, it is relatively specific for fat necrosis. However, if the microcalcification or the mass is spiculated, it is unspecific and sometimes biopsy is warranted.

4. Diagnostic mammogram with spot compression MLO and CC views or, if calcifications are the concern, workup with magnification ML and CC views. In some breast centers, all patients after lumpectomy receive diagnostic mammograms in the first place, which often times includes spot compression or magnification views in the first place.

5. The best test for questionable recurrent malignancy would be to perform breast MRI—however, there should be at least 6-month time interval between surgery and MRI; otherwise, it is difficult to distinguish

Pearls

• Fat necrosis is a benign inflammatory process, mostly related to prior surgery or trauma.
• Mammographic features of fat necrosis include the presence of lipid cysts, microcalcifications, coarse calcifications, and sometimes spiculated areas of increased density.
• Lipid cysts are round and oval lucent masses with thin rim that may or may not be calcified and are unequivocally benign.
• Fat necrosis can also present in the form of microcalcifications that might be even "pleomorphic" in shape and cannot be distinguished from malignancy and biopsy is warranted.
• If fibrosis is the dominant feature of fat necrosis, it can appear spiculated in shape.
• "Heterogenous and coarse" calcifications are common feature of fat necrosis but often times require additional monitoring and might be called "probably benign," depending on the morphology.

Suggested Readings

Hogge JP, Robinson RE, Magnant CM, Zuurbier RA. The mammographic spectrum of fat necrosis of the breast. *Radiographics.* 1995;15(6):1347-1356.

Taboada JL, Stephens TW, Krishnamurthy S, Brandt KR, Whitman GJ. The many faces of fat necrosis in the breast. *AJR Am J Roentgenol.* 2009;192(3):815-825.

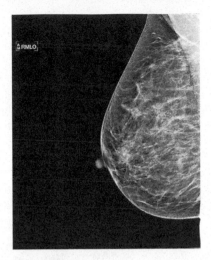

Right MLO.

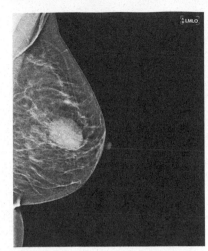

Left CC.

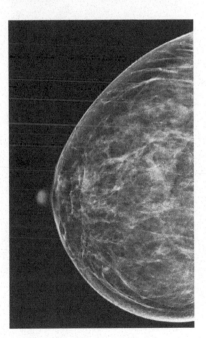

Right CC.

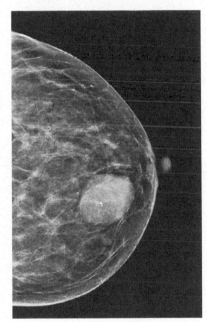

Left MLO.

1. What is the BI-RADS category for this diagnostic exam?

2. Which of the following are the Stavros benign criteria?

3. What is the risk of malignancy in a circumscribed mass in a woman younger than 25 years?

4. Which of the new technologies in breast imaging is likely to help our diagnosis of fibroadenoma?

5. What types of biopsies can make the diagnosis of fibroadenoma?

Case ranking/difficulty:

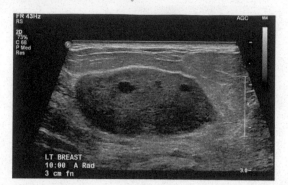

Ultrasound shows an "oval mass" with a "narrow zone of transition" (circumscribed). The echo texture is predominantly homogeneously hypoechoic, with some smaller cystic spaces within.

Answers

1. There are various approaches to a circumscribed benign-looking mass on both mammography and ultrasound. The patient is very young and the likely scenario is a fibroadenoma. Malignancy is very unusual in this age group, and some groups advocate using ultrasound only. According to BI-RADS, if this is the first visit, and the features are entirely benign (fulfill the Stavros criteria), then the patient may be given a BI-RADS 3 and 6-month ultrasound follow-up performed for stability. Some groups advocate for biopsy every solid mass at any age, and therefore would use the BI-RADS 4 category.

2. Stavros criteria for a benign lesion: (1) up to two or three gentle lobulations; (2) thin echogenic pseudo capsule; (3) intense hyperechogenicity; (4) ellipsoid shape; (5) the absence of malignant features.

3. The pretest probability of cancer in an under 25 years old is very low. A benign-looking mass that fulfills the criteria for a fibroadenoma on ultrasound can be safely followed with physical examination, and does not need a biopsy, if remains stable. Over the age of 25, the malignancy rate climbs to between 1% and 2% (BI-RADS 3) and therefore these lesions may be biopsied or followed with short-term follow-up.

4. Many of the new technologies are being investigated as an adjunct in characterization of lesions. There is frequently an overlap between findings in benign and malignant lesions with the same morphologic characteristics; therefore, none of these are currently used in the place of biopsy. Power Doppler helps to identify the blood vessels, which are said to be characteristically at the periphery. In young women, however, the fibroadenoma may be actively growing and contain large vascular channels.

5. If you have a trained breast cytologist (more common in Europe than in the United States), then a diagnosis of fibroadenoma can be made. All other types of biopsy can assist making the diagnosis of fibroadenoma, except perhaps an incisional biopsy, which takes superficial tissue (eg, in patients with inflammatory breast cancer with no known primary, or in suspect Pagets disease of the nipple).

Pearls

- Oval circumscribed mass in less than 25 years age group may be diagnosed on ultrasound alone. Biopsy is not required.
- Over 25 years, you can choose surveillance to determine stability, or if there are any suspicious features, proceed to ultrasound-guided core biopsy or diagnostic vacuum-assisted excision.

Suggested Readings

Hamilton L, Evans A, Cornford E, James J, Burrell H. Ultrasound diagnosis of fibroadenoma—is biopsy always necessary? *Clin Radiol.* 2008;63(9):1070-1071.

Stavros AT, Thickman D, Rapp CL, Dennis MA, Parker SH, Sisney GA. Solid breast nodules: use of sonography to distinguish between benign and malignant lesions. *Radiology.* 1995;196:123-134.

Tagaya N, Nakagawa A, Ishikawa Y, Oyama T, Kubota K. Experience with ultrasonographically guided vacuum-assisted resection of benign breast tumors. *Clin Radiol.* 2008;63(4):396-400.

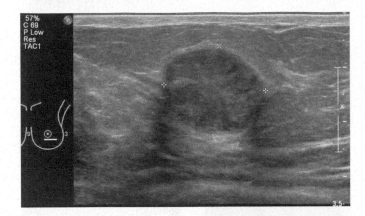
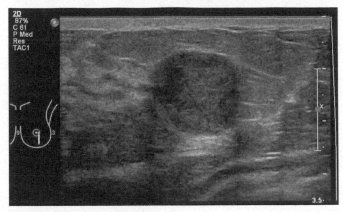
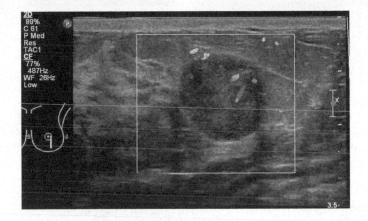

1. What is the reason to biopsy this mass that is palpable and circumscribed?

2. If this mass was an incidental finding on an ultrasound, what would be the next step?

3. What differentiates a phyllodes tumor from a fibroadenoma?

4. What would be the management if there are two masses like this—one palpable and one was an incidental finding?

5. What would be the management if there were multiple palpable benign-appearing masses?

Case ranking/difficulty: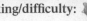

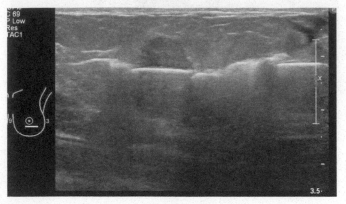

Ultrasound-guided core biopsy with 12-gauge needle.

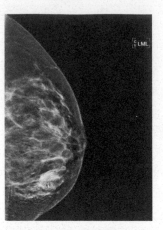

Mammogram of left ML view with mass and clip after biopsy.

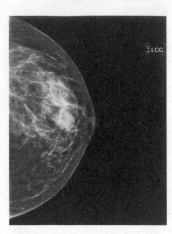

Mammogram of left CC view with mass and clip after biopsy.

Answers

1. Any new palpable mass can be considered suspicious due to the fact that it can be assumed that it has grown in size, since it was not palpable before. However, there are some radiologists who argue that a benign-appearing mass in a young patient is most likely a fibroadenoma, even if it is palpable and could be followed in 6 months. However, during the time of monitoring, any significant increase in size would then trigger biopsy.

2. It would be BI-RADS 3, "probably benign," and patient would be advised to return for ultrasound follow-up in 6 months, then, if finding is unchanged, 6 months later again, and then if stable, 1 year later. This results in time period of observation of 2 years. During that time, the finding remains "probably benign"—after 2 years, if the finding is unchanged, it can be classified as "benign" BI-RADS 2 and there is no need for further monitoring.

3. It shows in general histology with higher cellular activity and cellularity. Local recurrence rate is higher and in rare cases, there can be metastasis, for example, to the chest.

4. In this case, it would be reasonable to biopsy the palpable mass—again under the assumption that it has grown (was not palpable before) and follow the incidental, benign-appearing solid mass in 6 months.

5. It would not be unreasonable is in a young patient, where these well-circumscribed masses are most likely all fibroadenomas, to biopsy the largest of the findings and follow the rest in 6 months. MRI is not the first choice—unless there is a strong family history, then it might be considered as an additional "problem solving" modality in that particular case.

Pearls

- The histological appearance of phyllodes tumors may be the same as of large fibroadenomas—although they have greater cellularity and cell activity.
- Malignant behavior of phyllodes tumors, which can include metastasis to the lungs, is extremely rare. Most malignant phyllodes tumors reported in the literature had on histology an obvious sarcomatous element.
- Incomplete excision of phyllodes tumors has been stressed as a major determinant for local recurrence.

Suggested Readings

Barsky S, Gradishar W, Recht A, et al. *The Breast*. 4th ed. Saunders Elsevier USA; 2009.

Buchberger W, Strasser K, Heim K, et al. Phyllodes tumor findings on mammography, sonography and aspiration cytology in 10 cases. *AJR Am J Roentgenol*. 1991;157(4):715-719.

Guillot E, Couturaud B, Reyal F, et al. Management of phyllodes breast tumors. *Breast J*. 2011;17(2):129-137.

Palpable lump in the right breast

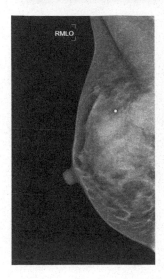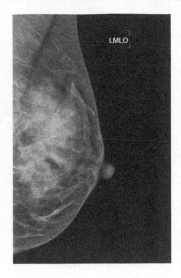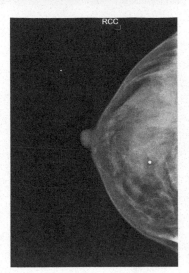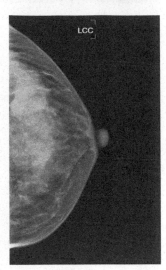

1. Why should a technical repeat be considered appropriate in this case?

2. What should be the next diagnostic imaging exam?

3. What is the likely pathology of a circumscribed mass?

4. Which of the following BI-RADS descriptors is supportive of a benign diagnosis?

5. Which findings favors phyllodes tumor over fibroadenoma?

Case ranking/difficulty: 🦠

Category: Diagnostic

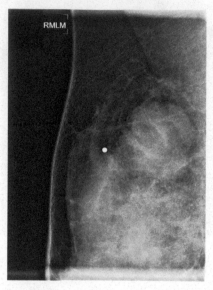

Right ML spot films show that this mass is circumscribed with gentle lobulations.

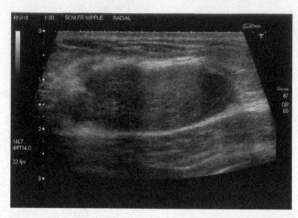

Targeted ultrasound shows a predominantly circumscribed mass with one edge that shows a lobulated area. Another view showed that this was artifactual, and the lesion was completely circumscribed.

Answers

1. This is a diagnostic workup and not a screening due to the age of the patient, and the palpable mass. A BI-RADS 0 is appropriate at this stage until further workup is performed, even though in reality the patient has not completed the mammographic workup.

2. As this patient is young, and there is a mass, you could go direct to ultrasound. If you wish to see the margins clearly to fully characterize the mass before ultrasound, then tomosynthesis or diagnostic mammograms with spot (+/− magnification) views are recommended. MRI will give a lot of information, but at this stage, it is not necessary. Some groups may consider PEM if the mass was not visualized, but there is a hard mass present. The downsides are the radiation dose from the isotope injection.

3. The key here is the "most likely" pathology. Cysts and fibroadenomas are common at this age. All the other diagnoses listed are in the differential diagnosis for this finding, but further workup is required. If this were a large and solid circumscribed mass, then phyllodes tumor is much higher in the list. Ductal carcinoma in situ (DCIS) can cause a noncalcified mass and can simulate a fibroadenoma, but it is rare in a radiologist's practice.

4. "Hypoechoic" is commonly used but does not help as a descriptor to differentiate benign from malignant morphology. "Acoustic enhancement" is more commonly found in benign solid masses and with cysts,

but also can occasionally be found in malignant lesions. A "narrow zone of transition" is the opposite of a hyperechoic rim you see around some cancers.

5. A phyllodes tumor may be identical to a large fibroadenoma, and have large vascular channels through it. Also, it may have wide channels where the ducts are not as distorted as they are in fibroadenomas, giving the leaf-like architecture seen on gross pathology.

Pearls

- "Circumscribed noncalcified mass."
- Likely cyst or fibroadenoma—confirm with diagnostic workup.

Suggested Readings

Chao TC, Lo YF, Chen SC, Chen MF. Sonographic features of phyllodes tumors of the breast. *Ultrasound Obstet Gynecol.* 2002;20(1):64-71.

Jacobs TW, Chen YY, Guinee DG, et al. Fibroepithelial lesions with cellular stroma on breast core needle biopsy: are there predictors of outcome on surgical excision? *Am J Clin Pathol.* 2005;124(3):342-354.

Veneti S, Manek S. Benign phyllodes tumour vs fibroadenoma: FNA cytological differentiation. *Cytopathology.* 2001;12(5):321-328.

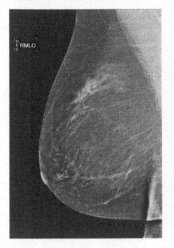 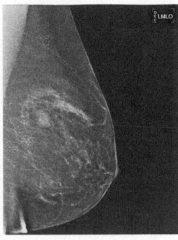 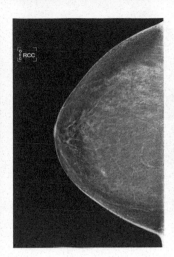 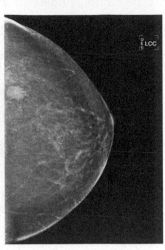

1. What is the BI-RADS category for this screening exam?

2. If no prior films are available, what BI-RADS category should you give?

3. On prior workup, an ultrasound shows a circumscribed oval mass with homogenous echo pattern. What is the diagnosis?

4. If this is a new mass on mammography, what would be your recommendations?

5. Core biopsy is reported as a fibroepithelial lesion. What is your recommendation?

Case ranking/difficulty:

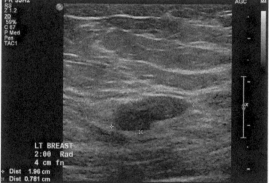

Ultrasound shows an oval circumscribed mass, which is parallel to the skin. There is an apparent notch on this single image, but on others, it was truly oval. If you see a notch, then you can turn on power Doppler and see a vessel going into the fatty hilum, which would confirm your suspicions that it was a lymph node.

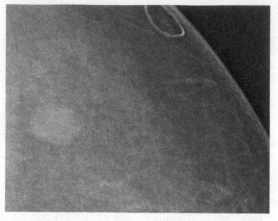

LCC spot magnification confirms that the lesion has a clean sharp margin. The overall descriptors are therefore "oval circumscribed mass."

Answers

1. This lesion was present on multiple prior examinations. It was stable in size and shape. The appearances are consistent with a cyst or fibroadenoma. If it has been present for over 3 years and stable, some readers would call this BI-RADS 1: negative.

2. This lesion has a low risk of malignancy, but if further examination confirms the presence of a cyst, then nothing further needs to be done. Some malignancies can present as a "benign" finding; therefore if a first visit, you need to recommend further workup. If it is solid and meets the Stavros criteria for a benign lump, then you can give it BI-RADS 3 and use short-term follow-up for a couple of years for stability.

3. The patient has no features of pregnancy or lactation-related change, and therefore the first two answers are unlikely. Phyllodes tumor is usually diagnosed in a growing "fibroadenoma" (ie, documented evidence of interval change). Mucinous carcinoma typically has slightly ill-defined margins on ultrasound, and may have a very heterogeneous echo pattern.

4. If you have tomosynthesis, then this may be the only tool you need to achieve analysis of the margins of the mass. If not, then spot (magnification) views to evaluate the mass margins should be performed. MRI is unlikely to add anything to the diagnosis at this point. Ultrasound-guided core biopsy is going to be required, as a developing mass has a much higher pretest probability for malignancy.

5. A fibroepithelial lesion is a high-risk lesion and may prove to be either fibroadenoma or phyllodes tumor at surgical excision. Age may be a factor in this patient being young, but there is a significant overlap between the risk of fibroadenoma and phyllodes based on age range.

Pearls

- Fibroadenomas are the most common finding in adolescent girls and young women.
- If not excised, they atrophy postmenopause, when they tend to calcify with characteristic dystrophic "popcorn" calcifications.
- If greater than 3 cm, often excised to exclude phyllodes tumor.
- Very rare risk of malignant phyllodes transformation.

Suggested Readings

Harvey JA, Nicholson BT, Lorusso AP, Cohen MA, Bovbjerg VE. Short-term follow-up of palpable breast lesions with benign imaging features: evaluation of 375 lesions in 320 women. *AJR Am J Roentgenol.* 2009;193(6):1723-1730.

Nishimura R, Taira N, Sugata S, Takabatake D, Ohsumi S, Takashima S. Suspicious calcifications in benign breast lesions: a radio-pathologic correlation. *Breast Cancer.* 2011;18(1):33-36.

Sabate JM, Clotet M, Torrubia S, et al. Radiologic evaluation of breast disorders related to pregnancy and lactation. *Radiographics.* 2007;27(Suppl 1):S101-S124.

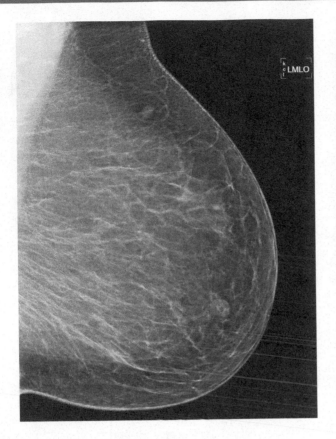
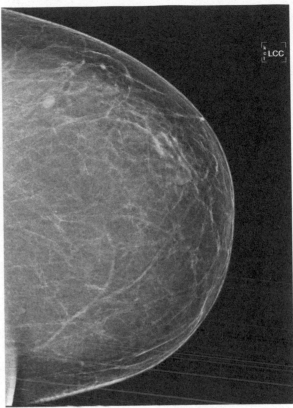

1. Why should a technical repeat be considered appropriate in this case?

2. What is the appropriate workup of the mass in the upper outer quadrant, if it is not a mole?

3. What are typical BI-RADS 3 lesions?

4. What is the management of a probably benign lesion?

5. What are other typical BI-RADS 3 lesions after diagnostic workup?

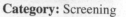
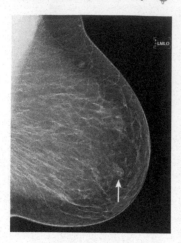

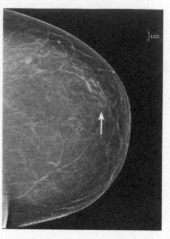

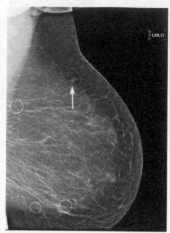

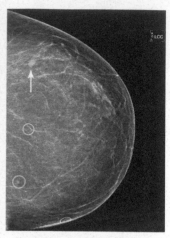

Screening mammogram of left MLO view of patient with moles. Noted are several benign-appearing masses. Nipple not in profile (*arrow*).

Screening mammogram of left CC view of patient with history of moles. Noted are several benign-appearing scattered masses. Nipple not in profile (*arrow*).

Screening mammogram of left MLO view with marker on multiple moles. However, one mass is not a mole.

Screening mammogram of left CC view with marker on multiple moles. One mass is not a mole. Nipple now is in profile.

Answers

1. Because the nipple is not in profile in both views.

2. The first step is a diagnostic mammogram that includes a spot compression MLO and CC view to assess the margin of the lesion.

3. There is no BI-RADS 3 on any screening exam! Screening exams should only result in BI-RADS 0 (recall)—BI-RADS 1 (normal) or BI-RADS 2 (benign). If there are masses like in this patient on a baseline exam and additional workup does not show any corresponding suspicious features and ultrasound is normal and does not show a corresponding finding, it is a classic example of a probably benign finding (BI-RADS 3).

4. The purpose of the "probably benign" category is to prove stability of a lesion defined as having a probability of malignancy of less than 2%. For that purpose, the most decisive images should be chosen as the follow up image. The follow-up should include magnification views, in case of calcifications, and spot compression views, in case of "mass" or "focal asymmetry." Follow-up should cover 2 years. The best approach is after the initial workup and next unilateral diagnostic mammogram in 6 months, then next bilateral diagnostic mammogram another 6 months later (12 months after the initial workup), and then the last follow-up diagnostic workup another 12 months later (24 months after initial workup). Each diagnostic workup needs to include the additional magnification or spot compression views.

5. The three classical mammogram BI-RADS 3 lesions are as follows: (i) a round and oval mass (as in our case) on a baseline mammogram after diagnostic workup, (ii) group of oval and round calcifications on a baseline mammogram after diagnostic workup, and (iii) focal asymmetry on baseline mammogram after diagnostic workup without suspicious finding on ultrasound. All of these lesions should be biopsied if new or if on further follow-up exams show any significant change. In addition, "complicated cyst" can also be followed as BI-RADS 3, or it can be aspirated.

Pearls

- Mole markers are helpful to differentiate real mass from mole(s).
- If there is mass on first mammogram and finding has "circumscribed margins" and is "round and oval" and ultrasound is unremarkable, finding is "probably benign," BI-RADS 3.
- According to the BI-RADS lexicon, probably benign finding will be monitored over 2 years or even 3 years with spot compression views to prove stability—after 2/3 years of being stable, it can be classified as "benign" BI-RADS 2 and patient can return to screening.

Suggested Reading

Sickles EA. Probably benign breast lesions: when should follow-up be recommended and what is the optimal follow-up protocol? *Radiology*. 1999;213(1):11-14.

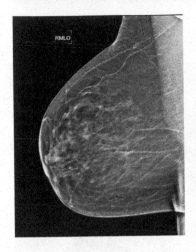 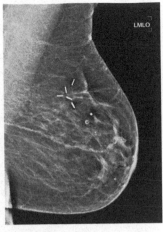 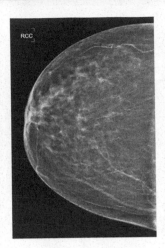 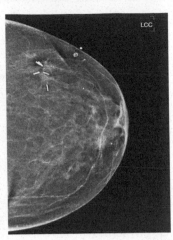

1. What BI-RADS classification should be used here?

2. What are causes of oil cysts in the breasts?

3. What is the next best imaging test?

4. What BI-RADS descriptors would you apply to this lesion?

5. What are the long-term sequelae of oil cysts?

Case ranking/difficulty: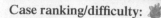

Category: Diagnostic

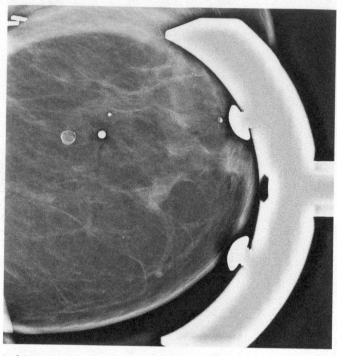

Left lateral spot magnification view with BB marker overlying the calcified oil cyst.

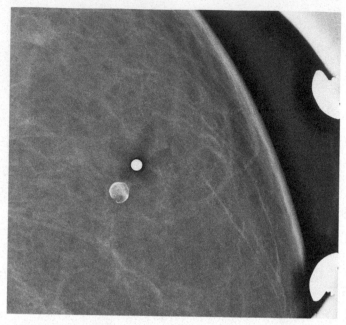

Left CC spot magnification view with BB marker. Palpable marker confirmed to lie immediately over the oil cyst. The imaging features are diagnostic.

Answers

1. Classical findings of a calcified oil cyst. A benign finding.

2. Well, we had to slip in an easier question. Oil cysts in the breast are very common. Just read a day of screening mammograms and you will observe your fair share. Minimal trauma, through seat belt injury and miscellaneous others.

3. No further workup is warranted when the findings like this are characteristic.

4. This is a type of fat necrosis and typically we talk about egg-shell calcifications, which BI-RADS refers to as "curvilinear." Linear calcifications are used in suspicious areas of calcifications. The actual calcific particles within the wall of the oil cyst can appear amorphous and pleomorphic, but the best fit to a diagnosis of oil cyst is "curvilinear."

5. There is no increased risk of breast cancer in a patient with underlying oil cysts. In most cases, oil cysts in screening populations are noted to resolve spontaneously. Rarely, they may go on to an established form of fat necrosis. Sarcomatous change does not occur. This is more likely in metaplastic carcinoma. Radial

scars have been associated with trauma, and it is not known if this is another post trauma variant process that causes both conditions.

Pearls

- Calcified oil cyst is diagnostic on mammography.
- No further tests required.
- If you perform ultrasound, you get a hard shadowing mass, which may make you call this harmless abnormality suspicious.

Suggested Readings

Bilgen IG, Ustun EE, Memis A. Fat necrosis of the breast: clinical, mammographic and sonographic features. *Eur J Radiol.* 2001;39(2):92-99.

Harvey JA, Moran RE, Maurer EJ, DeAngelis GA. Sonographic features of mammary oil cysts. *J Ultrasound Med.* 1997;16(11):719-724.

Mendelson EB. Evaluation of the postoperative breast. *Radiol Clin North Am.* 1992;30(1):107-138.

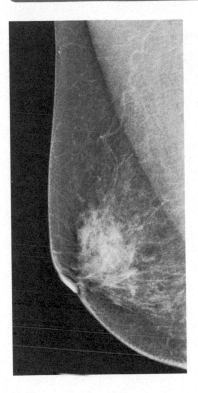
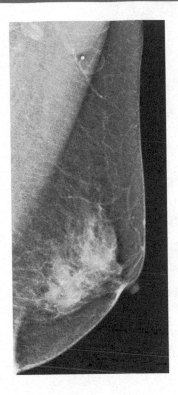
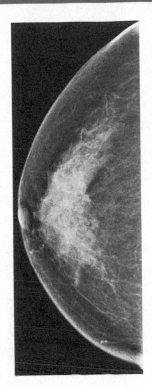
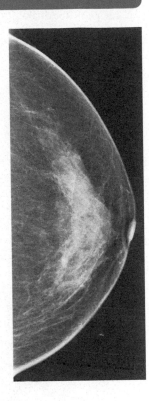

1. What BI-RADS classification should be used here?

2. What is the most likely pathology based on the imaging appearances?

3. What is the next best imaging test?

4. What type of biopsy should be performed?

5. Which radiological feature would lead you to suspect sarcomatous change in a fatty lump?

Case ranking/difficulty:

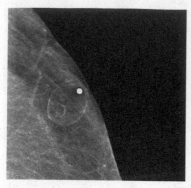

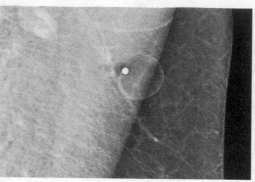

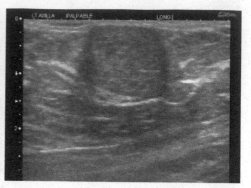

Spot left XCCL shows the palpable finding to be a "fatty density" lesion with a "thin sharply marginated" cortex.

Left MLO close-up—as of XCCL.

Ultrasound exam confirms an "isoechoic mass" consistent with a fatty mass—lipoma or epidermoid cyst.

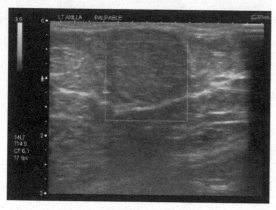

Ultrasound exam with power Doppler shows no evidence of abnormal flow.

4. This lesion is entirely harmless, and unless the patient requests that it be removed, the patient can safely be returned to routine screening. No biopsy need be performed.

5. Sarcomatous change in this type of lesion is very rare. The only thing you have to be aware of is an increase in solid component of the fatty mass, for example, if a lipoma that was completely lucent becomes more like a hamartoma, with both solid and lucent areas.

Pearls

- Classical appearances of lipoma or subdermal cyst.
- Ultrasound is not REQUIRED for the diagnosis, as this is typical enough on mammography.

Answers

1. This is a benign finding; therefore, a BI-RADS 2 assessment is appropriate. If the finding has been stable for more than 3 years, some would ignore the finding and give a BI-RADS 1 negative assessment.

2. The imaging appearances are similar in men and women, and in both entities. Sometimes, a lipoma can be felt as a soft lesion, whereas inclusion cysts are usually under high tension and are hard.

3. The images on mammography are characteristic enough to call this benign and leave alone. In this case, the lesion was palpable, and so completion of a diagnostic workup was performed, and also an ultrasound scan to confirm with the patient that what we were seeing was what was being felt. (The BB marker already told us this, but sometimes the patient asks for further confirmation that they can see for themselves.)

Suggested Readings

Adibelli ZH, Oztekin O, Gunhan-Bilgen I, Postaci H, Uslu A, Ilhan E. Imaging characteristics of male breast disease. *Breast J*. 2010;16(5):510-518.

Herreros-Villaraviz M, Mallo-Alonso R, Santiago-Freijanes P, Díaz-Veiga MJ. Epidermal inclusion cysts of the breast. *Breast J*. 2009;14(6):599-600.

Lam SY, Kasthoori JJ, Mun KS, Rahmat K. Epidermal inclusion cyst of the breast: a rare benign entity. *Singapore Med J*. 2010;51(12):e191-194.

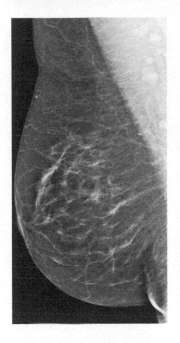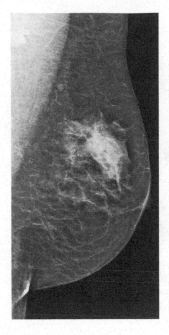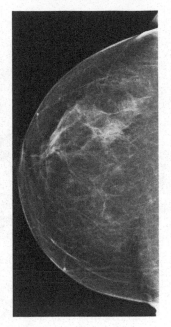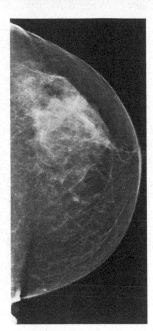

1. What is the finding on this first screening exam?

2. When can a global asymmetry be called benign?

3. What makes an asymmetry more concerning?

4. When patient returns for diagnostic workup, what is the first step?

5. What is the next step after ultrasound does not show any suspicious finding?

Case ranking/difficulty: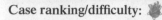

Category: Diagnostic

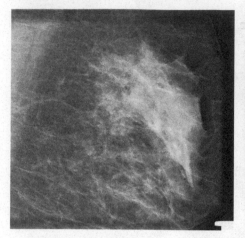

Diagnostic mammogram, spot compression left MLO view confirms the presence of focal asymmetry.

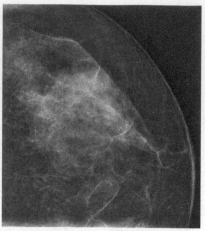

Diagnostic mammogram, spot compression left CC view confirms the presence of focal asymmetry.

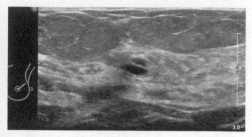

Ultrasound, left upper outer quadrant demonstrating incidental finding of simple cysts.

Answers

1. Mammogram demonstrates the left breast "focal asymmetry" in the upper outer quadrant. "Global asymmetry" would cover more than one quadrant. The small mass left superior breast on the MLO is small intramammary lymph node.

2. A global asymmetry is most likely normal fibroglandular tissue if on additional spot compression views there is no underlying distortion, calcifications, or mass and ultrasound is negative and there is no palpable mass associated with it. It can then be called BI-RADS 2 "benign" or if it remains still questionable, it could be called "probably benign" BI-RADS 3 and followed in 6 months and monitored over a time period of 2 years.

3. Any increasing asymmetry, any palpable abnormality, and any other morphological suspicious features are concerning and require biopsy. In case of a palpable abnormality in that area that correlates to the focal asymmetry, despite normal ultrasound, patient should in general receive stereotactic biopsy.

4. The first step is to perform left spot compression CC and MLO views. If there is no suspicious underlying distortion or other abnormality, patient needs additional ultrasound for further workup.

5. In case of negative ultrasound and negative diagnostic mammogram, this is a classical BI-RADS 3 lesion and patient needs to return in 6 months for left MLO and CC view and spot compression CC and MLO views to prove stability of this "most likely benign" finding. Small benign simple cysts as seen on ultrasound in this case do not change the approach—they are incidental benign findings.

Pearls

• If focal asymmetry does not show any underlying distortion or mass on spot compression views nor any abnormality on ultrasound and if patient does not feel lump in that area, finding is most likely normal fibroglandular tissue and can be classified as BI-RADS 3 and can be followed over a time period of 2 years.

• After monitoring for a period of 2 years, it can be called benign, BI-RADS 2.

• If the patient would feel a lump in that area, in general, the presence of corresponding focal asymmetry is more concerning and stereotactic biopsy is required.

Suggested Readings

Leung JW, Sickles EA. Developing asymmetry identified on mammography: correlation with imaging outcome and pathologic findings. *AJR Am J Roentgenol.* 2007;188(3):667-675.

Youk JH, Kim EK, Ko KH, Kim MJ. Asymmetric mammographic findings based on the fourth edition of BI-RADS: types, evaluation, and management. *Radiographics.* 2009;29(1):e33.

Palpable finding in the right breast

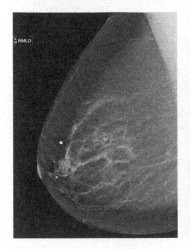 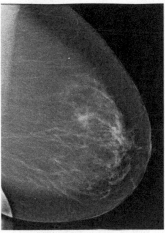 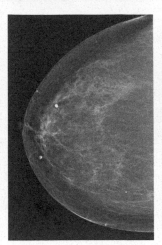 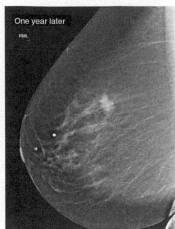

1. What BI-RADS classification should be used here?

2. What should be the next step if you perceive the mammogram as showing no significant finding?

3. The image from 1 year later can help you determine that abnormality on the original mammogram. What type of biopsy would you recommend?

4. The core biopsy comes back as fibrosis and plasma cells. What do you do next?

5. A developing focal asymmetry has what risk of malignancy associated with it?

Case ranking/difficulty: 🌰

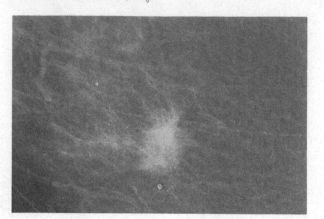

Spot magnification of the "focal asymmetry" reveals its true suspicious character.

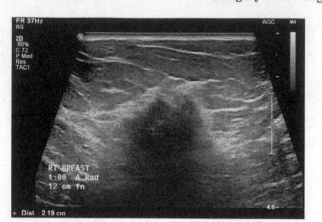

Targeted ultrasound shows an "irregular mass" with "angular margins" and dense "acoustic shadowing."

Answers

1. This is a diagnostic exam. There is a palpable marker over the area in the right upper outer quadrant at the site of patient complaint. If you do not see something underlying a palpable marker, then the next step should be to perform a targeted ultrasound to determine if there is a finding. The mammographic finding in this case is a subtle focal asymmetry with possible distortion. Spot views could have been performed to determine if there was any distortion, which would have confirmed a suspicious finding, prompting further investigation. A BI-RADS 4 assessment is the most appropriate in this situation.

2. The next best examination with a palpable finding is a targeted ultrasound, combined with careful palpation to determine if the palpation findings are a correlate to the ultrasound findings. If all examinations are normal, but you still are concerned, then a troubleshooting MRI may help. You have already determined that the mammograms are negative, so you would not do more mammograms.

3. You should be able to see the mass on ultrasound, especially as there is a palpable finding, and a BB or Sharpie marker may be on the patient's skin. Ultrasound remains the fastest, cheapest, and best type of biopsy for the patient to have in most settings bar calcifications or occult lesions. Ultrasound FNA may have a place if you have a breast cytopathologist, but this is not adequate for preoperative tissue markers that are needed.

4. The findings are not concordant, especially as this is a developing lesion and fibrosis does not explain the imaging findings. You are responsible for ensuring that this case is managed appropriately. In a quest for a preoperative diagnosis, and the original biopsy was not sampled

adequately, then repeating the biopsy may help to get accurate and representative tissue from the mass. If you used a 14-gauge core biopsy, it is time to bring out the "big guns" and go for vacuum-assisted biopsy. If the biopsy was already vacuum assisted, then surgical excision may be appropriate. A problem-solving MRI is unlikely to help, as your findings are already very suspicious.

5. Depending on the associated features, the average risk of malignancy of a developing focal asymmetry is around 20%. If there is associated segmental microcalcifications with a developing focal asymmetry, then this risk is more than 50%.

Pearls

- Always work up a "developing focal asymmetry" as high risk of malignancy compared with other mammographic findings.

Suggested Readings

Leung JW, Sickles EA. Developing asymmetry identified on mammography: correlation with imaging outcome and pathologic findings. *AJR Am J Roentgenol.* 2007;188(3):667-675.

Sickles EA. The spectrum of breast asymmetries: imaging features, work-up, management. *Radiol Clin North Am.* 2007;45(5):765-771, v.

Venkatesan A, Chu P, Kerlikowske K, Sickles EA, Smith-Bindman R. Positive predictive value of specific mammographic findings according to reader and patient variables. *Radiology.* 2009;250(3):648-657.

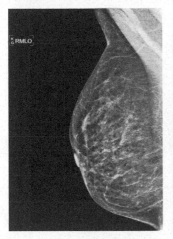
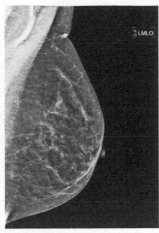
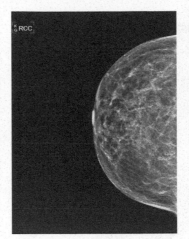
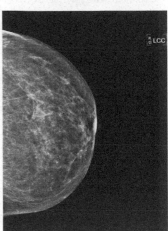

1. What is a diagnostic recall? Where is the abnormality?

2. What is the expected recall rate?

3. What is the target cancer detection rate in the United States in a screened population?

4. What will influence the cancer detection rate?

5. What are strategies to lower recall rate?

Case ranking/difficulty: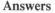

Category: Screening

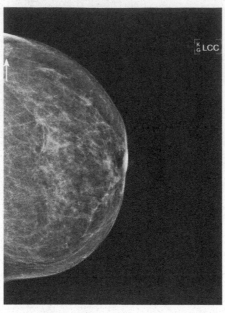

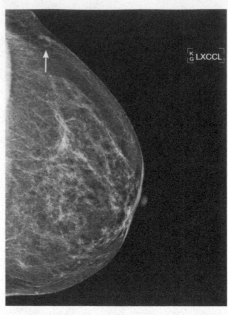

Screening mammogram, left CC view demonstrates uncertain density of lateral posterior breast.

Screening mammogram, left XCCL view shows that the density of left lateral breast is consistent with benign lymph node.

Answers

1. To work up an indeterminate abnormality seen on a good quality screening mammogram in general includes spot compression and/or magnification views. If screening mammogram is of not appropriate quality, additional views can be added as technical repeat and the patient can remain screening patient. In this particular case, if the patient has left the facility after screening, the exam can be called BI-RADS 0 and patient will be recalled for technical repeat and XCCL view will be obtained. There is a focal asymmetry seen on the left CC view, lateral posterior breast.

2. If a radiologist reads 100 screening mammograms and calls 10 patients back for workup of an abnormality, the radiologist has a recall rate of 10%.

3. The cancer detection rate in a screened population like in the United States is 3 to 5 cancers per 1000 screening mammograms.

4. The cancer detection rate depends on the skill of the radiologist, as well as the quantity of exams read per year, which may be reflected in the recall rate.

5. There are multiple efforts that can reduce recall rate. Besides training to recognize calcifications that can be called benign on standard views (oil cysts, dystrophic calcifications, etc.), it is extremely helpful to maximize the availability of old mammograms for comparison. Also helpful is to train to recognize densities that are caused by superimposed tissue.

Pearls

- "Focal densities" seen only on one view of concern, as they might be outside the field in the corresponding second view.
- In this particular case, a technical repeat with XCCL view, to include more tissue, did solve the issue.
- In the United States, the recall rate is supposed to be 10%. However, before a radiologist should adjust the recall rate, first it is crucial to make sure that the cancer detection rate is in the expected range.
- The recall rate depends on many factors, including screening penetration of the population, the presence of prior images, and reading setup (immediate vs. batch reading).

Suggested Readings

Carney PA, Sickles EA, Monsees BS, et al. Identifying minimally acceptable interpretive performance criteria for screening mammography. *Radiology*. 2010;255(2):354-361.

Ghate SV, Soo MS, Baker JA, Walsh R, Gimenez EI, Rosen EL. Comparison of recall and cancer detection rates for immediate versus batch interpretation of screening mammograms. *Radiology*. 2005;235(1):31-35.

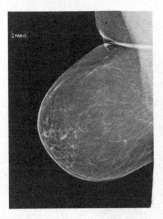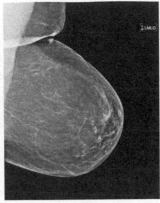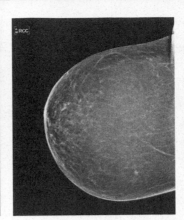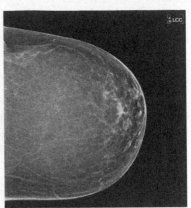

1. What is the BI-RADS category for this screening exam?

2. If this was a diagnostic exam, what descriptors would you use to describe the findings?

3. Based on the initial mammograms, where in the breast do you expect to find the mass?

4. What is the likely final pathology in this patient?

5. What additional mammographic views would you order?

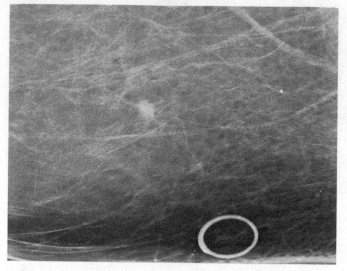

Close-up of the mass shows the "indistinct margins."

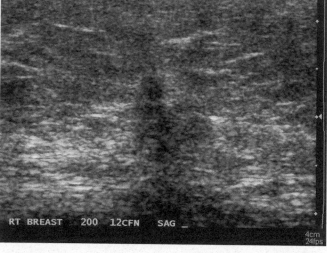

Ultrasound shows small mass as a correlate to the mammographic findings.

Answers

1. There is a finding that requires further workup, and therefore this should be a BI-RADS 0. Although your suspicion level may be high that this is a cancer, based on prior negative exams, it is possible that this might disappear on compression and further workup; therefore, to give it a BI-RADS 4 or 5 would commit the patient to having an unnecessary biopsy. It is always best to wait to get more images and complete the mammographic workup BEFORE you commit yourself to the final BI-RADS assessment.

2. The abnormality is seen on two views and is therefore a "focal asymmetry" (compared with a "one view asymmetry"). If you are sure that the lesion is space occupying, then you can use the term "mass." In this case, the margins are indistinct.

3. Remember that the images shown are not orthogonal, and obtaining a lateral film will assist you in estimating the position of the lesion for ultrasound exam. In the MLO projection, a medial lesion often moves up on the lateral, so although it currently appears at 3 o'clock, the lesion was actually seen at 2 o'clock on ultrasound.

4. It is in the correct position for a sebaceous cyst, but malignancy has to be excluded. Fibroadenomas generally do not appear as masses in older women, but usually as coarse dystrophic calcification, which in the early stages can be developing coarse heterogeneous and therefore prompt biopsy.

5. The lateral exam can be performed in two directions. It is best to choose the one that puts the lesion closest to the bucky to reduce geometric unsharpness. Hence, an LM versus an ML exam. Spot films should be performed. These can be magnified to increase the resolution, and the choice is dependent on the center you practice in. My approach is to ask that any spot films are always magnified, to get the best resolution possible from the exam, and to characterize mass margins and calcifications better.

Pearls

- Easy to spot mass in fatty breasts.
- The borders are not seen clearly enough to be given a negative or benign screening result.
- Diagnostic workup confirms that this is not a benign lesion.

Suggested Reading

Venkatesan A, Chu P, Kerlikowske K, Sickles EA, Smith-Bindman R. Positive predictive value of specific mammographic findings according to reader and patient variables. *Radiology*. 2009;250(3):648-657.

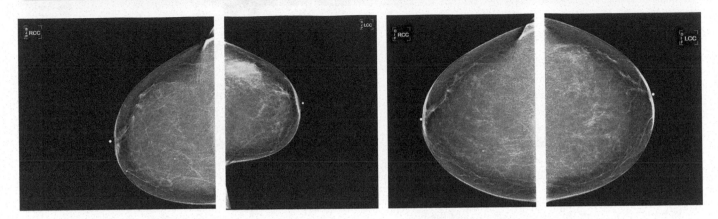

1. What is the BI-RADS category for this screening exam?

2. What is the next best examination you recommend?

3. What is the risk of malignancy in a regional asymmetry?

4. What type of biopsy should be performed?

5. When pregnancy has been completed, what happens to the asymmetry?

Case ranking/difficulty:

Answers

1. Findings were similar on the MLO films, with an asymmetric increase in breast density in the left upper half. No explanation is given for the recent increase in asymmetric breast density. The patient does not report any symptoms on her questionnaire. This is therefore a BI-RADS 0, needs further workup. If you think this is normal and had been stable, you could give it a BI-RADS 1, but we have evidence of developing change.

2. It is important to understand the reason for the increase in breast density in this young woman, and the best way to do this is a complete history and physical exam before giving her any more radiation. An ultrasound examination was performed first, as we believed her to be an unreliable historian, and wanted to rule out pregnancy first. Ultrasound showed normal glandular breast tissue.

3. The risk of malignancy is very low with a regional asymmetry. In this case, however, it is a new finding, and would be better described as a developing regional asymmetry, which is slightly more suspicious. The risk is nowhere near as great as in developing focal asymmetries, which have a high PPV for malignancy.

4. No treatment is required for physiological breast changes with pregnancy. If the area is palpable, some surgeons wish to follow up with interval physical exam and ultrasound.

5. The postpregnancy response is either none, staying stable, or a mild-to-marked reduction in fibroglandular volume as the physiological changes accompanying pregnancy diminish. This response can be quite dramatic in many women.

Pearls

- Normal physiological changes in pregnancy can give asymmetries (usually at least a regional asymmetry, to a global asymmetry).
- These are rapidly reversible following childbirth and cessation of breast feeding.
- In postmenopausal women, you can get similar changes with hormone replacement therapy.

Suggested Readings

Canoy JM, Mitchell GS, Unold D, Miller V. A radiologic review of common breast disorders in pregnancy and the perinatal period. *Semin Ultrasound CT MR*. 2012;33(1):78-85.

Kizer NT, Powell MA. Surgery in the pregnant patient. *Clin Obstet Gynecol*. 2011;54(4):633-641.

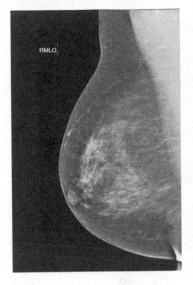 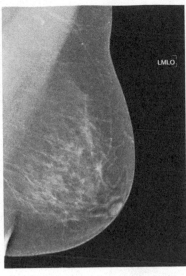 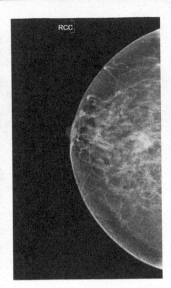 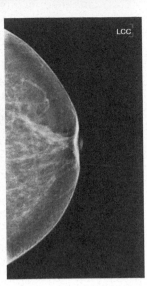

1. What BI-RADS classification should be used here?

2. What descriptors would you use for the calcifications present with the asymmetry?

3. What is the next best imaging test?

4. What type of biopsy should be performed?

5. If you see suspicious calcifications with an associated mass, what is the likely pathology?

Case ranking/difficulty: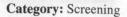

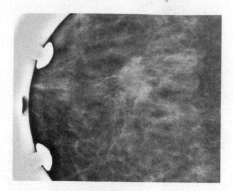

Right CC spot magnification views.

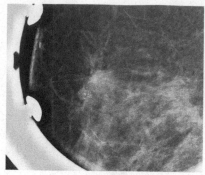

Right ML spot magnification views show an "ill-defined mass" with some possible "spiculation." There is also some associated "pleomorphic calcification" at one edge of the mass.

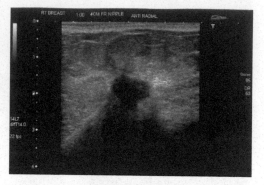

Targeted ultrasound shows a hypoechoic "mass" with "acoustic attenuation (shadowing)." The lesion is "parallel" and "sharply marginated," but those BI-RADS descriptors do not fit the suspicious assessment you are about to make, and therefore should not be used.

Answers

1. This is an abnormal screening exam, and so a BI-RADS 0 is appropriate as the finding requires further workup. A suspicious BI-RADS assessment should not be given as the finding could be due to superimposition or a benign finding, and a diagnostic workup is required.

2. At this stage, the patient is having a screening exam, and you do not have spot magnification views to characterize the calcific particles, so strictly you do not need to describe the calcifications. Best guess at this stage is that they are anything from "amorphous" through "coarse heterogeneous" to "fine pleomorphic."

3. Tomosynthesis has been proven to be good at differentiating masses and asymmetries, but its utility in characterizing calcifications has not been proven. Therefore, although tomosynthesis could be performed, you still need to perform spot magnification views to truly characterize the calcific particles.

4. The most important thing is to diagnose the invasive component of any disease, so ultrasound targeting of the mass is the way to go. You can still x-ray the specimens to see if you have harvested any calcifications. If you target the calcifications with stereotactic core biopsy, then you may miss the mass and the invasive disease.

5. The common pathological finding for highly suspicious calcifications associated with a mass is a high-grade invasive ductal cancer with high-grade DCIS. Low-grade DCIS is much more likely to be amorphous or like the benign calcifications associated with LCIS.

Pearls

- "Developing focal asymmetry" is high yield for a cancer.
- Full mammographic workup, followed by ultrasound if confirmed.
- You need to explain any developing focal asymmetry.

Suggested Readings

Leung JW, Sickles EA. Developing asymmetry identified on mammography: correlation with imaging outcome and pathologic findings. *AJR Am J Roentgenol.* 2007;188(3):667-675.

Sickles EA. Mammographic features of 300 consecutive nonpalpable breast cancers. *AJR Am J Roentgenol.* 1986;146(4):661-663.

Sickles EA. The spectrum of breast asymmetries: imaging features, work-up, management. *Radiol Clin North Am.* 2007;45(5):765-771, v.

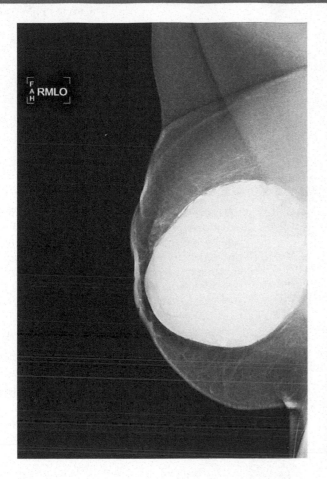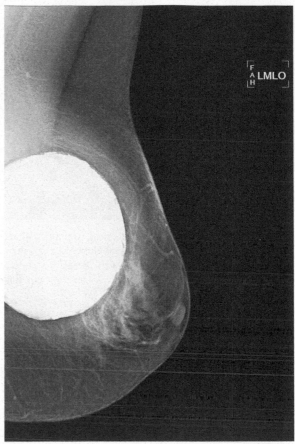

1. What BI-RADS classification should be used here?

2. What additional views do you need on a patient with implants?

3. What are the signs of implant rupture on ultrasound?

4. If there has been extracapsular rupture of the silicone implant, which of the following features are seen on ultrasound?

5. In intracapsular rupture of a silicone implant, which of the following are characteristic signs on MRI?

Case ranking/difficulty: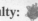

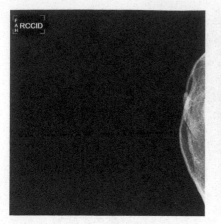

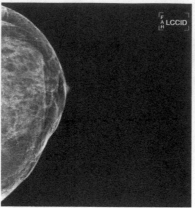

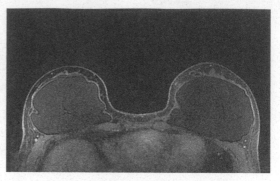

Right CC implant displaced (RCCID or Eklund). Virtually impossible to get good views of the right breast as the implant will not displace further.

Left CC implant displaced (LCCID or Eklund). We can see a little more of the breast tissue on this implant displaced view, but still not ideal.

MRI is the best examination to look for implant integrity, especially in women who have large volume implants relative to their remaining breast tissue. You can see the normal radial folds of the implants as wavy outlines to the implants. Silicone saturation sequences can also be performed if you are trying to determine whether a patient has a rupture.

Answers

1. This is a screening exam. There is no evidence of a malignancy. Describe the position of the implants and the lack of findings. As there is a finding, the appropriate assessment is BI-RADS 2: benign.

2. The implant displaced view, developed by Eklund, is the most common additional exam. For ultrasound readers, this means a difference between a diagnostic and a screening exam, as screening should be just CC and MLO views (with the exception of occasional XCCL views if needed to cover the breast tissue). However, as the patient has no other problem, some centers do all the views but still charge as a screening exam. Displacement views for screening are not routinely used in European screening programs.

3. The stepladder sign refers to multiple, discontinuous, parallel, linear echoes in the lumen. It is the most reliable ultrasound finding in intracapsular rupture. It is analogous to the linguine sign at MRI. A sidewinder is a type of missile. Neither serpentine or pasta signs help here. "Pasta" refers to the MRI "Linguine" sign.

4. Silicone disperses sound and you get a marked snowstorm, or white noise type of image. Frequently, granulomas may form that contain cyst-like fluid, but with foci of hyperechoic change with loss of posterior detail. Sensitivity of ultrasound for rupture with these signs ranges from 47% to 74% with a specificity of 55% to 96%.

5. There are two signs on MRI of intracapsular rupture. The first is the Linguine sign, where the capsule still contains the silicone, but the implant wall has deflated and fallen to the most dependent part of the capsule. The second is the teardrop sign, which refers to the presence of silicone both inside and outside of a radial fold, indicative of rupture. A dark fibrous capsule is a normal finding. Reactive fluid is commonly seen around textured implants, but is not a sign of rupture.

Pearls

- Silicone gel breast implants commonly used by cosmetic surgeons.
- Placement often prepectoral (subglandular) as easy to place.
- Capsule of prepectoral implant may calcify.
- May also occur with saline implants.

Suggested Readings

Friedman HI, Friedman AC, Carson K. The fate of the fibrous capsule after saline implant removal. *Ann Plast Surg*. 2001;46(3):215-221.

Peters W, Pritzker K, Smith D, et al. Capsular calcification associated with silicone breast implants: incidence, determinants, and characterization. *Ann Plast Surg*. 1998;41(4):348-360.

Peters W, Smith D, Lugowski S, Pritzker K, Holmyard D. Calcification properties of saline-filled breast implants. *Plast Reconstr Surg*. 2001;107(2):356-363.

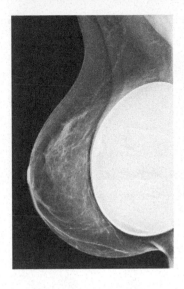 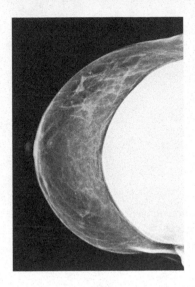 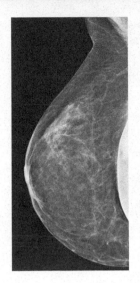 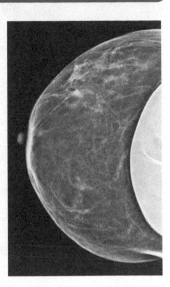

1. What is the workup in a patient with focal breast pain?

2. What is the best workup in a patient with breast implant and focal pain?

3. When is MRI indicated to work up implants for rupture?

4. What is the major difference between saline implants and silicone implants for imaging?

5. What is the likelihood of implant rupture due to spot compression view?

Case ranking/difficulty: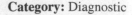

Category: Diagnostic

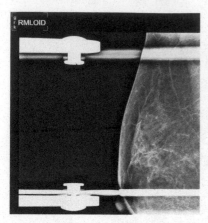

Diagnostic mammogram, right spot compression MLO view does not show any abnormality.

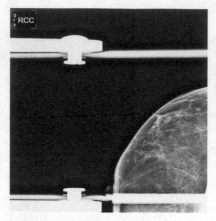

Diagnostic mammogram, right spot compression CC view does not show any abnormality.

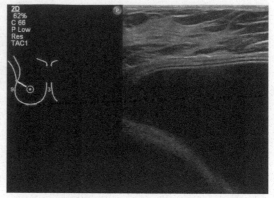

Ultrasound of right breast lateral outer quadrant is unremarkable as well.

Answers

1. In a patient with focal breast pain (patient can direct with index finger to a specific area), the patient needs diagnostic mammogram including spot compression views and workup with ultrasound targeted to the area of concern. In a patient younger than 30 years, ultrasound can be the first test, given the fact that in younger patients, radiation is more significant. If ultrasound is negative, as in most cases and in the absence of palpable lump, follow-up with mammogram can be an option at later time if the pain does not resolve.

2. Workup is the same. Mammograms and even spot compression views are part of the normal workup, even if patient has implant. Every patient with implants receives in addition to the standard MLO and CC views implant replacement MLO and CC views. This is crucial to expose as much tissue as possible, without overlap by the implant.

3. In saline implants, there is no need for MRI. Intracapsular rupture is not an issue. In silicone implants, dependent on the level of suspicion and the clinical situation, MRI is the best test to assess the integrity of the implant.

4. Saline implants can rupture, but then the saline will be absorbed by the tissue and the implant will completely collapse. Silicone implants can show intra- and extracapsular rupture. Extracapsular rupture indicates silicone leaking into the breast tissue and is in general an indication for replacement. It is easier to penetrate with mammography saline implants and detect abnormalities behind the implant.

5. Spot compression views ought to be performed with silicone and saline implants. Likelihood of rupture is extremely low, and the benefits of additional workup outweigh the very minimal chance of rupture in general. However, ultrasound in some cases can be a substitute replacing additional spot compression views, for example, if there is an obvious mass.

Pearls

- Diagnostic mammographic views should include implant displaced views as spot compression views to an area of concern, which should be marked with a BB.
- In this case, there is no abnormality identified. The next step in the workup is to perform an ultrasound directed to that particular area.
- Pitfall: Make sure to pay attention to the tissue behind the implant. In case of a saline implant, a mass or even small calcifications, if present, can often times be seen behind the implant.

Suggested Reading

Steinbach BG, Hardt NS, Abbitt PL, Lanier L, Caffee HH. Breast implants, common complications, and concurrent breast disease. *Radiographics*. 1993;13(1):95-118.

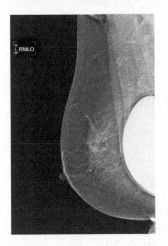 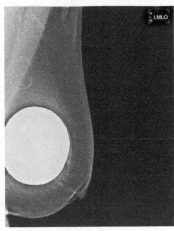 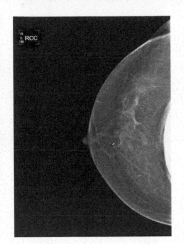 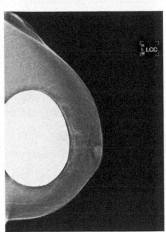

1. What is the BI-RADS category for this screening exam?

2. What type of implant is present?

3. What is the position of the implant?

4. What are the signs of a potential complication with prepectoral implants?

5. What are the radiological signs of silicone in the breast?

Case ranking/difficulty:

Answers

1. BI-RADS 2: benign. If you use the BI-RADS system and describe a finding in the breast, in this case, the implants, then you should give it a BI-RADS 2. If you choose to NOT give a finding, then BI-RADS 1 negative. This fits the European normal/benign category.

2. These are dense implants, and a valve is not seen, consistent with silicone implants.

3. Right retropectoral, left prepectoral.

4. Specifically, silicone granulomas present as soft tissue densities with indistinct margins around the implant capsule. They may arise from a previous implant rupture, for example, current saline implants following a ruptured silicone implant; therefore, the images may show potential silicone granulomas, BUT the patient has saline implants.

5. Extracapsular silicone can look very suspicious if there is no other evidence of prior implants on an exam. Silicone injections, common in Asia for augmentation, can give spiculate densities, and you can sometimes see the injection tracks. Most commonly, the free silicone gets walled off by inflammatory tissue, which explains the ill-defined margins.

Pearls

- Positioning of implants is in one of two tissue compartments, separated by the pectoral muscle.
- Frequently called retropectoral or prepectoral, sometimes subglandular is used, although the term is less specific.

Suggested Readings

Brower TD. Positioning techniques for the augmented breast. *Radiol Technol*. 1990;61(3):209-211.

Glicenstein J. History of augmentation mammoplasty [in French]. *Ann Chir Plast Esthet*. 2005;50(5):337-349.

Tebbetts JB. Breast augmentation with full-height anatomic saline implants: the pros and cons. *Clin Plast Surg*. 2001;28(3):567-577.

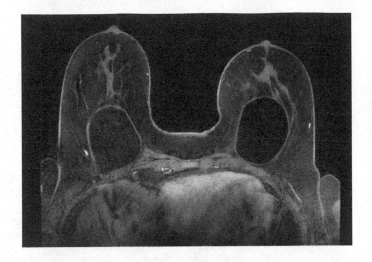 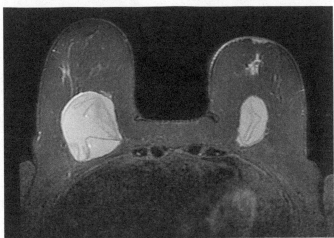

1. What BI-RADS classification should be used here?

2. What is the name given to the radiologic sign shown here?

3. In addition to normal sequences on MRI, what other sequences would you ask for to diagnose a rupture?

4. What is the risk of malignancy in patients with ruptured implants?

5. What is the average lifespan of a silicone implant?

Case ranking/difficulty: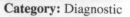

Category: Diagnostic

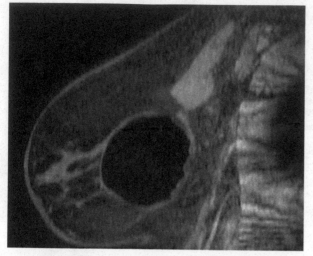

MRI—T1 postcontrast sagittal.

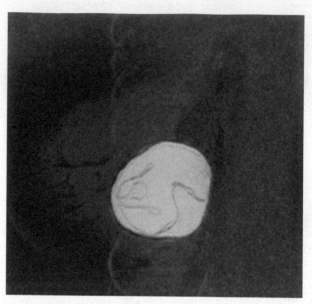

T2 sagittal silicone bright sequence. Note the coiled up inner capsule of the implant surrounded by silicone.

5. In a historic paper out of Baylor in the 1990s, the median lifespan of a silicone gel implant was estimated to be 16.4 years. (Goodman et al. 1998).

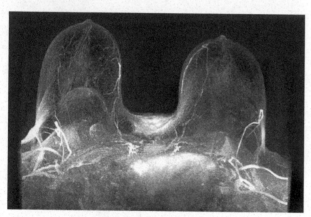

Subtracted axial MIP—note that the implant is subtracted out of the image, and if you do not deliberately look for it, you may miss the implant rupture.

Pearls

- Linguine sign is pathognomonic of intracapsular implant rupture.

Answers

1. These findings are benign; therefore, a BI-RADS 2 is appropriate.

2. Linguine sign—just like the pasta. Even if you just remember the pasta, it helps.

3. The silicone sequences are very helpful to spot the intracapsular rupture of an implant. Both silicone bright and silicone dark sequences may be performed. This may be particularly important in a patient with simple cysts when you suspect extracapsular silicone.

4. The same rate of malignancy is found as the general population at approximately 5 per 1000 women screened.

Suggested Readings

Goodman CM, Cohen V, Thornby J, Netscher D. The life span of silicone gel breast implants and a comparison of mammography, ultrasonography, and magnetic resonance imaging in detecting implant rupture: a meta-analysis. *Ann Plast Surg*. 1998;41(6):577-585; discussion 85-86.

Gorczyca DP, Gorczyca SM, Gorczyca KL. The diagnosis of silicone breast implant rupture. *Plast Reconstr Surg*. 2007;120(7, Suppl 1):49S-61S.

Juanpere S, Perez E, Huc O, Motos N, Pont J, Pedraza S. Imaging of breast implants—a pictorial review. *Insights Imaging*. 2011;2(6):653-670.

Mund DF, Farria DM, Gorczyca DP, et al. MR imaging of the breast in patients with silicone-gel implants: spectrum of findings. *AJR Am J Roentgenol*. 1993;161(4):773-778.

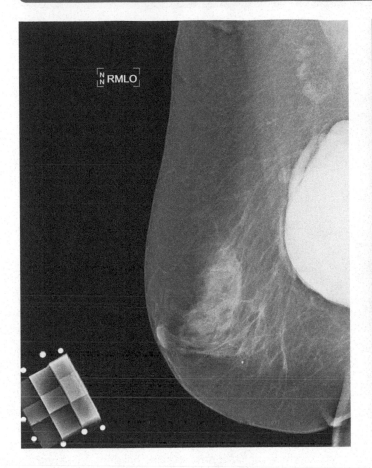 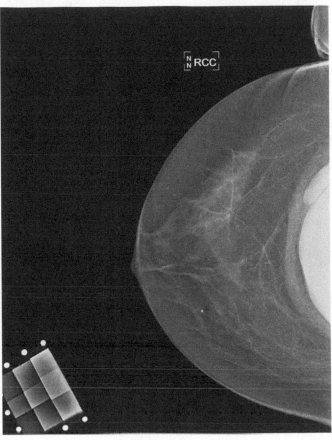

1. What BI-RADS classification should be used here?

2. What is the most likely cause for these appearances?

3. What is the next best imaging test?

4. What type of biopsy would you recommend?

5. When should the patient have her next mammography, if of screening age?

Case ranking/difficulty: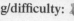

Category: Screening

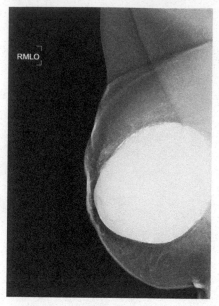

Right MLO—another implant with calcification of the capsule.

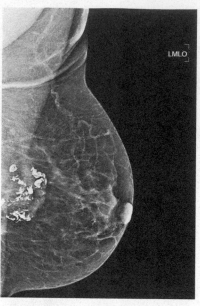

Left MLO of explanted prosthesis with residual calcified capsule.

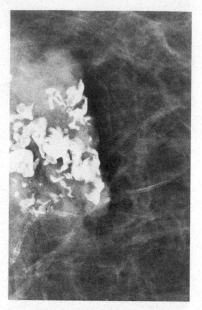

Left CC of explanted patient showing characteristic dystrophic calcifications.

Answers

1. These findings are characteristically benign. BI-RADS 2 is the most appropriate assessment to give.

2. There is a retropectoral silicone implant. There is also a circumscribed density around the implant. It is likely that prior implant had ruptured, and a new one placed.

3. Ultrasound and MRI are also good tools, but in the retropectoral placed implant, MRI would be the best tool to image the findings.

4. This is an obvious one, if you have already determined the diagnosis on imaging. No biopsy is required. If you have a potential silicone granuloma on ultrasound, then the features are not necessarily characteristic enough to avoid biopsy.

5. Depending on the guidelines in your country. In the United States, her next mammogram should be performed in 1 year. In Europe, in general, the screening interval is 2 years (United Kingdom, 3 years).

Pearls

- Coarse dystrophic contiguous calcifications are characteristic for implant capsule calcification.
- "Aunt Minnie" for board exams.

Suggested Readings

Juanpere S, Perez E, Huc O, Motos N, Pont J, Pedraza S. Imaging of breast implants—a pictorial review. *Insights Imaging.* 2011;2(6):653-670.

Peters W, Pritzker K, Smith D, et al. Capsular calcification associated with silicone breast implants: incidence, determinants, and characterization. *Ann Plast Surg.* 1998;41(4):348-360.

Peters W, Smith D. Calcification of breast implant capsules: incidence, diagnosis, and contributing factors. *Ann Plast Surg.* 1995;34(1):8-11.

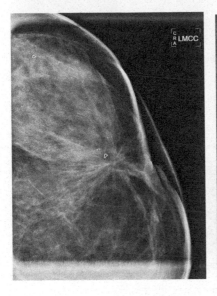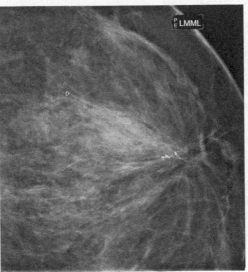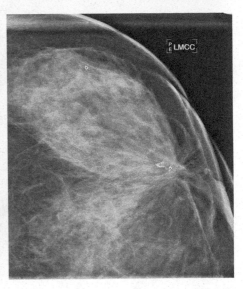

1. What are the findings on the spot compression views?

2. What is a typical time period where dystrophic calcifications develop after lumpectomy?

3. What would be good descriptors for benign calcifications after lumpectomy?

4. If there is concern of new calcifications in a lumpectomy bed, what could be the next step?

5. What would be the benefit of an MRI in this scenario?

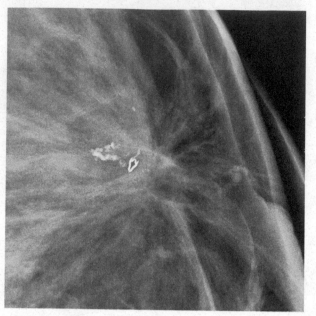

Left CC, additional electronic magnification demonstrating "coarse and heterogeneous" calcifications.

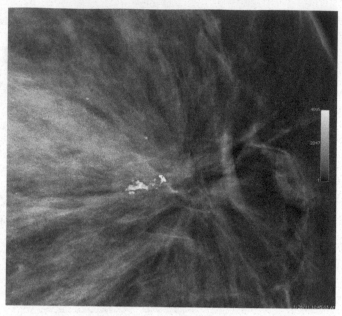

Left ML, additional electronic magnification demonstrating "coarse and heterogeneous" calcifications.

Answers

1. Spot compression views demonstrate architectural distortion. Noted is a clip due to prior benign biopsy. Noted is also development of dystrophic calcifications. They are "coarse" and are benign in nature.

2. Dystrophic calcifications develop, in general, between 2 and 44 months after lumpectomy.

3. The two types of benign calcifications that, in general, develop after lumpectomy could be related to fat necrosis and formation of oil cysts and have "egg shell" appearance with "lucent centers." Other typical benign calcifications would be dystrophic calcifications that are mostly macrocalcifications (larger than 1 mm) and coarse and plaque-like.

4. Depending on the level of suspicion, next steps could include 6-month follow-up, for example, to document the maturation of calcifications into an oil cyst, or MRI to see if there are any signs for abnormal enhancement in the scar area, or to repeat stereotactic biopsy.

5. MRI can be helpful to detect focal recurrent malignancy if performed about 6 months after lumpectomy. If the MRI is performed too early, it is impossible to distinguish between neogenesis of blood vessels due to tumor recurrence from postoperative changes.

Pearls

- Typical findings after lumpectomy on mammograms are skin thickening, "architectural distortion," and benign "dystrophic" calcifications and oil cysts.
- If there is concern that calcifications near lumpectomy bed are malignant, stereotactic biopsy should be performed.
- It is also helpful to compare the shape of the calcifications with the appearance of the initial preoperative calcifications that have been proven to be malignant.
- MRI can be useful to assess recurrent malignancy, but should be performed not early than 6 months after surgery.

Suggested Readings

Krishnamurthy R, Whitman GJ, Stelling CB, Kushwaha AC. Mammographic findings after breast conservation therapy. *Radiographics*. 1999;19 (Spec no.):S53-S62; quiz S262-S263.

Pinsky RW, Rebner M, Pierce LJ, et al. Recurrent cancer after breast-conserving surgery with radiation therapy for ductal carcinoma in situ: mammographic features, method of detection, and stage of recurrence. *AJR Am J Roentgenol*. 2007;189(1):140-144.

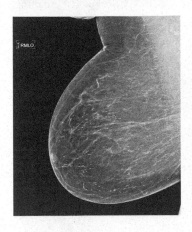
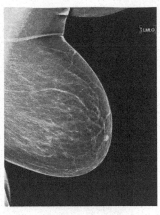
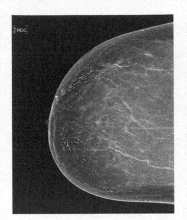
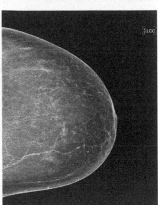

1. What is the appropriate descriptor for these calcifications?

2. What is an important differential diagnosis and why?

3. What is the typical appearance of calcifications in comedocarcinoma?

4. What is the assessment of the mammogram?

5. What is the consequence of the assessment?

Case ranking/difficulty:

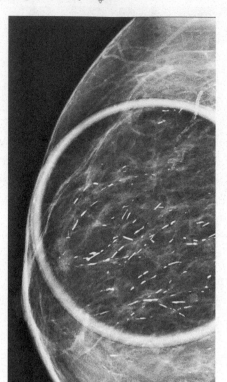

Diagnostic mammogram, right MLO magnification view demonstrates "rod-like calcifications."

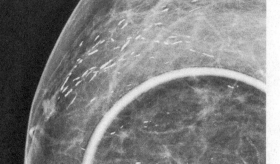

Right CC magnification view demonstrates "rod-like" calcifications.

Answers

1. These are typical "large rod-like" calcifications in bilateral and symmetric distribution. Secretory calcifications are large (more than 1 mm in general), rod-like, and bilateral and symmetric.

2. An important differential diagnosis is "casting" (Tabar) calcifications as seen in high-grade DCIS (comedocarcinoma).

3. Comedocarcinoma shows typical "casting" (Tabar) calcifications in segmental distribution that are more fine and pleomorphic in form and are in general consistent with fast progressive high-grade DCIS.

4. These calcifications are BI-RADS 2: benign.

5. These are benign calcifications and patient can return for next screening exam in 1 year.

Pearls

- "Large rod-like" calcifications are typical benign calcifications also called secretory calcifications.
- They affect the larger and intermediate ducts in mostly older and asymptomatic patients.
- Secretory calcifications are most often bilateral, but when present unilateral can be confused with comedocarcinoma.
- Unlike comedocarcinoma calcifications, secretory calcifications are solid and smoothly marginated and sometimes more than 1 cm in size and widely spaced and usually not branching.

Suggested Readings

Bland KI, Copeland EM. The Breast: Comprehensive Management of Benign and Malignant Diseases. 4th ed. Philadelphia, PA: Saunders Elsevier; 2009.

D'Orsi CJ, Bassett LW, Berg WA, et al. *Breast Imaging Reporting and Data System: ACR BI-RADS–Mammography.* 4th ed. Reston, VA: American College of Radiology; 2003.

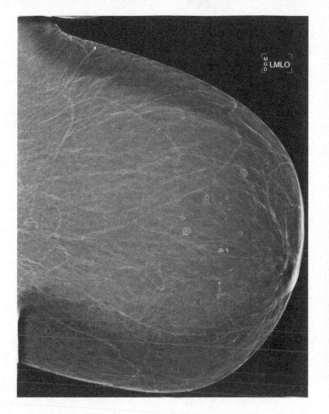
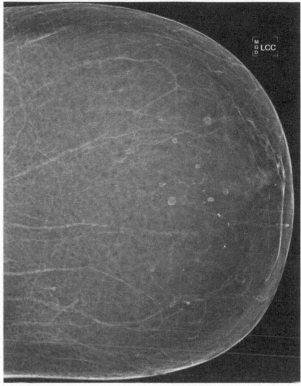

1. What are BI-RADS descriptors for benign calcifications?

2. What is the name of these calcifications and the assessment?

3. What is the difference between "milk of calcium" and an "oil cyst"?

4. If you suspect the presence of skin calcifications, how can you prove it?

5. How can you obtain a tangential view?

Case ranking/difficulty: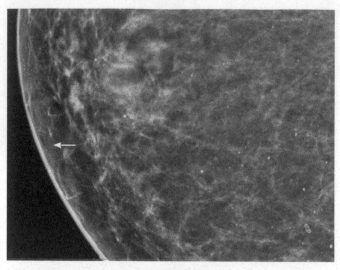

Magnification right CC view, demonstrating skin calcifications (*arrow*) and scattered oil cysts.

Answers

1. "Amorphous" and "coarse and heterogeneous" are descriptors for calcifications of intermediate concern. "Eggshell or rim" calcifications are benign calcifications related to oil cysts. "Rod-like" calcifications are benign calcifications related to plasma cell mastitis. "Coarse or popcorn-like" calcifications are benign calcifications related to fibroadenoma.

2. These are typical benign (BI-RADS 2) calcifications consistent with diagnosis of oil cysts. They are round and often times in multiple locations and have a characteristic appearance with "eggshell or rim" calcification with lucent center. There is no need for follow-up or biopsy.

3. The etiology of oil cysts is fat necrosis. The etiology of "milk of calcium" are proliferative changes of the breast parenchyma with formation of multiple small cysts related to the lobules of the parenchyma with small collection of liquid calcium within the cysts causing typical layering as seen on the ML view. Both are "benign" finding according to the BI-RADS lexicon.

4. If there is a group of calcifications that are likely within the skin, tangential views are the way to prove it.

5. A tangential view is obtained by putting the patient in a mammogram unit using a paddle with window (like for a needle localization)—mark the calcifications with BB. Then, patient is put into position in which the BB is tangential at the edge of the scan field (tangential view). If the calcifications are not seen within the subcutaneous fat, the view is either not really tangential to the calcifications and needs to be adjusted or the calcifications are not in the skin.

Pearls

- Most breast calcifications are benign and this includes "lucent-centered" skin calcifications, "coarse and popcorn" type calcifications, "tram-like" vascular calcifications, and "milk of calcium" type calcifications.
- For diagnostic workup of calcifications, never perform magnification MLO view, but always perform magnification ML view to maximize chance to detect benign "milk of calcium."
- To prove location of calcifications within the skin, it is prudent to obtain tangential views.
- "Eggshell"-type calcifications are typical for oil cysts.

Suggested Reading

D'Orsi CJ, Bassett LW, Berg WA, et al. *Breast Imaging Reporting and Data System: ACR BI-RADS–Mammography*. 4th ed. Reston, VA: American College of Radiology; 2003.

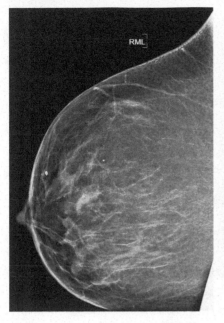 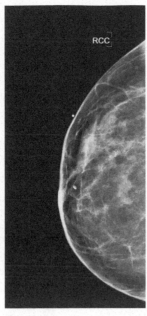 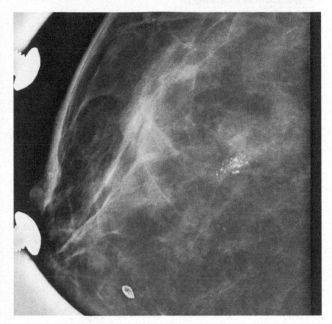

1. What BI-RADS classification should be used here?

2. What is the most likely pathology based on the imaging?

3. What further imaging would you recommend?

4. In determining extent of disease, what tools should be considered?

5. What type of biopsy would you perform?

Case ranking/difficulty:    **Category:** Screening

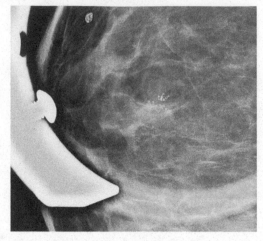

Right ML spot magnification. Note the distribution of the calcifications, which is segmental toward the nipple.

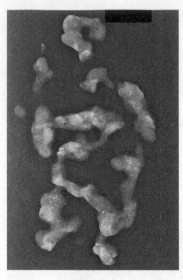

Specimen x-ray–extensive coarse "pleomorphic" calcifications in most cores—evidence of good sampling. "Fine pleomorphic" calcifications on mammograms often appear coarse on specimen x-ray, which illustrates limitations in our current technology for analyzing calcification morphology in situ.

Answers

1. This is a diagnostic workup; therefore, BI-RADS 4 is the best fit, as the finding has at least a 50% risk of malignancy with this type and distribution of calcifications.

2. High-grade calcifications typically present with these features. Low-grade DCIS is often "punctate" or "amorphous." It may be faint and difficult to see. Sometimes referred to as "powdery" calcifications, likely arising in the TDLU rather than the ducts.

3. At this stage, the diagnostic workup needs to be completed and the calcifications characterized. A lateral view helps localization within the breast. Spot views are not good enough on their own without the increased resolution of magnification. Tomosynthesis has not yet shown to have any utility in microcalcification characterization. MRI may be used later in the workup when proven DCIS for extent of disease.

4. Ultrasound may be used, especially if there is an associated density with the calcifications. Also, when the patient has dense breasts, ultrasound can more easily visualize a mass associated with DCIS. DCIS can be found among diffuse benign calcifications, and sometimes multiple stereotactic core biopsies need to be used to determine extent. MRI has utility with high-grade DCIS, although some groups also say it has value in ALL types of DCIS. PEM and BSGI may be useful in dense breast tissue when there are multiple invasive cancers, but there are no data on disease extent with DCIS.

5. If there is an associated mass with the microcalcifications, there is a 50% chance of invasive disease, and that is the area that needs targeting, as it will direct the performance of a sentinel node biopsy as part

of treatment. Adding a specimen x-ray to the procedure helps to improve the specificity of the test. Stereotactic core biopsy is the standard type of biopsy with this finding. MRI biopsy should not be needed at this stage. PEM biopsy is helpful in patients with dense breasts and occult mammographic disease, but not in DCIS.

Pearls

- Fine pleomorphic calcifications are suspicious and require biopsy (BI-RADS 4C according to the 5th edition) (risk of malignancy >50%).
- Stereotactic core with specimen x-ray.
- If visible on ultrasound, biopsy and include specimen x-ray.

Suggested Readings

Burnside ES, Ochsner JE, Fowler KJ, et al. Use of microcalcification descriptors in BI-RADS 4th edition to stratify risk of malignancy. *Radiology.* 2007;242(2):388-395.

Hofvind S, Iversen BF, Eriksen L, Styr BM, Kjellevold K, Kurz KD. Mammographic morphology and distribution of calcifications in ductal carcinoma in situ diagnosed in organized screening. *Acta Radiol.* 2011;52(5):481-487.

Yamada T, Mori N, Watanabe M, et al. Radiologic-pathologic correlation of ductal carcinoma in situ. *Radiographics.* 2010;30(5):1183-1198.

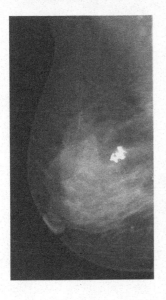 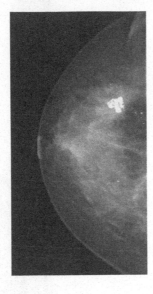 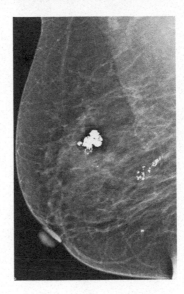 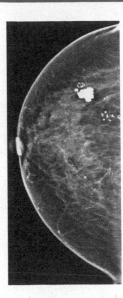

1. What is the appropriate description of these calcifications?

2. What is the next step?

3. What is the description of the increasing group of calcifications in the new screening mammogram?

4. What is the assessment of the second mammogram?

5. What is the significance of new/increasing calcifications in general?

Case ranking/difficulty:

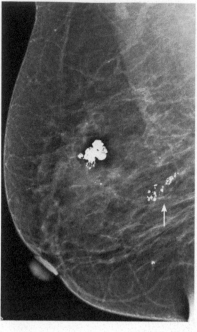

Right MLO view with increasing group of calcifications in posterior lateral breast.

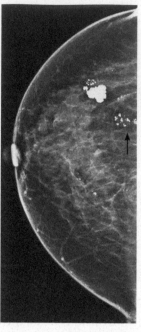

Right CC view with increasing group of calcifications in lateral posterior breast.

Answers

1. This is a typical case of "coarse and popcorn-like" calcifications that are characteristic for fibroadenoma.

2. This is a benign mammogram and patient can return in 1 year for next mammogram.

3. These new calcifications are of the same characteristics. They are "coarse" and "popcorn like" as well. They appear to have increased in number since prior study. However, the area was not well covered on the prior exam.

4. These calcifications are of the same characteristics as the other calcifications in the anterior breast and are also consistent with benign calcifications—despite the fact that they are new.

5. It depends on the morphology of the calcifications. There are benign calcifications that can develop over time and that need no further workup.

Pearls

- "Coarse and popcorn-type" calcifications are typical for involuting fibroadenoma. Finding is benign (BI-RADS 2).
- Fibroadenoma is the most frequently seen mass in young patients and this is because of proliferation of lobular, epithelial, and mesenchymal elements under estrogen stimulation.
- Fibroadenomas develop, in general, in young patients and involute during older age due to withdrawal of estrogens and the process of hyalinization and subsequent calcification.
- In early stage of involution, calcifications may not be easy to differentiate from "pleomorphic" or "casting" (Tabar)-type calcifications.

Suggested Reading

Nussbaum SA, Feig SA, Capuzzi DM. Breast imaging case of the day. Fibroadenoma with microcalcification. *Radiographics*. 1998;18(1):243-245.

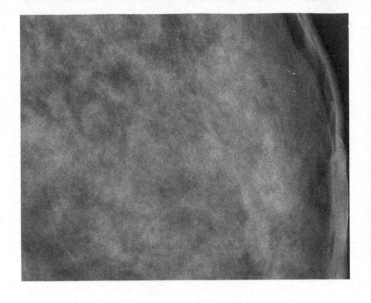 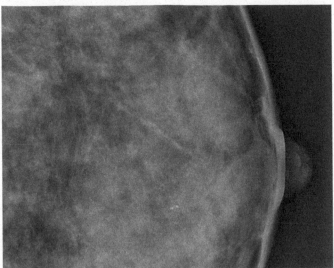

1. What is the best description of the group of calcifications?

2. What is the next step if the group is new?

3. What is the technique with the highest specificity for milk of calcium?

4. What is "milk of calcium"?

5. What is the appropriate final assessment?

Case ranking/difficulty: 🎖

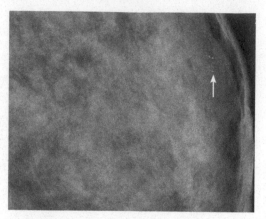

Diagnostic mammogram, left ML magnification view demonstrating layering and "tea cup shape" of some of the calcifications within the concerning group.

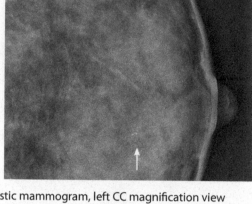

Diagnostic mammogram, left CC magnification view demonstrating group of "amorphous" calcifications.

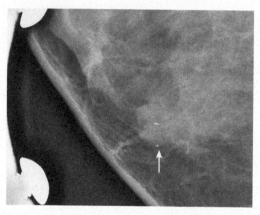

Diagnostic mammogram, right ML magnification view demonstrating group of calcifications with "milk of calcium."

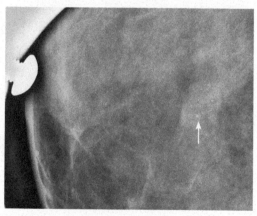

Diagnostic mammogram, right CC magnification view demonstrating group of "amorphous" calcifications.

Answers

1. Given the presence of layering and tea cup formations on ML view, the group is consistent with milk of calcium.

2. If there is layering seen, the group is benign and consistent with milk of calcium—patient can return for next exam in 1 year.

3. Perpendicular magnification views are the appropriate technique to document milk of calcium. There is never a need to perform a MLO magnification view. All magnification views should be performed in ML and CC plane—in particular, if milk of calcium is suspected.

4. Milk of calcium is a form of proliferative breast change with accumulation of calcium containing fluid in microcysts.

5. This is a typical benign finding: BI-RADS 2.

Pearls

- This is a nice example to demonstrate that all magnification views should be performed in perpendicular angle (ML and CC) to each other to maximize the effect of layering.
- There is no need ever to perform a MLO magnification view, except there is no other way to reach most posterior areas of the breast near the chest wall.

Suggested Reading

Imbriaco M, Riccardi A, Sodano A, et al. Milk of calcium in breast microcysts with adjacent malignancy. *AJR Am J Roentgenol.* 1999;173(4):1137-1138.

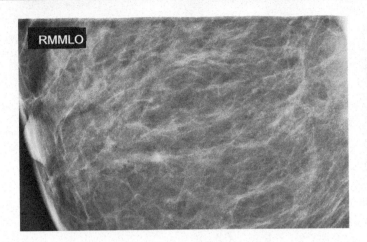 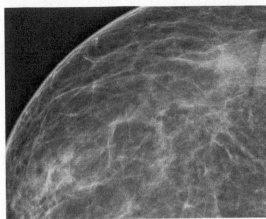

1. What BI-RADS classification should be used here?

2. Which of the following calcification distribution modifiers are most suspicious for malignancy?

3. What is a special type of calcifications that you need to avoid using suspicious descriptors for?

4. What type of intervention would you recommend?

5. What type of pathology could amorphous microcalcifications represent?

Category: Diagnostic

Answers

1. The calcifications are made up of three separate clusters, but form a segmental distribution giving an approximate risk of malignancy of 30%. According to the 5th edition of BI-RADS, this is a BI-RADS 4B classification.

2. Some linear and branching calcifications are seen in classically benign findings such as "secretory" calcifications of duct ectasia, and are featured as a special case in the BI-RADS manual. All special cases featured in the BI-RADS manual are typical board questions, and you should be able to recognize these entities and differentiate them from suspicious calcifications.

3. The special type referred to here is "secretory" calcifications that are a result of duct ectasia or periductal mastitis. These calcifications are characteristic, but are otherwise LINEAR, and may be BRANCHING. The distribution may be "SEGMENTAL." All of these BI-RADS descriptors and their distribution modifiers are suggestive of malignancy, and therefore should not be used. A simple description of secretory calcifications is enough.

4. Standard mammographic workup including spot magnification views is needed to characterize the calcific particles. Critical examination of any prior exams also needed to determine whether these calcifications are developing. If stability is greater than 3 years, they are more likely to be either benign or possibly low-grade DCIS, of no emergent need for intervention. However, this is controversial. If the patient has not been worked up before, and the calcifications look suspicious, recommend biopsy, with specimen x-ray to determine satisfactory sampling.

5. High-grade DCIS are often denser calcifications, seen best when analyzing specimen x-rays. Tabar classifies these as variants of crushed stone. "Amorphous" calcifications can be due to a spectrum of normal to disease, from milk of calcium seen in the CC view, to low/intermediate-grade DCIS. ADH and LCIS are frequently picked up on stereotactic core biopsy. The calcifications in LCIS are not related to the LCIS itself, as the calcifications are normally benign.

Pearls

- Analysis of microcalcifications requires the use of spot magnification views or "fine" settings on photon counting systems.
- Determine the individual shapes of the calcifications. If they are difficult to describe, then they can be called "amorphous."
- Determine the most suspicious distribution of the calcifications—"scattered," through "grouped" and "clustered" to "segmental."

Suggested Readings

Bent CK, Bassett LW, D'Orsi CJ, Sayre JW. The positive predictive value of BI-RADS microcalcification descriptors and final assessment categories. *AJR Am J Roentgenol.* 2010;194(5):1378-1383.

Burnside ES, Ochsner JE, Fowler KJ, et al. Use of microcalcification descriptors in BI-RADS 4th edition to stratify risk of malignancy. *Radiology.* 2007;242(2):388-395.

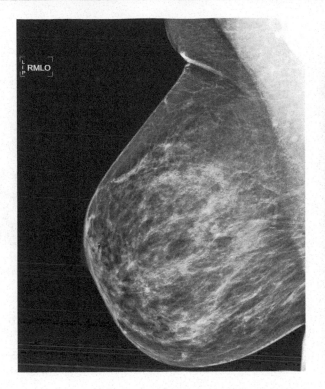

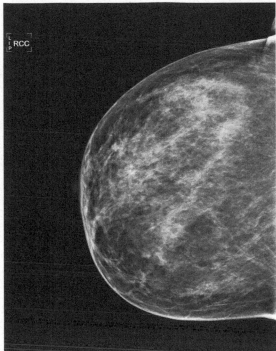

1. What is the finding on screening mammogram?

2. What is the next step?

3. What is the appropriate first step of workup?

4. What is the next step?

5. What would be the benefit of MRI?

Case ranking/difficulty: 🐾   **Category:** Screening

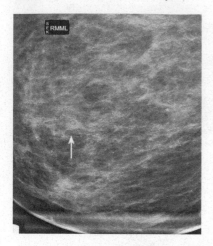

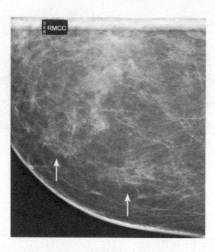

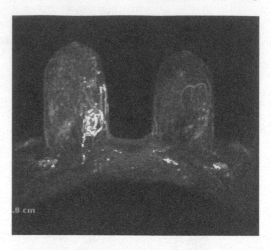

Diagnostic mammogram, right ML magnification view demonstrating group of "pleomorphic" calcifications, in "linear" distribution.

Diagnostic mammogram, right CC magnification view demonstrating group of "pleomorphic" calcifications in "linear" distribution.

MRI, MIP image, after IV contrast, demonstrates different enhancement kinetic patterns, including washout enhancement.

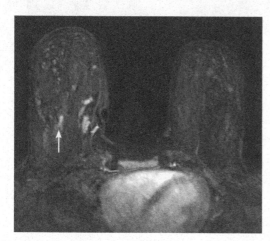

MRI after IV contrast and subtraction demonstrating linear enhancement and second area more laterally (*arrow*).

Answers

1. Noted are "pleomorphic" calcifications right medial breast in "segmental" distribution.

2. Patient needs to be called back BI-RADS 0 for additional workup with diagnostic mammogram.

3. The first step is magnification ML and CC views. There is almost never a reason to perform MLO magnification views—except where the ML projection might not be able to cover the posterior tissue. On ML and CC magnification views, it is easier to detect milk of calcium. Then ultrasound is recommended to assess patient for solid component.

4. In this patient, first step is stereotactic biopsy to obtain pathology, which did show intermediate-grade DCIS. Then additional MRI was performed to assess for multicentric and multifocal disease.

5. MRI did show additional linear enhancement in lateral right breast, which did not correlate to any calcifications and would have been missed. This could be confirmed with MRI-guided biopsy and patient was treated with mastectomy because of the presence of multicentric disease (disease in more than one quadrant). MRI in this case did change surgical management.

Pearls

• Large group of "pleomorphic and linear" calcifications in "segmental" distribution could be classified as BI-RADS 5: "highly suspicious."

• Given the extent of more than 7 cm in antero-posterior (AP) diameter and the additional MRI biopsy-proven area of additional DCIS lateral right breast, mastectomy was performed.

Suggested Reading

Virnig BA, Tuttle Tm, Shmliyan T, et al. Ductal carcinoma in situ of the breast: a systematic review of incidence, treatment and outcomes. *J Nat Cancer Inst.* 2010;102(3):170-178.

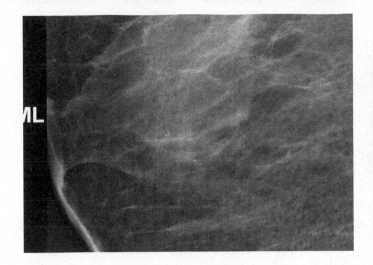
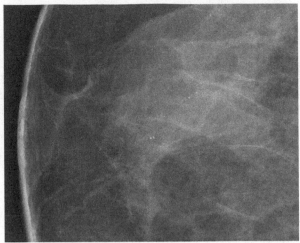

1. What it the appropriate BI-RADS descriptor for the calcification?

2. This was a new group of calcifications—what is the next step?

3. If the calcifications are seen on first screening mammogram, what would be reasonable?

4. What is the appropriate workup of a group of calcification?

5. What is the final assessment based on the magnification views, if the calcifications are new?

Case ranking/difficulty: 🐾

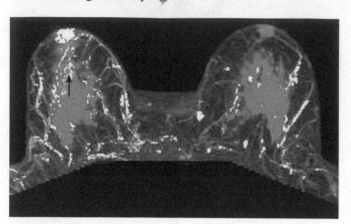

MRI, T1-weighted sequence after IV contrast with MIP technique demonstrates corresponding area of strong enhancement with washout kinetics right breast.

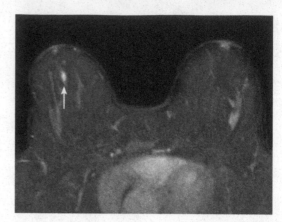

MRI, T1-weighted sequence after IV contrast demonstrating linear area of increased enhancement in the right breast, corresponding to the mammogram finding.

Answers

1. This is a group of "round and oval" calcifications in the right retroareolar breast.

2. If this was a new group of calcifications, patient needs to be biopsied with stereotactic biopsy device. The calcifications are relatively benign, since "round and oval"—but the fact that they are new is a red flag.

3. On screening exam, patient should never be categorized as BI-RADS 3; it had to be BI-RADS 1 or BI-RADS 2 or BI-RADS 0 "incomplete" like in this case. In this case, the finding needed to be worked up with magnification views.

4. For calcifications, an ML and CC view should be performed, NEVER a MLO magnification view. This is true, since milk of calcium is much better characterized on two perpendicular views (ML and CC) than on MLO and CC view.

5. BI-RADS 4 if this is a new group of calcifications and was not seen on prior mammogram. BI-RADS 3, if it is the first mammogram, would be appropriate and then they should be followed over 2 years. Follow-up should be performed with the images with being most sensitive and specific to detect change, with magnification views—not with standard views.

Pearls

- If group of calcifications is seen on a first screening mammogram and on subsequent diagnostic mammogram with magnification views and is described as "round and oval," it can be called "probably benign."
- However, if the group is new, like in this case, biopsy is mandatory.
- Follow-up diagnostic mammograms should include magnification views, since any change, such as new amorphous calcifications during the follow-up time period of 2 years, would trigger biopsy.
- The BI-RADS lexicon gives the option of 2 or 3 years follow-up; during that time period, the calcifications remain "probably benign."

Suggested Readings

Rosen EL, Baker JA, Soo MS. Malignant lesions initially subjected to short-term mammographic follow-up. *Radiology*. 2002;223(1):221-228.

Sickles EA. Breast calcifications: mammographic evaluation. *Radiology*. 1986;160(2):289-293.

Sickles EA. Probably benign breast lesions: when should follow-up be recommended and what is the optimal follow-up protocol? *Radiology*. 1999;213(1):11-14.

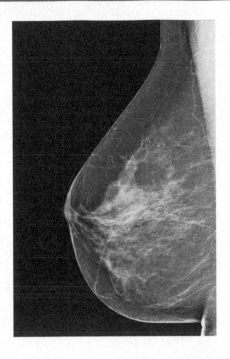 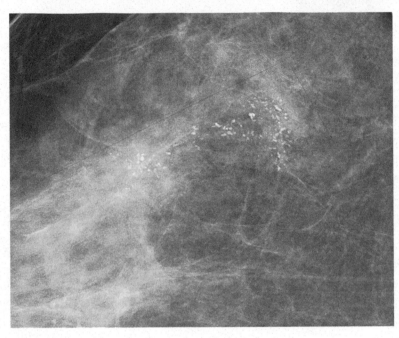

1. What is the BI-RADS category for this diagnostic exam?

2. What is the next best examination you recommend?

3. What is the best description for the distribution of calcifications?

4. What other imaging test would you recommend?

5. What type of biopsy would you recommend?

Case ranking/difficulty: 🌑

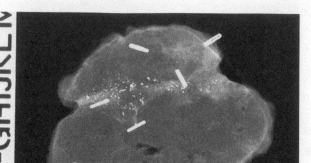

Operative specimen containing calcifications and margin markers.

Answers

1. It is a diagnostic workup, so a BI-RADS 0 is not applicable. The calcifications have between a 50% and 99% risk for DCIS, so it encompasses both the BI-RADS 4C and BI-RADS 5 categories.

2. Further spot magnifications views should be performed to further characterize the calcific particles.

3. This is a segment of calcifications; although it may be orientated down a duct system, it is not strictly linear.

4. The first test I would recommend if you see any density associated with calcifications is a targeted ultrasound. First to see if there is a mass associated with the calcifications, which gives you a likely risk of invasive disease, and therefore metastatic potential. Some surgeons do sentinel node biopsy in high-grade DCIS just in case there is an occult focus of invasive disease in the breast. MRI is best suited for determining both the extent of the DCIS and also if there is an associated mass to indicate invasion. There is no need for ultrasound staging of the axilla, as so far there is no evidence of invasive disease. Same argument for PET/CT.

5. Cytology no longer has a place in the diagnosis of DCIS. Fourteen-gauge or vacuum-assisted core biopsy can be used under ultrasound (if visible, and especially if there is a mass). Stereotactic core biopsy if there is no ultrasound finding. The risk of upstaging—going from ADH to DCIS, or DCIS to invasive disease—is lessened by increased numbers of cores and increased volume of cores, so many radiologists would recommend large gauge core biopsy (vacuum assisted) for DCIS.

Pearls

- High-grade DCIS has a good chance of being upstaged to invasive disease.
- Diligently search for evidence of possible invasion.
- Take a good amount of tissue to reduce the risk of undersampling.
- Remember that we are only seeing the calcified part of the disease, and there may be more noncalcified disease that we are not seeing.
- MRI is the best imaging modality for extent.

Suggested Readings

Hayward L, Oeppen RS, Grima AV, Royle GT, Rubin CM, Cutress RI. The influence of clinicopathological features on the predictive accuracy of conventional breast imaging in determining the extent of screen-detected high-grade pure ductal carcinoma in situ. *Ann R Coll Surg Engl.* 2011;93(5):385-390.)

Kropcho LC, Steen ST, Chung AP, Sim MS, Kirsch DL, Giuliano AE. Preoperative breast MRI in the surgical treatment of ductal carcinoma in situ. *Breast J.* 2012;18(2):151-156.

Rahbar H, Partridge SC, Demartini WB, et al. In vivo assessment of ductal carcinoma in situ grade: a model incorporating dynamic contrast-enhanced and diffusion-weighted breast MR imaging parameters. *Radiology.* 2012;263(2):374-382.

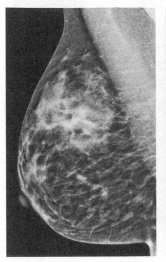 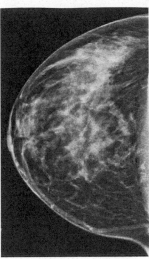 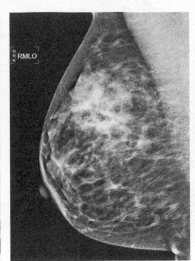 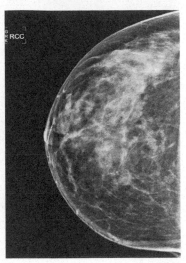

1. What is the finding on the mammogram?

2. What is the assessment based on the magnification views?

3. What is the preferred next step in the workup?

4. Why can it be helpful to have ultrasound first?

5. What would be the next step after the ultrasound-guided biopsy?

Case ranking/difficulty: 🐞

Category: Diagnostic

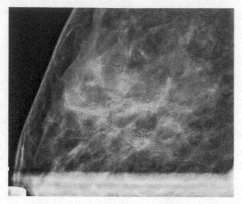

Diagnostic mammogram, right magnification ML view. Noted is group of "pleomorphic" calcifications in "segmental" distribution.

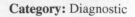
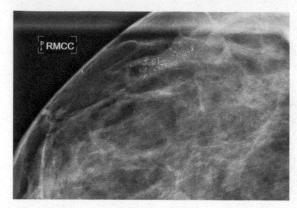

Diagnostic mammogram, right magnification CC view. Noted is group of "pleomorphic" calcifications in "segmental" distribution.

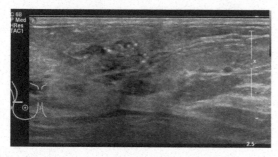

Ultrasound of right breast upper outer quadrant demonstrates hypoechoic mass with associated calcifications.

Answers

1. This is typical appearance of group of "pleomorphic" calcifications in "segmental" distribution.

2. This is a typical appearance of a BI-RADS 5 finding—it is "highly suspicious" for malignancy.

3. Ultrasound is the preferred next step to further assess for possible invasive solid component. However, to perform stereotactic biopsy without prior ultrasound would also be reasonable but not the preferred next step.

4. Ultrasound is helpful for further evaluation to find a possible associated solid part of the malignancy, which would likely be the invasive component of the process. Also, even if there is no solid part, ultrasound might be able to visualize the calcifications and ultrasound-guided biopsy might be an alternative approach to stereotactic biopsy. Ultrasound-guided biopsy is in general more convenient to the patient.

5. Specimen x rays are always helpful to confirm the presence of calcifications in the tissue. A clip should be placed in all circumstances. MRI may better define the extent of the pathology.

Pearls

- In some situations such as this, it is important to perform specimen mammogram of the cores obtained under ultrasound-guided biopsy to make sure that the calcifications are within the specimen.
- Abnormalities can be classified as BI-RADS 5—"highly suspicious" for malignancy. The consequence is that if pathology would show benign finding, such as "focal fibrosis and benign calcifications," this would not be concordant and the biopsy had to be repeated or the patient had to go directly to surgery.
- If abnormality is called BI-RADS 4—"suspicious," it is assumed that it could still be a benign underlying pathology.

Suggested Reading

Soo MS, Baker JA, Rosen EL. Sonographic detection and sonographically guided biopsy of breast microcalcifications. *AJR Am J Roentgenol.* 2003;180(4):941-948.

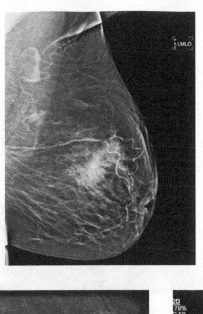
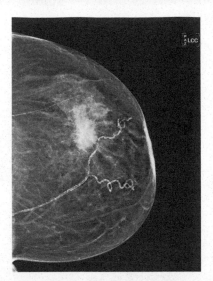
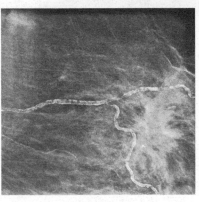
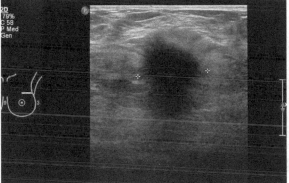

1. What is the best description of the pertinent abnormality?

2. What is the most likely final assessment after diagnostic workup?

3. What is the difference between BI-RADS 4 and BI-RADS 5?

4. What is the description of the abnormality on ultrasound?

5. If there are suspicious lymph nodes, is biopsy with FNA helpful?

Case ranking/difficulty: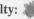

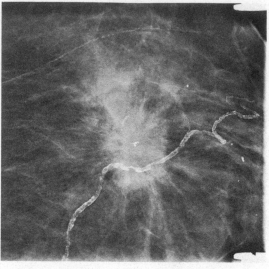

Diagnostic mammogram, left spot compression CC view demonstrating "spiculated" mass.

On ultrasound with duplex, no abnormal flow is identified.

Answers

1. This is an example of a highly suspicious finding, consistent with "mass" with "spiculated margin" with "high density."

2. BI-RADS 5 is the most likely assessment—however, first, additional diagnostic workup is required.

3. BI-RADS 4 has the meaning of abnormality being suspicious—according to BI-RADS lexicon edition 4, it can be divided into BI-RADS 4a, b, and c depending on the level of suspicion. However, all BI-RADS 4 lesions could represent benign pathology and it would still be concordant. BI-RADS 5, however, indicates that this is highly suspicious, and even if pathology comes back as benign, it is not concordant and patient needs to go to surgery.

4. This mass can be described as "hypoechoic mass" with "nonparallel orientation" (taller than wide) and posterior "acoustic shadowing" and "spiculated" margin.

5. Ultrasound-guided FNA of morphologically suspicious lymph nodes is not only helpful to provide the surgeon with more information before surgery replacing the sentinel lymph node procedure, but it is also cost-effective. The likelihood of the presence of pathological axillary lymph nodes correlates to the size of the malignancy.

Pearls

- According to the BI-RADS lexicon 4th edition, the group 4, "suspicious" can be divided into subgroups 4a, small; 4b, moderate; and 4c, substantial likelihood of malignancy.
- Also, category BI-RADS 5 exists that indicates "highly suspicious" for malignancy.
- To differentiate between BI-RADS 4 and BI-RADS 5 does have significant impact on the decision process, since BI-RADS 5 lesion does need surgical excision if stereotactic biopsy is technically not feasible or if the pathology results demonstrate benign finding.

Suggested Readings

Lazarus E, Mainiero MB, Schepps B, Koelliker SL, Livingston LS. BI-RADS lexicon for US and mammography: interobserver variability and positive predictive value. *Radiology*. 2006;239(2):385-391.

Stavros AT, Thickman D, Rapp CL, Dennis MA, Parker SH, Sisney GA. Solid breast nodules: use of sonography to distinguish between benign and malignant lesions. *Radiology*. 1995;196(1):123-134.

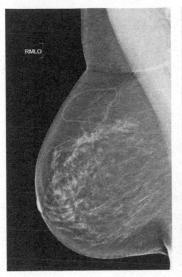 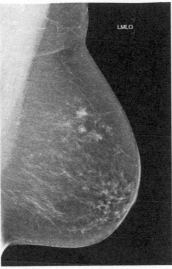 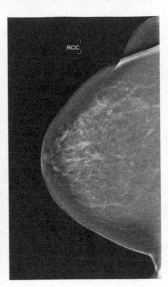 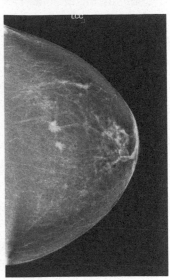

1. What BI-RADS classification should be used here?

2. What is the most likely pathology based on the imaging?

3. What is the next best imaging test?

4. Do these findings fulfill the multiple masses test of BI-RADS?

5. What should be considered if a patient is insistent on breast conservation?

Case ranking/difficulty: 🌸

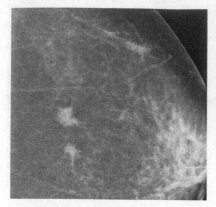

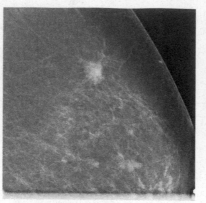

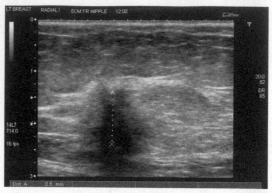

Left CC spot magnification. The three potential masses are now seen with "spiculate" margins.

Left ML spot magnification.

Ultrasound measurement of the distance between two of the masses.

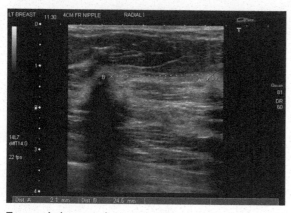

Targeted ultrasound.

Answers

1. This is a screening exam that has a potential abnormality and therefore by definition needs further workup. The appropriate BI-RADS assessment is therefore 0.

2. Potentially, these appearances before workup could be either invasive ductal carcinoma or fat necrosis. DCIS usually presents with microcalcifications, but may be seen as a circumscribed mass, mimicking a fibroadenoma in a young woman. Mucinous carcinoma usually presents as a mass with indistinct margins, sometimes difficult to differentiate from a simple cyst.

3. The mammographic workup should be completed before further imaging tests. A lateral exam, with spot or spot magnification views, will help to characterize the margins of the masses and characterize any calcific particles associated.

4. The answer is a clear NO. The "multiple masses" note should be used to reflect your opinion of multiple

bilateral noncalcified fibroadenomas or cysts. You need to have at least two masses on one side and at least one in the contralateral breast to use this rule of benignity.

5. MRI is a prerequisite in multifocal disease, especially if the patient does not have large volume breasts, as it may be difficult to achieve a good cosmetic result. However, MRI may distinguish between multifocal and multicentric disease, determine whether the pectoral muscle is involved, the absence of contralateral findings, and finally for surgical planning to give a roadmap of the disease.

Pearls

- If you spot one suspicious lesion, suggestive of malignancy, look for a second lesion—usually in the line of the milk duct up to the nipple.

Suggested Readings

Bauman L, Barth RJ, Rosenkranz KM. Breast conservation in women with multifocal-multicentric breast cancer: is it feasible? *Ann Surg Oncol.* 2010;17(Suppl 3):325-329.

Howe HL, Weinstein R, Alvi R, Kohler B, Ellison JH. Women with multiple primary breast cancers diagnosed within a five year period, 1994-1998. *Breast Cancer Res Treat.* 2005;90(3):223-232.

Rezo A, Dahlstrom J, Shadbolt B, et al. Tumor size and survival in multicentric and multifocal breast cancer. *Breast.* 2011;20(3):259-263.

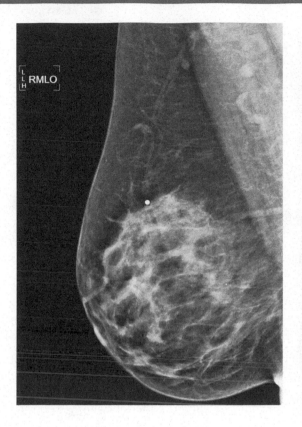
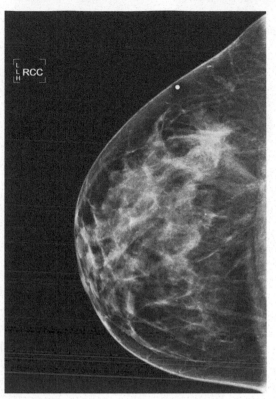

1. What is the first step of workup of a 40-year-old female with palpable abnormality?

2. In case of normal ultrasound, what is the next step?

3. How appropriate is MRI as a problem-solving modality to address inconclusive findings on mammogram?

4. How would you describe the finding on the mammogram?

5. What do you expect to see on ultrasound?

Case ranking/difficulty: 🌸

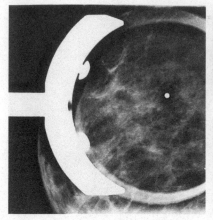

Spot compression, right MLO view with BB marker on area of palpable abnormality.

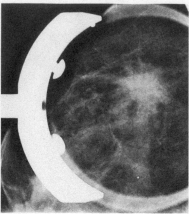

Spot compression, right CC view with BB marker on area of palpable abnormality demonstrating "focal asymmetry" with "spiculated" margin.

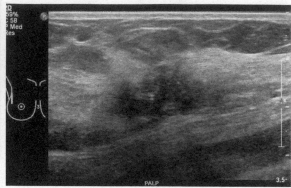

Ultrasound of right breast shows corresponding "hypoechoic spiculated mass."

Answers

1. Workup includes diagnostic mammogram including spot compression views and ultrasound.

2. Next step then would be to perform stereotactic biopsy. Another option could be to perform MRI and call mammogram BI-RADS 0—this might in particular apply to an inconclusive mammogram in the situation of a palpable abnormality.

3. To use breast MRI as a problem-solving tool in case of inconclusive mammogram findings is controversial. It does not eliminate the need for a thorough workup with additional views and ultrasound. If the finding is suspicious on mammogram and normal on ultrasound, MRI cannot eliminate the need for biopsy. However, in selected cases, MRI can help to further make the case that an inconclusive mammogram finding, which otherwise would be called BI-RADS 3, does not need to be biopsied—however, follow-up with mammography in 6 months is still warranted despite negative MRI. While the negative predictive value of MRI is high, it is not 100% and, for example, low-grade DCIS can appear normal on breast MRI.

4. The best descriptor is "focal asymmetry" with "spiculated" margin or "mass" with "spiculated" margin. Asymmetry is preferred, since it is not well seen on the other projection and has concave borders.

5. The mass is hypoechoic in comparison with the fat layer above; it is "irregular" in shape and has "spiculated" margins. It is "wider than tall" (Stavros). It does not show significant "posterior acoustic shadowing."

Pearls

- In case of normal ultrasound, in particular, if there is a palpable abnormality and if there is abnormal morphology seen on mammogram, stereotactic biopsy should be performed.
- If the finding on mammography is inconclusive, breast MRI can be helpful in selected cases as problem-solving modality to determine the level of concern, because of extremely high negative predictive value.

Suggested Reading

Moy L, Elias K, Patel V, et al. Is breast MRI helpful in the evaluation of inconclusive mammographic findings? *AJR Am J Roentgenol.* 2009;193(4):986-993.

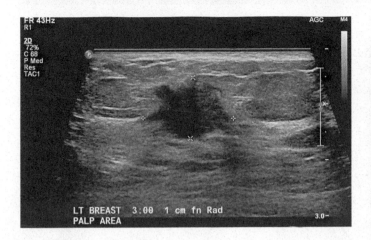 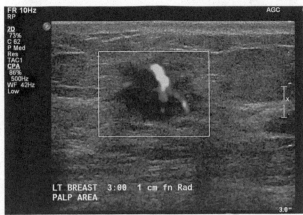

1. What descriptors can be applied to this finding?

2. What BI-RADS category would you place this lesion in?

3. If the patient is younger than 30 years, what is the likely pathology?

4. If the patient is younger than 25 years, do you need to do a mammogram?

5. What pathologies cause increased vascularity inside a mass?

Case ranking/difficulty: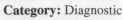

Category: Diagnostic

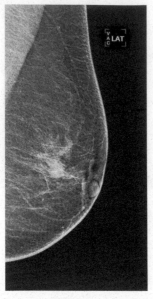

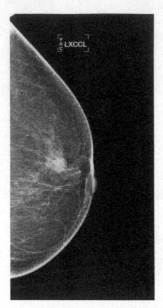

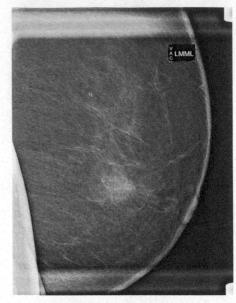

Because of her age, an ultrasound was the first imaging exam. Lateral, there is an irregular, partially obscured mass in the upper half of the breast.

XCCL performed, as mass is in outer half.

Spot magnification shows that the mass is ill defined. Based on both the mammogram and ultrasound findings, a biopsy is now recommended. Final pathology: IDC Gd2 ER/PR+ HER2−.

Answers

1. If the mass is not a good geographic fit for round or oval, the shape should be called IRREGULAR.

2. The findings are not classical of malignancy, and extremes of age can give atypical radiological findings. It is certainly in the 90% and above risk of invasive cancer, and some may give it a BI-RADS 5, as it is a cancer until proven otherwise.

3. It is still most likely to be a cancer, with these features, although fat necrosis and an early abscess can all give the same appearances.

4. Regardless of age, the patient has suspicious ultrasound findings and a mammogram should be performed. MRI is likely to have an important role, but may not visualize any associated DCIS.

5. Vascularity is not confined to invasive cancers. Young women with a fibroadenoma will often have very large vascular channels, and only a biopsy will help in distinguishing between a fibroadenoma and a phyllodes tumor. Vascularity is seen in developing abscesses before liquefaction in a phlegmon. Cysts usually have peripheral vascularity if inflamed.

Pearls

- Regardless of age, a suspicious ultrasound should prompt a mammogram for correlation, unless there is a classic abscess, in which case the mammogram should be delayed.
- Key here is the irregular mass on ultrasound that makes it malignant until proven otherwise.
- Associated DCIS often found with the tumor, seen as reflective particles within the hypoechoic mass itself, or in a dilated duct associated with the tumor.

Suggested Readings

Kim JH, Ko ES, Kim do Y, Han H, Sohn JH, Choe du H. Noncalcified ductal carcinoma in situ: imaging and histologic findings in 36 tumors. *J Ultrasound Med*. 2009;28(7):903-910.

Park JS, Park YM, Kim EK, et al. Sonographic findings of high-grade and non-high-grade ductal carcinoma in situ of the breast. *J Ultrasound Med*. 2010;29(12):1687-1697.

Tozaki M, Fukuma E. Does power Doppler ultrasonography improve the BI-RADS category assessment and diagnostic accuracy of solid breast lesions? *Acta Radiol*. 2011;52(7):706-710.

61-year-old patient with palpable abnormality in the left upper outer quadrant (left two images are the 2 year prior study. Current study on the right)

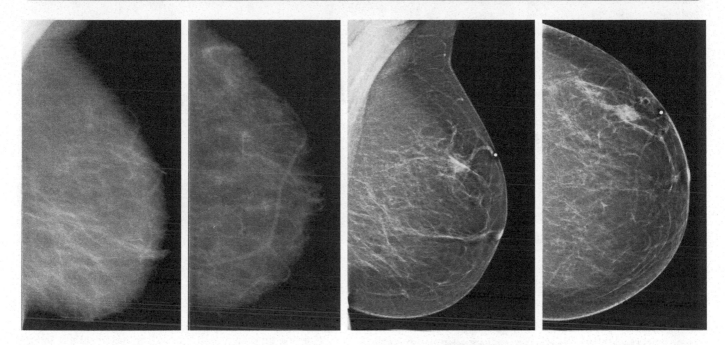

1. Why could the lesion on spot compression views be called "mass" and not "asymmetric density"?

2. What etiology could explain a developing mass?

3. Why is fibroadenoma not a likely differential diagnosis?

4. What would you do if ultrasound does not show any abnormality?

5. What would you do if patient cannot tolerate to lie on the stereotactic biopsy table and no ultrasound finding is detected?

Case ranking/difficulty: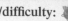

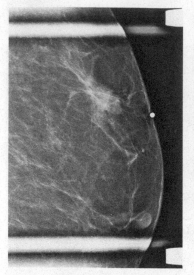

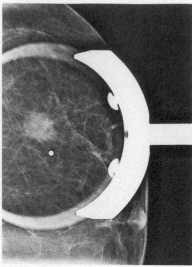

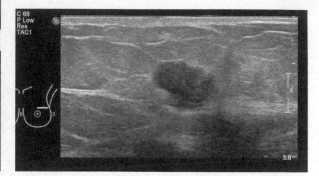

Diagnostic mammogram, left spot compression MLO view demonstrating mass with "lobular shape" and partially "obscured margin."

Diagnostic mammogram, left spot compression CC view demonstrating mass with "irregular shape."

Ultrasound demonstrates associated "hypoechoic mass" with "irregular" shape and "angular" margin.

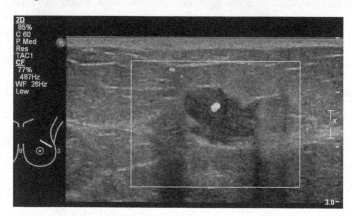

Ultrasound with duplex demonstrates some flow in the center of the mass.

Answers

1. This is a case where the pictures would support the term "mass" over "asymmetric density," since it is seen on two images and has convex shape on spot compression views.

2. Any new mass raises concern, in particular, if it is associated with palpable abnormality. There are also benign findings, such as cyst, fibroadenoma, hematoma, or fat necrosis that can explain new mass. However, any developing mass needs to be biopsied, unless it is a simple cyst or other definitely benign etiology on ultrasound. In the appropriate clinical setting, if there is history of trauma, hematoma could also explain the presence of new mass on mammography.

3. In a 61-year-old patient, it is very unlikely that there will be a new fibroadenoma. Fibroadenomas usually develop in younger age group under the influence of estrogen.

4. Any new mass is concerning, unless consistent with a simple cyst or other clearly benign finding as seen on ultrasound. With the appropriate history, hematoma could explain benign mass. If mass does not correlate to any benign ultrasound finding, patient needs stereotactic biopsy. Any suspicious abnormality on imaging, in general, should be biopsied first, before sending the patient to breast surgeon.

5. Patient then should get surgical excision. Any lesion seen on two planes can be localized with needle and send to surgical excision.

Pearls

- Ultrasound finding of "hypoechoic," solid mass (flow on duplex) with "angular margin" that correlates to palpable abnormality is suspicious (BI-RADS 4) and ultrasound-guided biopsy should be performed.

Suggested Readings

Piccoli CW, Feig SA, Plazzo JP. Developing asymmetric breast tissue. *Radiology.* 1999; 211(1):111-117.

Youk JH, Eun-Kyung K, Kung HK, et al. Asymmetric mammographic findings based on the fourth edition of BI-RADS: types, evaluation and management. *Radiographics.* 2009;29(1):e33.

Lump in left axillary tail

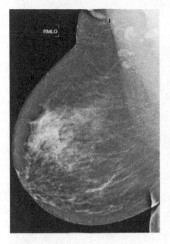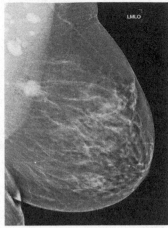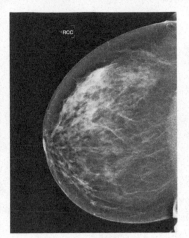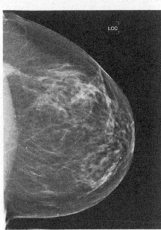

1. What BI-RADS classification should be used here?

2. What is the most likely pathology based on the imaging?

3. What is the next best imaging test?

4. What type of biopsy would you recommend?

5. If the axillary nodes are palpable on this patient, what is the likelihood of nodal metastases?

Case ranking/difficulty: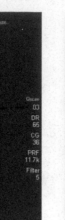

Category: Diagnostic

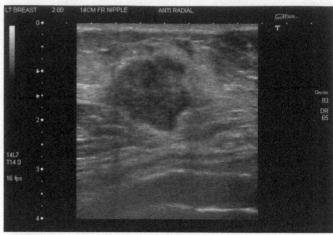

Ultrasound of mass with power Doppler shows no significant flow in an "oval" mass.

Ultrasound—in the orthogonal plane, the mass is seen to have angular margins and possibly some duct extension.

Answers

1. A BI-RADS 4 or 5 is appropriate in this case that turned out to be a high-grade invasive ductal carcinoma.

2. This is an ill-defined mass in an older patient with no history of trauma or surgery at that site; so, fat necrosis and fibroadenoma are not in the differential diagnosis. An infected sebaceous cyst is usually around the bra line, but in theory it can occur on the skin anywhere in the breast. A complex sclerosing lesion usually presents with architectural distortion, +/− a mass, and may have a dark center. This should be regarded as a carcinoma until proven otherwise.

3. Strictly, a full mammographic workup needs to be completed before proceeding to ultrasound, which could be with spot views or tomosynthesis. However, if there are no calcifications associated with the mass, some would go on directly to perform targeted ultrasound scanning. Ultrasound core biopsy will be needed following the diagnostic workup. MRI may be helpful if the pectoral muscle is thought to be involved, or if other foci are seen separate from the index mass.

4. Ultrasound is the easiest and cheapest way to perform biopsy in this situation, under direct vision. In very dense breasts, or in circumstances where the lesion is occult to conventional tests, MRI biopsy or PEM biopsy (if avid) may be used.

5. With a known primary cancer, palpable nodes are extremely likely to contain metastases UNLESS the patient has recently had a breast biopsy. In that situation, only ultrasound staging of the nodes is likely to confirm suspicious nodes. In a recent paper, patients with palpable nodes and suspicious ultrasound exams had a greater than 75% chance of positive nodes.

Pearls

Differential diagnosis:
- High-grade malignancy.
- Metastases to the breast.
- Fibroadenoma.

Suggested Readings

Bode MK, Rissanen T. Imaging findings and accuracy of core needle biopsy in mucinous carcinoma of the breast. *Acta Radiol.* 2011;52(2):128-133.

Choi YJ, Seong MH, Choi SH, et al. Ultrasound and clinicopathological characteristics of triple receptor-negative breast cancers. *J Breast Cancer.* 2011;14(2):119-123.

Surov A, Fiedler E, Holzhausen HJ, Ruschke K, Schmoll HJ, Spielmann RP. Metastases to the breast from non-mammary malignancies: primary tumors, prevalence, clinical signs, and radiological features. *Acad Radiol.* 2011;18(5):565-574.

Palpated lump in the left breast

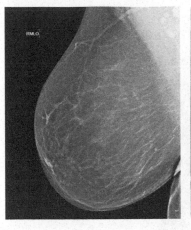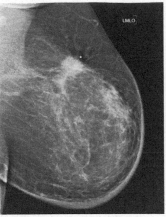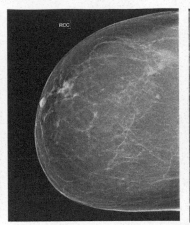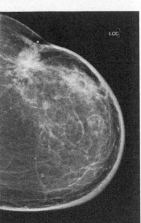

1. What BI-RADS classification should be used here?

2. What is the most likely pathology based on the imaging?

3. What is the next best imaging test?

4. What type of biopsy would you recommend?

5. What is the medical differential of unilateral edema of the breast?

Case ranking/difficulty:

Category: Diagnostic

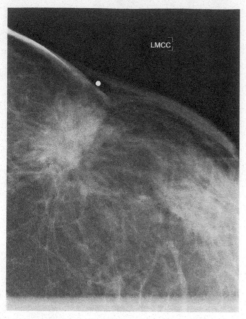

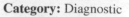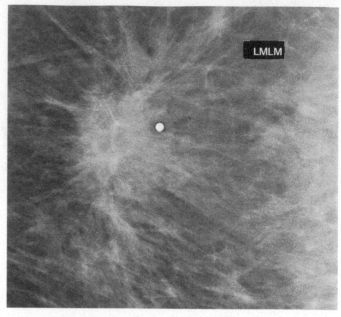

Left CC spot magnification. Note the "spiculate" margins and the "linear microcalcification" associated with the tumor. Calcifications appear to be growing down the spicules.

Left LM spot magnification view shows similar appearances.

Answers

1. This is a diagnostic examination as the patient has a palpable finding. The findings are sufficient for extremely high confidence for malignancy, in that the probability of malignancy is near 100%; therefore, a BI-RADS 5 is appropriate. The only other setting where these imaging appearances occur is post–lumpectomy and radiation therapy, but you do not see microcalcifications unless there is residual disease, or developing fat necrosis with "dystrophic" calcifications.

2. Yes, there is DCIS present, but this is associated with a spiculate mass. Masses are rarer in lobular cancer, where the findings may be subtle, and present as mild distortion or a shrinking breast.

3. The patient is likely to need chemotherapy in the neoadjuvant setting to make surgery possible, so accurate staging of the disease is important. This includes staging of the nodes in the axilla, as they are often the first to disappear with chemo.

4. In this case, the mass is visible, so an ultrasound biopsy is best. If no underlying mass is seen, then MRI needs to be performed first to identify any underlying mass, followed by second look ultrasound of any abnormality found that might represent the primary disease. Sometimes, incisional biopsy is required to confirm that this is malignant infiltration rather than simple unilateral

lymphedema. As of the time of writing, there is no tomosynthesis-guided biopsy technique.

5. Unilateral lymphedema has been reported secondary to primary cardiac failure, renal failure, and brachiocephalic vein occlusion.

Pearls

- Skin thickening is a sign of radiological "inflammatory" breast cancer.
- There may not be any associated clinical signs of inflammatory change.
- Systemic disease can give similar appearances. Do not forget heart failure.
- Inflammatory cancer can occur in the presence or absence of an obvious primary (index) cancer.

Suggested Readings

Alunni JP. Imaging inflammatory breast cancer. *Diagn Interv Imaging*. 2012;93(2):95-103.

Dilaveri CA, Mac Bride MB, Sandhu NP, Neal L, Ghosh K, Wahner-Roedler DL. Breast manifestations of systemic diseases. *Int J Womens Health*. 2012;4(4):35-43.

Uematsu T. MRI findings of inflammatory breast cancer, locally advanced breast cancer, and acute mastitis: T2-weighted images can increase the specificity of inflammatory breast cancer. *Breast Cancer*. 2012;19(4):289-294.

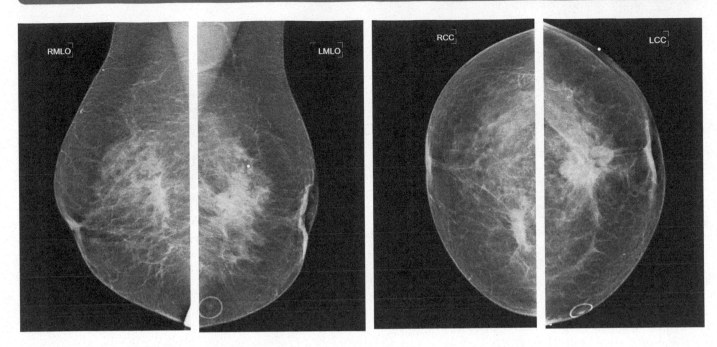

1. What BI-RADS classification should be used here?

2. What is the most likely pathology based on the imaging?

3. What should be the next imaging investigation?

4. There is a palpable finding in the left axilla. You find a node on ultrasound. What is the chance that this is metastatic?

5. What type of biopsy would you recommend?

Case ranking/difficulty: 🌑

Category: Diagnostic

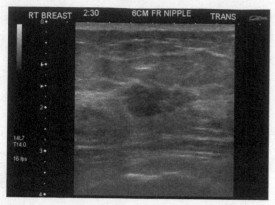

Right breast—"irregular mass" identified. There are few supporting signs of malignancy, with the absence of acoustic shadowing.

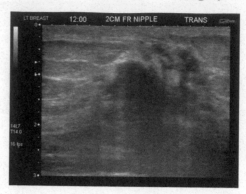

Left breast ultrasound. Much more obvious on ultrasound compared with the right breast as an "irregular mass" with "heterogeneous echo pattern" and "complex acoustic attenuation." "Duct extension" is seen, extending from the tumor.

Answers

1. Bilateral findings either a BI-RADS 4 or 5 depending on how convinced you are that they are malignant. It is alright to call a BI-RADS 5 on the left and a BI-RADS 4 on the right. You are allowed to give a separate BI-RADS assessment for each side.

2. The most common cancer is invasive ductal cancer. Lobular cancer tends to present with distortion or shrinking breasts, which can be difficult to pick up when symmetrical.

3. The patient may have additional diagnostic films, especially spot magnification views if the patient has calcification associated with either lesion, but the next other workup is ultrasound to characterize both masses and stage the axilla. MRI may be used later, but in this situation, the patient is likely to have a bilateral mastectomy; therefore, unless there is concern about involvement of the pectoral muscle, MRI may not be required.

4. An abnormal node in the presence of a palpable lymph node finding on clinical exam has been shown to significantly correlate to involvement with metastases. One paper has the rate higher than 75%. There are various published criteria for suspicious lymph nodes requiring biopsy:

   • Cortical thickening >3 mm (4 mm if recent biopsy);
   • Irregular thickening of cortex, for example, "hump"; and
   • Length versus width ratio approaching 1:1.

5. Ultrasound-guided core biopsy of the breast masses is important as tissue biomarkers including ER, PR, and HER2 receptors need to be evaluated. These cannot be easily done on FNA cytology. Also new multigene

DNA subtyping arrays are frequently performed to inform decision making about treatment and risk of recurrence (recurrence index), which make tissue cores more appropriate. Stereotactic FNA cytology is historic, having been used in the past, particularly in Europe, but it has no real use today.

Pearls

• Bilateral findings if not circumscribed round or oval masses and without calcifications are not obviously benign, and need further workup.
• Symmetry is usually your friend.
• Use first principles and analyze the findings to determine suspicion.

Suggested Readings

Girardi V, Carbognin G, Camera L, et al. Multifocal, multicentric and contralateral breast cancers: breast MR imaging in the preoperative evaluation of patients with newly diagnosed breast cancer. *Radiol Med.* 2011;116(8):1226-1238.

Nichol AM, Yerushalmi R, Tyldesley S, et al. A case-match study comparing unilateral with synchronous bilateral breast cancer outcomes. *J Clin Oncol.* 2011;29(36):4763-4768.

Tonyali O, Tufan G, Benekli M, Coskun U, Buyukberber S. Synchronous bilateral breast cancer in a patient with kindler syndrome. *Clin Breast Cancer.* 2012;12(2):145-146.

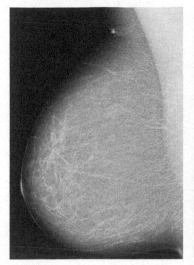
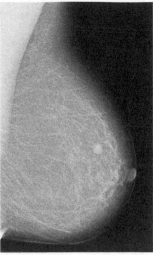
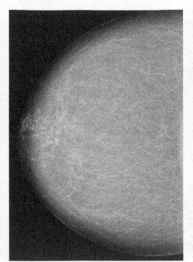
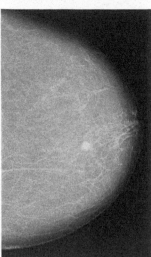

1. What is the BI-RADS category for this screening exam?

2. What is the background breast density?

3. If you want to recall this patient, what are your recommendations?

4. What is the risk of invasive cancer in this patient?

5. If you were to describe the margins of the mass on this mammogram, which terms would you use?

Case ranking/difficulty: 🌸

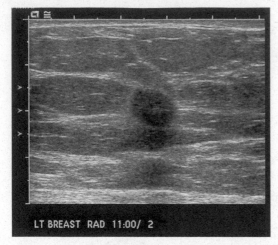

Ultrasound scan—"circumscribed" hypoechoic mass that would appear benign in a different setting, although the margin is not as sharp as you would expect for something like a fibroadenoma.

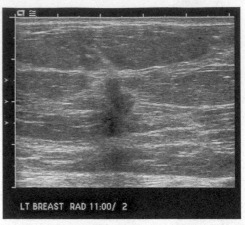

Ultrasound—satellite lesion shows more malignant-looking characteristics, being taller than wide (Stavros) with "irregular margins" and some "acoustic shadowing."

Answers

1. There is clearly an abnormality in the left breast that was perceived to be benign (BI-RADS 2) by the reading radiologist, despite not having any prior exams. The margins are irregular with some suspicion of distortion/spiculation, and the patient should have been given a BI-RADS 0 and recalled for extra views and ultrasound scanning. If you believe that the findings are clearly suspicious, Sickles advises against calling it BI-RADS 4 or 5 from screening due to many patients going directly to surgery rather than being worked up first. (Do not forget that BI-RADS 5 is more than 95% risk of malignancy, and there are still up to 5% of those cases that eventually turn out to be benign.)

2. There is virtually no residual breast tissue in this screened woman, and so the accurate descriptor is "almost entirely fat."

3. There are different approaches to an obvious breast mass. Some people do direct ultrasound as the first test on recall. BI-RADS, however, recommends completing the diagnostic workup mammographically BEFORE proceeding with ultrasound. There are several reasons for this, including doing the lateral film, so that you can triangulate where the lesion will be found on targeted ultrasound. The addition of spot (+/– magnification) compression is used by many groups to

   (a) further characterize the margins of the mass and
   (b) to determine if there are any associated calcifications, representing DCIS either in or more importantly outside of the index cancer, as this has management implications.

4. If you can determine the spiculations associated with this mass, you can give this a category 5 assessment, as it is characteristic of malignancy. Many people prefer to call this suspicious and give it a BI-RADS 4 (although in the upper end of the BI-RADS 4 category).

5. This is an "irregular mass" but with "indistinct margins." Possibly even "spiculate." Irregular describes the shape of the mass, but not the margin. This was initially described as a round mass, but that is a benign descriptor and does not apply here. Circumscribed is a margin descriptor, but does not apply to this case.

Pearls

- Never ignore a mass in otherwise fatty breasts.
- Check prior films for stability.
- If never worked up, then do diagnostic workup.
- If any suspicious features, then biopsy.

Suggested Readings

Colleoni M, Rotmensz N, Maisonneuve MG, et al. Outcome of special types of luminal breast cancer. *Ann Oncol.* 2012;23(6):1428-1436.

Garne JP, Aspegren K, Linell F, Rank F, Ranstam J. Primary prognostic factors in invasive breast cancer with special reference to ductal carcinoma and histologic malignancy grade. *Cancer.* 1994;73(5):1438-1448.

Lacroix-Triki M, Suarez PH, MacKay A, et al. Mucinous carcinoma of the breast is genomically distinct from invasive ductal carcinomas of no special type. *J Pathol.* 2010;222(3):282-298.

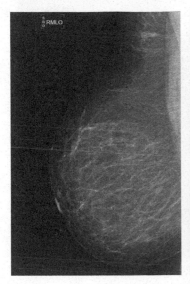 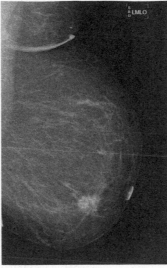 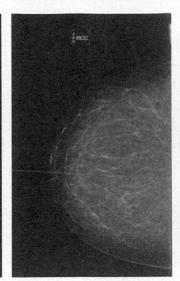 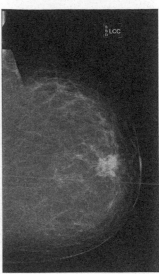

1. What BI-RADS descriptor would you use for the shape of this mass?

2. Why is it important to identify the associated DCIS?

3. What diagnostic tests should you recommend?

4. What type of biopsy should you do?

5. If the biopsy comes back as fat necrosis, what is the next step?

Case ranking/difficulty: 🌸

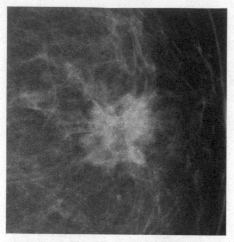

Spot magnification view (LSMCC) of spiculate mass with calcifications inside and outside the tumor.

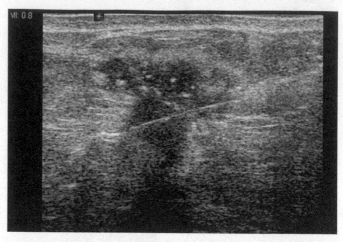

Targeted ultrasound examination—irregular mass containing calcification. In this image, you can identify the biopsy needle passing through the inferior aspect of the tumor. More anterior passes will be required, along with specimen x-rays, to determine harvesting of calcification associated with the mass.

Answers

1. This is an irregular mass. If there are spicules arising from the mass that are easily visible, then a spiculate mass would be applicable.

2. In dense breast tissue, the suspicious calcification may be the only clue that you have a tumor growing in the breast. DCIS associated with invasive cancer is very commonly found, but may be calcified on noncalcified. The density associated with the calcification on mammography or ultrasound is the trigger to think about associated invasive disease. Calcification outside of the tumor due to DCIS may have an impact of the management of the patient. This is called extra invasive component and is associated with a high risk of local recurrence, even after radiation treatment.

3. Spot magnification views should be performed of the mass and calcium to get a better idea of the spread of the calcifications in the breast and to measure extent. Ultrasound will help to evaluate the presence of invasive disease. In this sort of case, MRI may give a better estimate of extent of disease. PET/CT and PEM have no role in the diagnostic workup of this patient, unless there is evidence of metastatic disease.

4. Although all are theoretically correct, the best type of biopsy is the fastest and cheapest to get a diagnosis. Since we require tissue typing and biomarkers, core biopsy should be performed. If you have trouble seeing the lesion on ultrasound, then stereotactic core biopsy may be used. MRI biopsy gives the highest reimbursement, but it is not optimal in this patient. FNA is used, particularly in Europe, and I believe it still has

a place for rapid diagnosis of malignancy. But tissue is required to personalize treatment, so core biopsy has become the default method of biopsying the breast.

5. If you gave it BI-RADS 5, then the finding of fat necrosis is not concordant, and you have to recommend surgical excision. If it was a BI-RADS 4 with more dystrophic calcifications, you could do almost all of the above. At the end of the day, you need more tissue in a lesion that has so many suspicious findings.

Pearls

- High-grade tumors in older women may present as pseudocircumscribed masses.
- A combination of mammography and ultrasound may be required to prompt biopsy.

Suggested Readings

Atalay C, Irkkan C. Predictive factors for residual disease in re-excision specimens after breast-conserving surgery. *Breast J*. 2012;18(4):339-344.

Barbalaco Neto G, Rossetti C, Fonseca FL, Valenti VE, de Abreu LC. Ductal carcinoma in situ in core needle biopsies and its association with extensive in situ component in the surgical specimen. *Int Arch Med*. 2012;5(1):19.

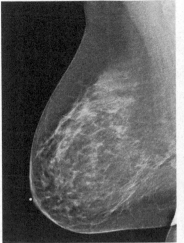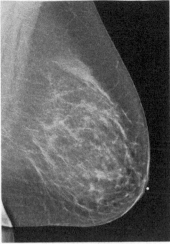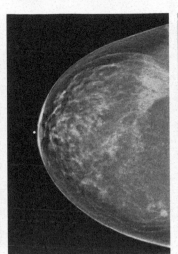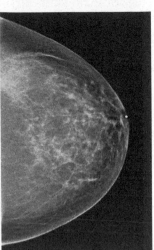

1. What BI-RADS classification should be used here?

2. What is the risk of malignancy with a focal asymmetry in this position?

3. What further imaging would you recommend?

4. What type of biopsy should be performed?

5. The patient states she has a skin lesion on the inner part of the right breast. What do you do?

Case ranking/difficulty:

Category: Screening

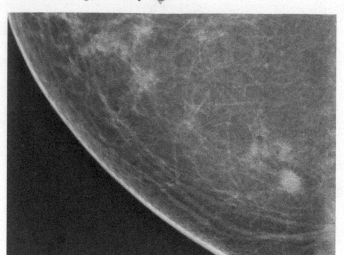

RCC spot magnification confirms an "ill-defined" soft tissue "mass" in the inner half of the CC film.

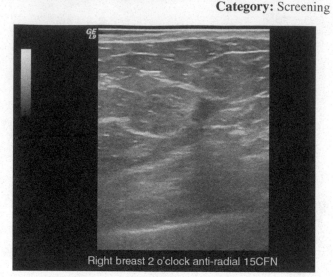

Right breast 2 o'clock anti-radial 15CFN

Ultrasound confirms a correlate of an "irregular mass" at the site of the mammographic abnormality.

Answers

1. This is a screening examination; therefore, a BI-RADS 0 assessment should be rendered with a recommendation for further films. Further workup should include lateral and spot magnification views to determine if there is a mass. If truly a mass, then ultrasound may be required.

2. Same question but in a different format, as you do not make the risk of malignancy until you have done the diagnostic workup. There is a focal asymmetry in one of the danger areas in the medial aspect of the CC film. This increases the risk of malignancy, similar to a developing focal asymmetry.

3. Diagnostic mammograms or tomosynthesis should be performed to complete the diagnostic workup before targeted ultrasound being performed. The mass is usually visible on ultrasound.

4. Cytology is useful for a rapid diagnosis of malignancy when you have a trained breast cytopathologist available. Core biopsy with placement of a marker clip is the best way to get a diagnosis and tissue biomarkers BEFORE surgery. Stereotactic core biopsy is technically difficult in this location. MRI biopsy not warranted. Surgical excision should not be carried out before a preoperative diagnosis is obtained.

5. Repeating the relevant right mammograms with a skin marker may demonstrate clearly that the mammographic finding is in fact in the skin and projected over the breast. You can risk introducing infection by doing a punch biopsy of a sebaceous cyst.

Pearls

- Small breast cancers can appear like normal breast tissue.
- DANGER area such as the immediately posterior medial aspect of the CC films is one place, as is the inferior mammary fold on the MLO view, where cancers occur simulating normal entities.

Suggested Readings

Leung JW, Sickles EA. Developing asymmetry identified on mammography: correlation with imaging outcome and pathologic findings. *AJR Am J Roentgenol.* 2007;188(3):667-675.

Sickles EA. The spectrum of breast asymmetries: imaging features, work-up, management. *Radiol Clin North Am.* 2007;45(5):765-771, v.

Venkatesan A, Chu P, Kerlikowske K, Sickles EA, Smith-Bindman R. Positive predictive value of specific mammographic findings according to reader and patient variables. *Radiology.* 2009;250(3):648-657.

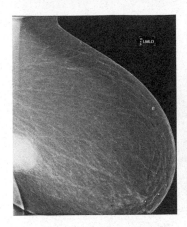 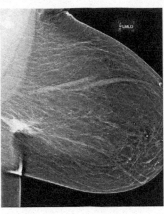 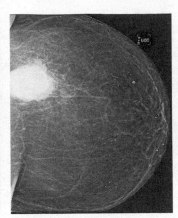 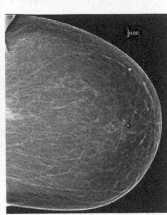

1. Why is there a difference between the sets of images?

2. What BI-RADS category would you place this lesion in?

3. What is the most likely pathology?

4. What tissue biomarkers are routinely measured in a patient with breast cancer?

5. The patient has now completed treatment. What is your role now to direct the surgeon?

Case ranking/difficulty: 🌑

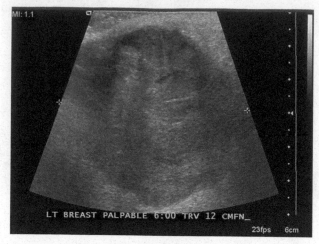

Ultrasound of mass pretreatment. Mainly uniphasic mass.

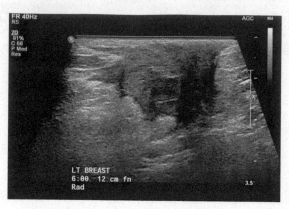

Ultrasound of mass posttreatment. There is a mix of solid and fluid (necrotic debris).

Answers

1. Sometimes, postsurgery films can look like this, BUT there are no supporting signs that the patient has had surgery, for example, a scar, surgical clips, skin thickening, and so on. If the patient is unfit for surgery, sometimes they are offered neoadjuvant hormone therapy, as often you can obtain control and avoid surgery. The usual reason for these appearances is due to the patient having neoadjuvant chemotherapy (NAC) for the cancer. The only reason for NAC in this patient was that the tumor was stuck to the pectoral muscle, and deforming surgery would have to have taken place if chemo was not considered first.

2. In this case, the patient was not a screener, and therefore not BI-RADS 0. If anything, it would be a BI-RADS 4 or 5 depending on your suspicion of malignancy. However, in this patient, she has a known diagnosis of breast cancer (BI-RADS 6), and is now presenting following NAC with a lesion that has shrunk significantly to allow successful surgery.

3. Mucinous carcinomas typically appear semicystic or with evidence of enhancement on ultrasound. Tubular cancers tend to present as spiculate masses with LONG SPICULES. Lobular cancer is usually subtle and presents as vague distortion, or developing asymmetry. DCIS typically presents with calcifications.

4. The routine biomarkers used on all breast cancer patients are ER, PR, and HER2 status. This assists in breaking down appropriate treatment by identifying the biological type of breast cancer. Ki-67 is a proliferation index that assists with recurrence risk, but not routinely measured. However, things are changing rapidly, and various gene panels such as Oncotype Dx and MammaPrint are being used more and more to subtype tumors and stratify chemotherapy.

5. The surgeons need accurate marking of the position of the lesion now that the mass in no longer palpable. Because you placed a marker clip before neoadjuvant chemotherapy, you can now find the clip for the surgeon. It is the patient's decision, not yours, to decide whether, having shrunk the tumor, she will have a mastectomy or not. Injection of dye is done in the OR as it rapidly moves to the nodes. Injection of tracer for sentinel node can be done at the time of the needle localization or in the OR ready room.

Pearls

- Response to neoadjuvant chemotherapy can be marked, with many patients having a pathological complete response.
- MRI is a good tool to monitor response to chemotherapy, both with volume measurements and in determining the type of response (due to enhancement patterns).
- If MRI is not available, ultrasound has also been successfully used for monitoring response, as well as molecular breast imaging and other new techniques.

Suggested Readings

de Bazelaire C, Calmon R, Thomassin I, et al. Accuracy of perfusion MRI with high spatial but low temporal resolution to assess invasive breast cancer response to neoadjuvant chemotherapy: a retrospective study. *BMC Cancer.* 2011;11(11):361.

Lyou CY, Cho N, Kim SM, et al. Computer-aided evaluation of breast MRI for the residual tumor extent and response monitoring in breast cancer patients receiving neoadjuvant chemotherapy. *Korean J Radiol.* 2011;12(1):34-43.

Shin HJ, Baek HM, Ahn JH, et al. Prediction of pathologic response to neoadjuvant chemotherapy in patients with breast cancer using diffusion-weighted imaging and MRS. *NMR Biomed.* 2012;25(12):1349-1359.

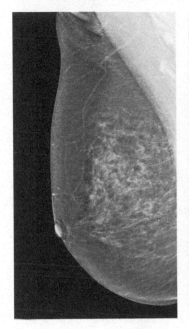
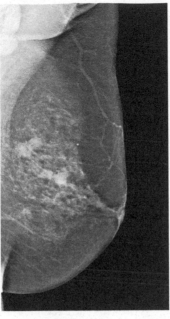
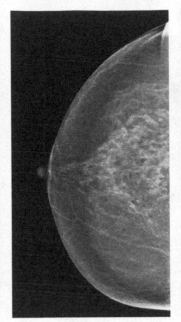
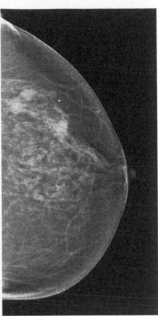

1. What BI-RADS classification should be used here?

2. What is the frequency of multiple findings in a breast with a known primary breast cancer?

3. Patients with multifocal breast cancer have an increased risk of which of the following?

4. What should be the next imaging investigations?

5. What type of biopsy would you recommend?

Case ranking/difficulty: 🌸

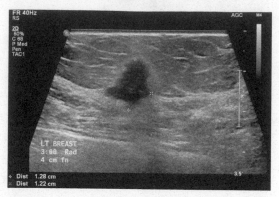

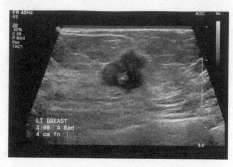

Ultrasound: Lesion 2—This shows the mass has a central reflective area. Check back with the mammogram to determine if there is any potential for associated DCIS.

Ultrasound: Lesion 1—"Ill-defined" "irregular" mass that is "nonparallel" (taller than wide). It has low level echoes inside and there is a minor degree of "acoustic attenuation."

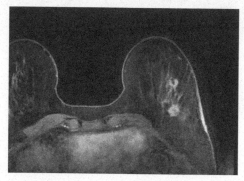

MRI—Subtracted axial MIP. This is often the best way of showing the relationships of the various masses in 3D space, plus it allows for staging and assessment of the extent of the mass and distance from the nipple.

4. If you have tomosynthesis, then it can replace the diagnostic workup for multiple masses. Targeted ultrasound can then be performed to document the masses and evaluate for locoregional spread. MRI will also need to be performed as the best method to establish extent of disease, especially if breast conservation is being considered. Techniques such as breast specific gamma imaging (BSGI) and positron emission mammography (PEM) may be used in dense breasts for suspected multifocality.

5. Ultrasound is the best biopsy tool if the masses can be easily found. Rarely, the masses are hard to visualize on mammography and stereotactic core biopsy of two of the masses, furthest apart may need to be done.

Pearls

- When you see one cancer, look for the second.
- If you see two, look even harder for more.
- Determine whether in same segment (multifocal) or not.
- MRI should be performed for staging, especially if the patient wishes to consider breast conservation.

Answers

1. This is not a screening exam. There are multiple irregular masses containing microcalcification, suggesting DCIS, and spot magnification is needed to characterize the calcific particles.

2. The data vary on this, with estimates of between 10% and 20%. With the advent of regular MRI scans for staging purposes, more second ipsilateral and also contralateral second primaries are being detected, suggesting that the real number is yet unknown.

3. The larger tumor burden and likelihood of locoregional spread means that nodal involvement and systemic metastases are more likely with multiple cancers. Several authors have suggested that tumor size should be aggregated for the patients to receive appropriate therapy. Currently, only the largest of the tumors is used for prognosis calculations.

Suggested Readings

Ustaalioglu BO, Bilici A, Kefeli U, et al. The importance of multifocal/multicentric tumor on the disease-free survival of breast cancer patients: single center experience. *Am J Clin Oncol.* 2011;35(6):580-586.

Spanu A, Chessa F, Battista Meloni G, et al. Scintimammography with high resolution dedicated breast camera and mammography in multifocal, multicentric and bilateral breast cancer detection: a comparative study. *Q J Nucl Med Mol Imaging.* 2009;53(2):133-143.

Yang WT. Staging of breast cancer with ultrasound. *Semin Ultrasound CT MR.* 2011;32(4):331-341.

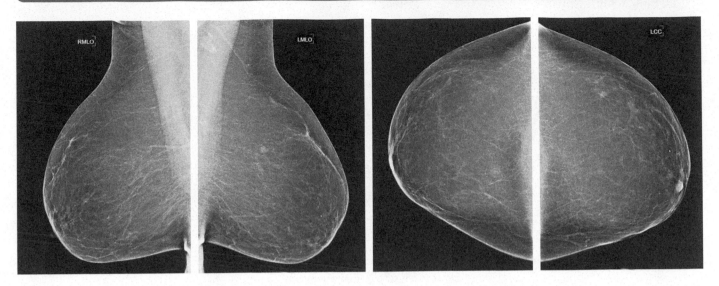

1. What BI-RADS classification should be used here?

2. The prior exams are now available. Stable since 3 years earlier. What is your BI-RADS assessment?

3. If found to be benign, what is the likely pathology?

4. If found to be malignant, what is the likely pathology?

5. What type of biopsy would you recommend?

Case ranking/difficulty: 🏵

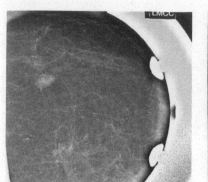

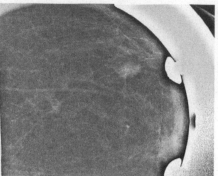

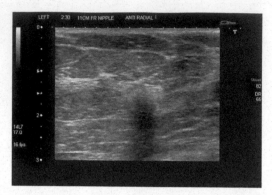

Left CC: current exam close-up. This demonstrates an "irregular mass" with "spiculate" margins.

Left CC: 2009 exam close-up. On the prior exam, the radiologist decided the finding was due to an intramammary lymph node, and because it was "stable" did not recall it. Just because it is stable, does not mean it is benign—use margin characteristics to determine whether the finding needs further workup.

Ultrasound—looked similar in 2009 to 2011, but just smaller.

Answers

1. This is an abnormal screening mammogram, and the appropriate BI-RADS category to use is therefore BI-RADS 0: Further workup needed.

2. There is no change since the prior exam. It is a solitary mass seen in fatty breasts. Some would give this a BI-RADS 2, benign, as the lesion has been stable for several years, but the lesion is too small and the margins not well enough seen to leave alone without a full diagnostic workup. For that reason, a BI-RADS 0, needs further imaging, would be appropriate.

3. Isolated papillomas tend to be central. Multiple papillomas tend to be peripheral. Fibroadenoma and simple cysts can give these appearances. If a cyst has been present for 3 years, there is likely to be proteinaceous secretions within and is therefore more likely to be a complicated cyst than a simple cyst. *Note*: The BI-RADS lexicon dropped the term "complex cyst" in the 4th edition (2003) as there was confusion, and the only term that should be used is "complicated cyst." An ectopic intramammary node is possible, but there is no notch seen or fatty hilum to indicate this.

4. High- and intermediate-grade invasive ductal carcinoma is unlikely to have been relatively stable for 3 years. It is far more likely to be a low-grade tumor or possibly a special type of invasive ductal, such as a mucinous cancer. Phyllodes tumors can be found in older patients, but one feature is rapid growth, even the benign end of the spectrum of PT.

5. This mass is not palpable. Ultrasound-guided FNA cytology or core biopsy is appropriate, depending on the availability of a breast pathologist. Stereotactic biopsy can be used when not visible on ultrasound scanning. Surgical biopsy is historical in this situation, when a preoperative diagnosis can be made by needle biopsy.

Pearls

- Small mass in fatty breasts, suspicious until proven otherwise.
- Do full diagnostic workup.
- Have a low threshold for biopsy in this situation.

Suggested Readings

Esserman LJ, Shieh Y, Rutgers EJ, et al. Impact of mammographic screening on the detection of good and poor prognosis breast cancers. *Breast Cancer Res Treat.* 2011;130(3):725-734.

Tamaki K, Ishida T, Miyashita M, et al. Correlation between mammographic findings and corresponding histopathology: potential predictors for biological characteristics of breast diseases. *Cancer Sci.* 2011;102(12):2179-2185.

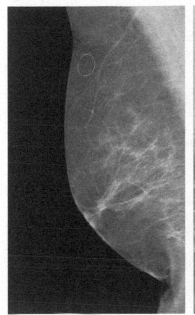 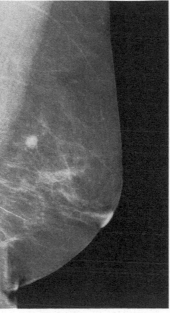 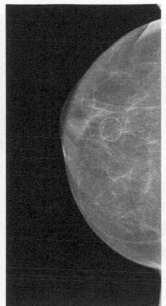 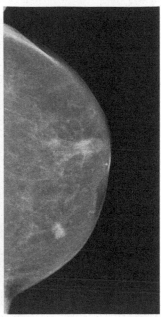

1. What BI-RADS classification should be used here?

2. What is the most likely pathology based on the imaging?

3. What is the next best imaging test?

4. This is a special type of IDC called mucinous (colloid). What are the ultrasound features that you expect to see?

5. What is the most common age group to find this special type of tumor?

Case ranking/difficulty: 🍁

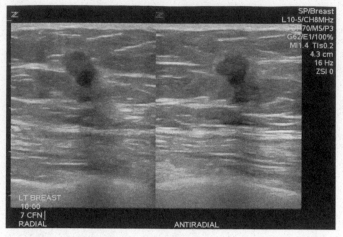

Ultrasound confirms a "nonparallel" or taller than wide mass with irregular margins.

Answers

1. This is clearly not a benign finding within fatty breasts, and requires further workup. Therefore, BI-RADS 0.

2. The findings are typical for a developing invasive ductal carcinoma, and sometimes a special subtype that does not have specific unique imaging features.

3. Diagnostic workup that may include spot (magnification) views and ultrasound, but may include tomosynthesis in place of regular diagnostic mammograms. Ultrasound should be performed when you have completed the mammographic workup.

4. This lesion is often seen as a solid mass with acoustic enhancement on ultrasound. It has either irregular or indistinct margins. The echogenicity is rarely anechoic, unless your ultrasound machine settings are incorrect. Spiculation is much rarer due to the lesion being very slow growing and not attracting a strong desmoplastic reaction.

5. This is more common in the elderly, with a peak incidence in the 70s.

Pearls

- Special type of IDC.
- Good prognosis.
- Mucin containing, therefore, can have acoustic enhancement on ultrasound.

Suggested Readings

Bode MK, Rissanen T. Imaging findings and accuracy of core needle biopsy in mucinous carcinoma of the breast. *Acta Radiol.* 2011;52(2):128-133.

Lacroix-Triki M, Suarez PH, MacKay A, et al. Mucinous carcinoma of the breast is genomically distinct from invasive ductal carcinomas of no special type. *J Pathol.* 2010;222(3):282-298.

Lam WW, Chu WC, Tse GM, Ma TK. Sonographic appearance of mucinous carcinoma of the breast. *AJR Am J Roentgenol.* 2004;182(4):1069-1074.

Lump for 3 years—diagnostic exam

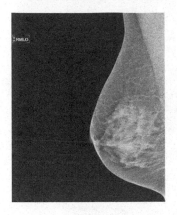 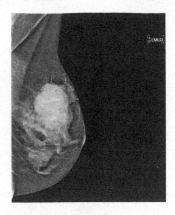 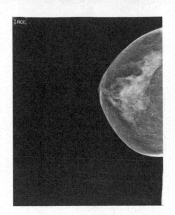 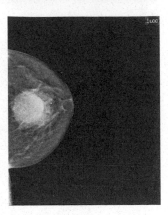

1. What BI-RADS classification should be used here?

2. What should be the next diagnostic imaging exam?

3. What type of biopsy would you consider with this lesion?

4. Pathology shows DCIS high grade with no invasion. What is your recommendation?

5. The finding shows Gd 3 IDC ER–PR–HER2–. What is this finding called?

Case ranking/difficulty: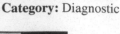

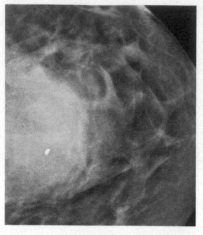

LCC spot compression shows that the mass margins are "microlobulated" and "ill defined." The mass contains a marker clip from a biopsy.

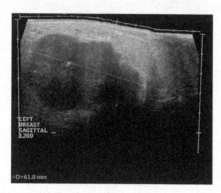

Ultrasound—compound imaging in an attempt to show the size of the mass.

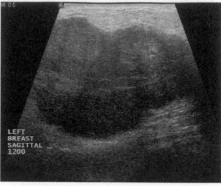

Ultrasound shows a predominantly "oval mass" with "circumscribed margins" and two gentle lobulations. The mass is larger than the width of the probe. The ultrasound appearances are therefore benign, and are trumped by the mammographic appearances.

Answers

1. This is not a screening examination as the patient has palpable findings. Although the lesion is suspicious of malignancy, the margins being so smooth and circumscribed means that I would give a BI-RADS 4 rather than a 5 in this situation.

2. Tomosynthesis, if you have it, would likely have already been used. Diagnostic mammograms have lesser value unless you can see associated microcalcifications inside or outside of the tumor (extensive intraductal component), which would have an additional impact on treatment. MRI for large tumors, especially if lobular, or those associated with DCIS, is very helpful for extent of disease and surgical planning. Also good for detecting involved internal mammary nodes and Rotters (interpectoral) nodes. If the mass is locally advanced, then PET/CT for staging is recommended.

3. Palpation-guided biopsy is not as accurate as ultrasound-guided core biopsy. Core biopsy is the best type of tissue

to obtain, as we need tissue biomarkers preoperatively in a patient who could potentially go on to have neoadjuvant chemotherapy. Surgical excision without preoperative biopsy is not standard care.

4. The patient has a finding that is highly unlikely to be DCIS; therefore, the finding is nonconcordant. You need to have an invasive cancer that is ER/PR negative before chemotherapy can be justified. Treatment of DCIS is surgical. Either you need to repeat the core biopsy and target a margin of the lesion or get an excisional biopsy.

5. The lack of estrogen or progesterone-receptor positivity, plus the lack of c-ERB (HER) 2 overexpression, means that this is a triple negative.

Pearls

- Large tumors have increased risk of locoregional spread.
- MRI should be considered for staging to visualize internal mammary and Rotter's node involvement.

Suggested Readings

Croshaw R, Shapiro-Wright H, Svensson E, Erb K, Julian T. Accuracy of clinical examination, digital mammogram, ultrasound, and MRI in determining postneoadjuvant pathologic tumor response in operable breast cancer patients. *Ann Surg Oncol.* 2011;18(11):3160-3163.

Singer L, Wilmes LJ, Saritas EU, et al. High-resolution diffusion-weighted magnetic resonance imaging in patients with locally advanced breast cancer. *Acad Radiol.* 2012;19(5):526-534.

Uematsu T. MRI findings of inflammatory breast cancer, locally advanced breast cancer, and acute mastitis: T2-weighted images can increase the specificity of inflammatory breast cancer. *Breast Cancer.* 2012;19(4):289-294.

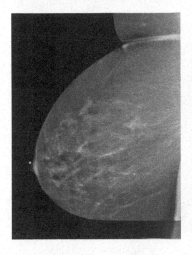 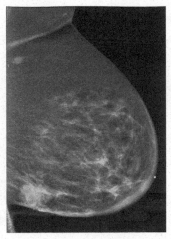 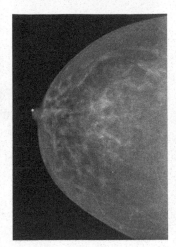 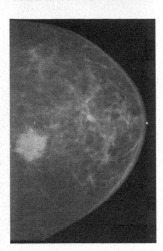

1. What BI-RADS classification should be used here?

2. What is the most likely pathology based on the imaging?

3. The patient has had an ultrasound confirming the mass. What is the next diagnostic test?

4. Biopsy shows IDC. What is the next imaging test you would recommend?

5. The patient has now completed treatment. What is your role now to direct the surgeon?

Case ranking/difficulty:

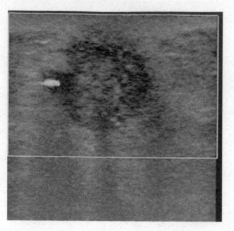

Irregular mass containing calcifications.

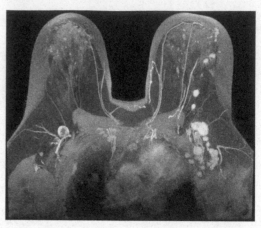

MRI—Thin MIP showing mass plus intramammary and also axillary nodes, not appreciated on mammography.

Answers

1. This is a diagnostic examination. The findings are characteristic, allowing you to give a B-RADS 5 assessment.

2. Inflammatory breast cancer is usually invasive ductal cancer, although sometimes it is seen with a DCIS mass, and no proven invasive focus on biopsy. Invasive lobular usually presents late with a hard nodular and shrunken breast. Infection should not present with this type of appearance. An infected sebaceous cyst will be obvious on physical examination. If this were postlumpectomy, the features are more compatible with an inflammatory recurrence.

3. When a patient with a likely malignancy is already having a diagnostic ultrasound, it is easy to perform axillary staging at the same visit, to speed up the diagnostic process. It has the added benefit of determining whether any nodes look abnormal, and you can then recommend biopsy of the node(s). Ultrasound core biopsy needs to be done to confirm the diagnosis and also to allow the measurement of tissue biomarkers to determine the subtype of the tumor. Ultrasound FNA cytology can be performed, but that limits the diagnosis to malignancy only rather than tissue required pre-neoadjuvant chemotherapy. There is no place for surgical excision to make a diagnosis of breast cancer in this setting.

4. The first imaging test should be MRI to determine the extent of the disease, to screen the contralateral breast, and to image the locoregional lymphatic drainage. In many centers, a PET/CT is also used at this stage for staging purposes. PEM and BSGI are sometimes useful to find other tumors in dense breasts. Surgical incisional biopsy is not required, as lymphatic involvement can be seen on core biopsy.

5. A repeat MRI to see the current playing field is an important part of presurgical intervention after chemo. Similar comments for PET/CT, although this may vary by center. The tumor will be analyzed when excised surgically. Patients may go on to axillary dissection regardless of you finding a normal axilla at this stage.

Pearls

- Cancer that causes edema of the breast and skin thickening is called inflammatory breast cancer, but this does not necessarily mean that there is clinical inflammatory cancer.
- We can identify early changes of inflammatory cancer better on imaging than on physical exam.
- Watch for additional foci of disease.
- Evaluate nodes before neoadjuvant chemotherapy.

Suggested Readings

Alunni JP. Imaging inflammatory breast cancer. *Diagn Interv Imaging.* 2012;93(2):95-103.

Boisserie-Lacroix M, Debled M, Tunon de Lara C, Hurtevent G, Asad-Syed M, Ferron S. The inflammatory breast: management, decision-making algorithms, therapeutic principles. *Diagn Interv Imaging.* 2012;93(2):126-136.

Uematsu T. MRI findings of inflammatory breast cancer, locally advanced breast cancer, and acute mastitis: T2-weighted images can increase the specificity of inflammatory breast cancer. *Breast Cancer.* 2012;19(4):289-294.

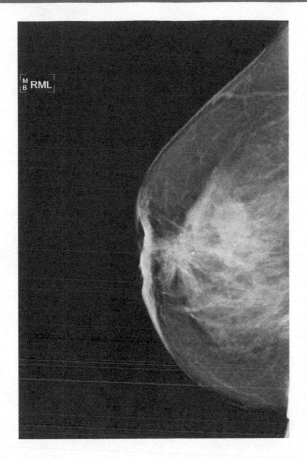
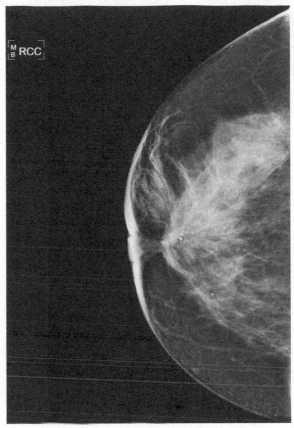

1. Which of the BI-RADS descriptors most accurately represents the findings?

2. What is the most common type of tumors giving these appearances?

3. What BI-RADS score is appropriate in this case?

4. What are the likely findings on physical examination?

5. What are the radiologic features of "inflammatory" cancer?

Case ranking/difficulty:

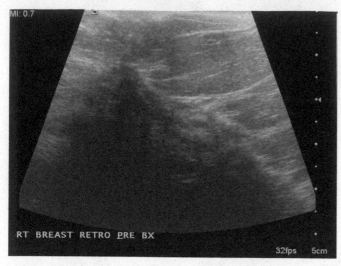

MI: 0.7

RT BREAST RETRO PRE BX

32fps   5cm

Ultrasound of subareolar region showing distortion and shadowing.

Answers

1. Although a mass is present, it is difficult to see because of the surrounding dense breast tissue, the retroareolar nature of the lump, and the associated distortion. It would be accurate to report distortion as the major finding in this case, and say a "possible" mass is present.

2. Tubular carcinoma typically has LONG spicules with a small central mass. Lobular carcinomas are frequently difficult to see because of their growth pattern, and may present as an asymmetry or distortion. Invasive ductal carcinoma (no special type) may cause distortion due to degree of invasion.

3. This is typical of a central/subareolar cancer causing distortion, so a BI-RADS 5 should be appropriate. If you think there is a possibility of another cause, then give a BI-RADS 4.

4. Most of the above findings may be seen in a patient with this type of mammogram. Occasionally, a subareolar malignancy may not present with any physical finding.

5. Radiological "inflammatory" carcinoma frequently is seen before any physical findings of skin redness or "peau d'orange." Blockage of skin lymphatics by tumor emboli causes the radiological features of inflammatory carcinoma. There is a higher likelihood of involved axillary nodes in inflammatory carcinoma.

Pearls

- Skin thickening with increased density of supporting structures of the breast is often due to inflammatory carcinoma.

Suggested Readings

Caumo F, Gaioni MB, Bonetti F, Manfrin E, Remo A, Pattaro C. Occult inflammatory breast cancer: review of clinical, mammographic, US and pathologic signs. *Radiol Med*. 2005;109(4):308-320.

Harrison AM, Zendejas B, Ali SM, Scow JS, Farley DR. Lessons learned from an unusual case of inflammatory breast cancer. *J Surg Educ*. 2012;69(3):350-354.

Uematsu T. MRI findings of inflammatory breast cancer, locally advanced breast cancer, and acute mastitis: T2-weighted images can increase the specificity of inflammatory breast cancer. *Breast Cancer*. 2012;19(4):289-294.

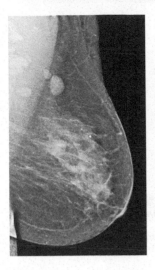 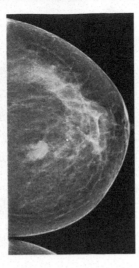 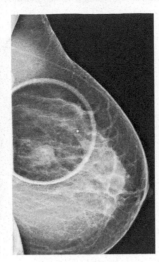 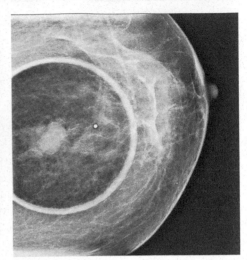

1. What is included in the diagnostic workup of a palpable mass?

2. What is the significance of the lymph nodes seen on the mammogram?

3. How can the mass be described on the mammogram?

4. What would be the next step after the spot compression views?

5. If the mass is not seen on ultrasound, what would be the next step?

Case ranking/difficulty:

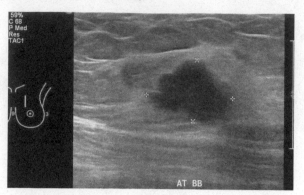

Gray-scale ultrasound of left breast hypoechoic mass with "lobulated" shape and "angulated margin."

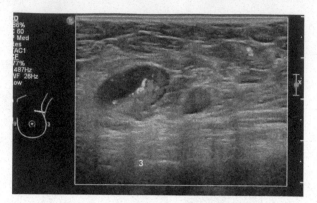

Gray-scale ultrasound with duplex demonstrating increased central flow.

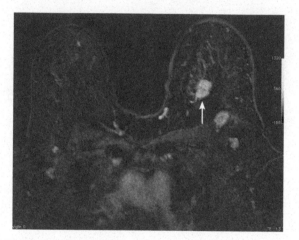

MRI, T1-weighted image after IV contrast, subtraction technique, demonstrating mass corresponding to index lesion (*arrow*) and lymph nodes.

"indistinct," or "spiculated"), and by their density ("high," "equal," or "low density"). This mass has "lobular" shape and partially "obscured" margin and is of "equal" density in comparison with the fibroglandular tissue.

4. Ultrasound would be the next step to work up the mass and the lymph nodes.

5. If the mass is not seen on ultrasound, stereotactic biopsy is the next step to obtain tissue.

Answers

1. Workup includes standard mammogram and spot compression views with BB marker on the area of concern. In addition, ultrasound should be performed. Thermography is a technique that uses infrared sensors to detect heat and is not recognized as being part of evidenced-based breast imaging.

2. The lymph nodes as seen in the upper outer quadrant and axilla are relatively small, none is larger than 1.5 cm, but they are relatively dense and no fatty hilum is recognized. Given the presence of a palpable abnormality, the presence of lymph nodes makes the palpable mass even more suspicious and raises concern for possible metastatic disease.

3. Masses are described by shape ("round" and "oval"— "lobular" or "irregular"), by the appearance of their margin ("circumscribed," "microlobulated," "obscured,"

Pearls

- After ultrasound-guided biopsy of suspicious finding in the breast, it is helpful to search for lymph nodes and perform biopsy, if suspicious lymph nodes can be detected.
- The biopsy of the lymph node can be performed as fine needle aspiration or as core biopsy with a 14-gauge needle or even with larger-core biopsy needle, depending on the location of the lymph node.
- Pathology demonstrated in this case presents invasive ductal carcinoma and metastatic carcinoma in the suspicious lymph node.

Suggested Readings

Abe H, Schmidt RA, Kulkarni K, Sennett CA, Mueller JS, Newstead GM. Axillary lymph nodes suspicious for breast cancer metastasis: sampling with US-guided 14-gauge core-needle biopsy—clinical experience in 100 patients. *Radiology.* 2009;250(1):41-49.

Abe H, Schmidt RA, Sennett CA, Shimauchi A, Newstead GM. US-guided core needle biopsy of axillary lymph nodes in patients with breast cancer: why and how to do it. *Radiographics.* 2007;27(Suppl 1):S91-S99.

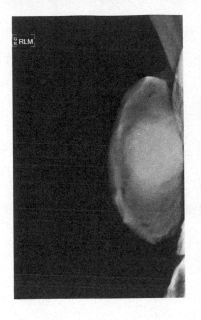
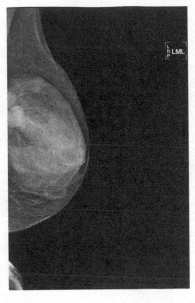
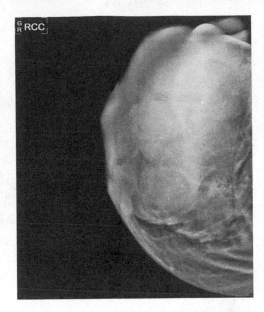

1. What BI-RADS classification should be used here?

2. What should be the next diagnostic imaging exam?

3. Core biopsy shows ER–PR–HER2+ IDC. What is your recommendation?

4. MRI and PET/CT both show nodes to level 2 in the axilla and interpectoral space. What do you recommend?

5. Three months posttreatment, follow-up imaging is now normal. What is your BI-RADS assessment?

Case ranking/difficulty: 🌸

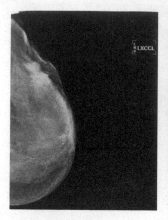

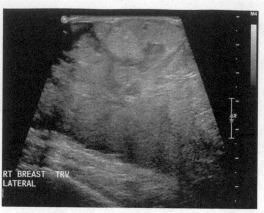

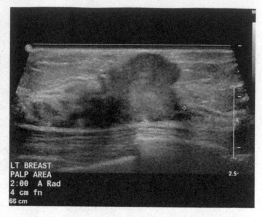

LXCCL shows possibly two separate masses in the outer left breast.

Right breast ultrasound—the tumor takes up the whole field.

Left breast ultrasound confirms the presence of another cancer in the contralateral breast.

Answers

1. Hopefully, with a fungating mass, you would be happy to give this lesion a BI-RADS 5. Always watch for second cancer.

2. With such a large tumor, further diagnostic mammograms of tomosynthesis would be futile. Ultrasound scanning to determine areas of viable tissue, away from large blood vessels for biopsy, is one of the most important next tasks. While scanning, it is worth staging the axilla for lymphadenopathy. MRI will be used later for staging the disease and potential for resectability. PEM does not add anything to the diagnosis in this type of case.

3. Initial staging for a presumed stage 4 tumor is to perform an MRI (if technically possible) for chest wall invasion and mapping of lymph nodes. PET/CT gives additional information in the thorax, especially if the patient is unable to lay prone for the MRI. Surgery may not be possible until the lesion has been shrunken down, and then is likely to be a "toilet" mastectomy post–neoadjuvant chemotherapy.

4. While the patient may need neoadjuvant chemotherapy, staging of the nodes with either FNA or core biopsy has become important, especially as more patients are getting complete pathological response to chemotherapy. Evidence that at least one node was involved helps in the determination of appropriate treatment postchemotherapy. Some groups prefer small-gauge core biopsy to get tissue biomarkers from the metastatic node.

5. As there is no evidence of malignancy, you could use BI-RADS 1, but there is likely to be a residual biopsy clip, so BI-RADS 2 would be more appropriate.

HOWEVER, the patient has had biopsy-proven malignancy and has not had surgery to excise the "cancer" and therefore the appropriate BI-RADS category is 6: known malignancy. Surgical treatment is recommended. You could edit the report to say that it is a BI-RADS 6: known TREATED malignancy.

Pearls

- Dense breast due to fungating locally advanced breast cancer.
- Ultrasound and MRI have a major role in assessing the extent of the disease and performing staging, as well as monitoring the response to neoadjuvant chemotherapy.

Suggested Readings

Croshaw R, Shapiro-Wright H, Svensson E, Erb K, Julian T. Accuracy of clinical examination, digital mammogram, ultrasound, and MRI in determining postneoadjuvant pathologic tumor response in operable breast cancer patients. *Ann Surg Oncol.* 2011;18(11):3160-3163.

Singer L, Wilmes LJ, Saritas EU, et al. High-resolution diffusion-weighted magnetic resonance imaging in patients with locally advanced breast cancer. *Acad Radiol.* 2012;19(5):526-534.

Uematsu T. MRI findings of inflammatory breast cancer, locally advanced breast cancer, and acute mastitis: T2-weighted images can increase the specificity of inflammatory breast cancer. *Breast Cancer.* 2012;19(4):289-294.

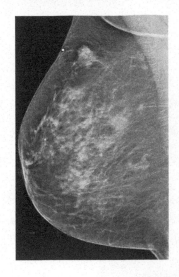
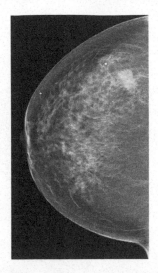
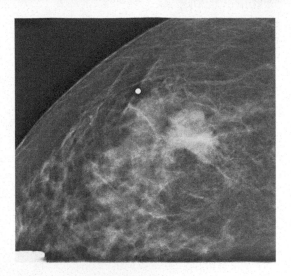

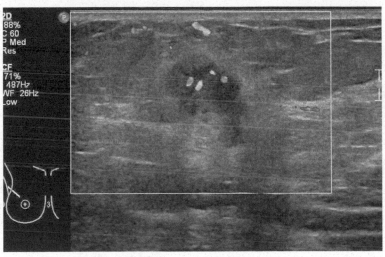

1. What should be included in workup for palpable mass?

2. What would be the next step if mammogram and ultrasound are normal?

3. Patient had recent normal mammogram 3 months ago and is referred for workup of lump. What is the workup?

4. What is the abnormality in this case?

5. What is the appearance of the abnormality on ultrasound?

Case ranking/difficulty:

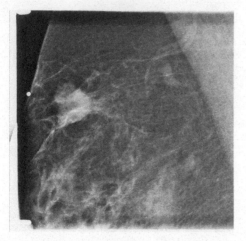

Spot compression of right MLO view with BB on palpable abnormality.

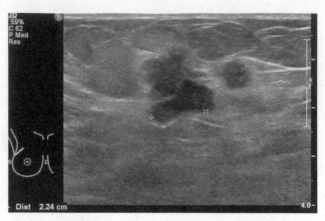

Ultrasound B mode image demonstrates corresponding "spiculated" mass.

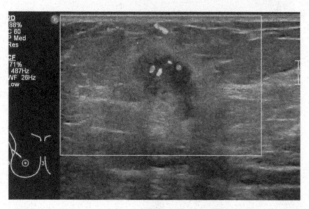

Ultrasound with duplex of the palpable abnormality.

Answers

1. For patients older than 30 years, the first step is a mammogram with BB marker over the area of palpable lump. Mammogram also includes spot compression views with BB marker. Next step—regardless of the outcome of the mammogram—is to perform an ultrasound. Ultrasound is important not only for characterization of the mass if seen on mammogram but also for the choice for possible biopsy.

2. Despite normal imaging, there is a possibility of the presence of a malignancy in the scenario of palpable abnormalities. Further management should be based on clinical grounds, meaning that usually the gynecologist or the primary care physician who refers the patient has to decide if the palpable finding is worrisome enough to send the patient to a breast surgeon. Based on the clinical evaluation of the breast surgeon, a biopsy might be performed without imaging guidance.

3. Given the presence of a normal mammogram 3 months ago, it is not unreasonable, after reviewing the old images, to start with an ultrasound first. If ultrasound does not show any abnormality— depending on the situation, and also the density of the recent mammogram—workup can be stopped or repeat mammogram can be performed. If mammogram is more than 6 months old, the first step is to repeat the mammogram for the symptomatic side.

4. Noted is the mass right upper outer quadrant that is better evaluated on the submitted spot compression view. On spot compression view, the mass is irregular and lobulated and of increased density.

5. Ultrasound demonstrates "irregular" marginated mass with increased flow and in part "posterior acoustic enhancement."

Pearls

- The consequence of classifying mass as BI-RADS 5 instead of BI-RADS 4 is that in case pathology would show a benign finding such as fibrosis, the finding would not be concordant.
- Any BI-RADS 5 finding is highly suspicious, and if core biopsy results in benign histology, surgical excision is the next step.
- Any BI-RADS 4 finding that has benign histology on core biopsy can be concordant, depending on the situation, and follow-up might be appropriate.

Suggested Reading

Parikh JR. ACR appropriateness criteria on palpable breast masses. *J Am Coll Radiol.* 2007;4(5):285-288.

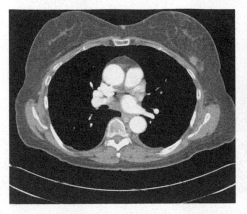
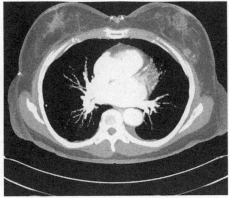
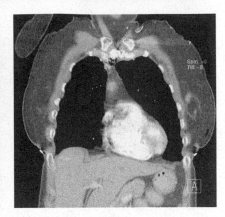

1. What BI-RADS classification should be used here?

2. What is the next best imaging test?

3. If you know that this patient has primary colon cancer, what would be the most likely appearances of breast metastases?

4. Why should you perform a mammogram if there is a finding on CT?

5. What CT features may assist in characterizing a primary breast mass on CT?

Case ranking/difficulty: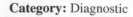

Category: Diagnostic

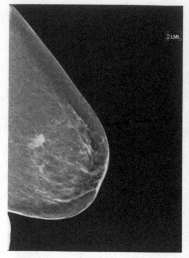

Left ML.

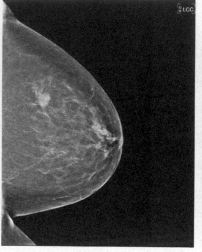

Left CC.

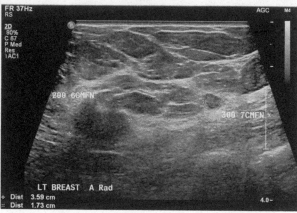

Ultrasound scanning shows second tumor toward nipple.

Answers

1. This is a trick question, as BI-RADS does not apply to incidental breast findings on CT scans. Appropriate mammographic and ultrasound workup needs to be performed.

2. This patient needs diagnostic mammograms to determine the nature of the lesion seen on CT.

   If confirmed, then an ultrasound scan can be performed. A screening exam only allows for CC and MLO views (in the United States). As a result, diagnostic mammography is the best next test.

3. Breast metastases are rare, but frequently present as circumscribed masses.

   Calcifications within breast masses, especially if dystrophic, have a benign connotation—usually due to degenerating fibroadenomas. Irregular masses can be found, as in this case. See case of melanoma metastases for comparison.

4. Mammography is the gold standard for breast imaging, and a suspicious finding on CT (or other modality) should trigger a diagnostic workup. Calcifications are best seen with mammography. Mass margins can be characterized by the use of spot (magnification) films. If cancer is present in one breast, you need to screen the contralateral breast.

5. Ultimately, it is not easy to characterize a mass on CT findings only. However, dense dystrophic calcification within fibroadenomas can help in the diagnosis.

Correlation with recent mammograms is important. A 2011 paper in *European Journal of Radiology* demonstrated increased enhancement in malignant masses on CT, but the bottom line is that a finding on CT should be worked up in the conventional manner.

Pearls

- Margins are the most important CT finding.
- If circumscribed, likely benign, except for a patient with a known primary who may present with oval circumscribed metastases.

Suggested Readings

Adejolu M, Huo L, Rohren E, Santiago L, Yang WT. False-positive lesions mimicking breast cancer on FDG PET and PET/CT. *AJR Am J Roentgenol.* 2012;198(3):W304-W314.

Nakamura N, Tsunoda H, Takahashi O, et al. Frequency and clinical significance of previously undetected incidental findings detected on computed tomography simulation scans for breast cancer patients. *Int J Radiat Oncol Biol Phys.* 2012;84(3):602-605.

Surov A, Fiedler E, Wienke A, Holzhausen HJ, Spielmann RP, Behrmann C. Intramammary incidental findings on staging computer tomography. *Eur J Radiol.* 2011;81(9):2174-2178.

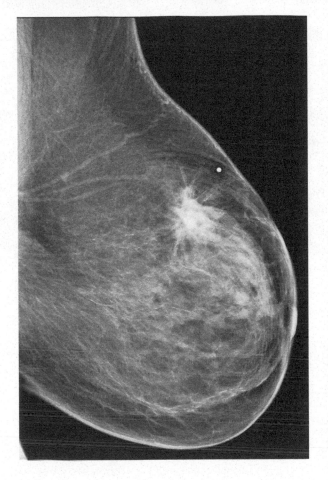

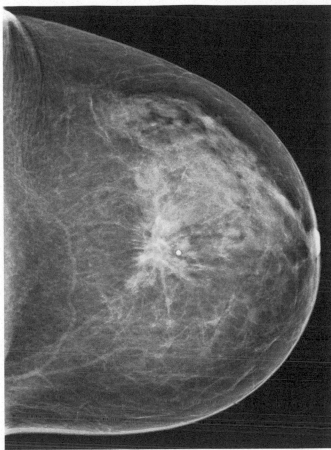

1. What BI-RADS score should be given in this case?

2. What is the most likely pathology given these appearances?

3. What is the next important investigation?

4. A solid mass is identified at ultrasound. What should you do next?

5. Apart from H&E stains of the core biopsy, what other investigations would you order?

Case ranking/difficulty:

Category: Diagnostic

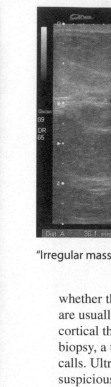

Prior mammogram—can you see the cancer in retrospect?

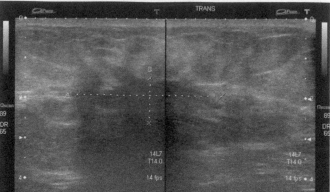

"Irregular mass" ultrasound correlate.

Answers

1. This is not a screening examination, and so a definitive diagnosis can be made. The features include spiculation and distortion, which should at least trigger a BI-RADS 4, and more likely BI-RADS 5, as you would not accept a nonmalignant biopsy as being concordant with these appearances.

2. Invasive ductal carcinoma of no special type (NST) is the most common carcinoma giving these appearances. If the question was worded "what are the possible pathologies giving these appearances," then both tubular carcinoma (which normally has long spicules) and invasive lobular carcinoma (which presents mainly as distortion, and rarely as a mass) are possibilities.

3. Physical exam and targeted ultrasound are the most important next steps. Tomosynthesis could help if you perceived distortion possibly due to superimposition. MRI is likely to be an important part of this patient's management, but not just yet.

4. If a highly suspicious mass is seen on ultrasound, it is worth scanning the ipsilateral axilla to determine whether there are any pathological lymph nodes. These are usually composed of irregular nodes or have focal cortical thickening of >3 mm. If they have had a recent biopsy, a threshold of >4 mm will reduce false-positive calls. Ultrasound-guided core biopsy is indicated for a suspicious mass seen on ultrasound.

5. ER, PR, and HER2 status are essential for the tailored treatment of breast cancer, as treatment varies by subtype. Ki-67 could be ordered, which is a proliferation index. Other tests such as 20 or 70 gene tests are frequently performed on patients who have neoadjuvant chemotherapy.

Pearls

- Subtler signs of early breast cancer.
- Developing focal asymmetry.
- Possible dense superimposition.

Suggested Readings

Biganzoli L, Wildiers H, Oakman C, et al. Management of elderly patients with breast cancer: updated recommendations of the International Society of Geriatric Oncology (SIOG) and European Society of Breast Cancer Specialists (EUSOMA). *Lancet Oncol.* 2012;13(4):e148-e160.

Zbar AP, Gravitz A, Audisio RA. Principles of surgical oncology in the elderly. *Clin Geriatr Med.* 2012;28(1):51-71.

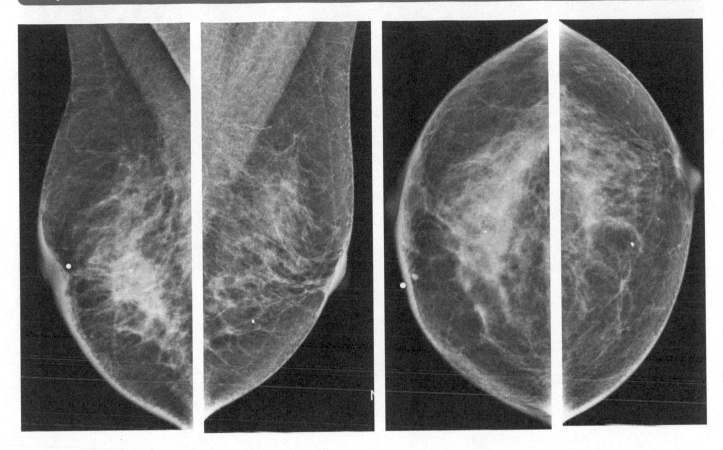

1. What is the pertinent finding?

2. What would be the next step of workup?

3. What is the significance of skin thickening?

4. If you have skin thickening but no other suspicious lesion in the breast, what can be the next step of workup?

5. What is the distribution of the calcifications in the right breast?

Case ranking/difficulty: **Category:** Diagnostic

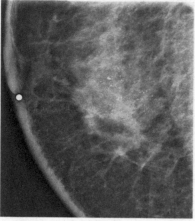

Diagnostic mammogram, right spot compression ML view, demonstrating "pleomorphic" calcifications in "regional distribution" (>2 cm).

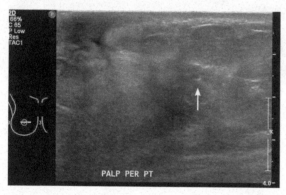

Ultrasound of right inferior retroareolar breast demonstrates mass and also demonstrates the presence of the microcalcifications (*arrow*).

Answers

1. Noted are indeterminate calcifications of the right breast that, on additional magnification views, are consistent with "pleomorphic" calcifications in "regional (>2 cm area) distribution." There is also thickening of the skin and mild retraction of the nipple.

2. Next step is workup of the calcifications with magnification ML and CC view and ultrasound of the retroareolar breast.

3. Skin thickening can be seen in case of invasive lymphatic involvement of the skin, like in this case; it can reflect inflammatory component in case of mastitis or it can be due to prior radiation treatment; however, this would likely be not as focal as in this case.

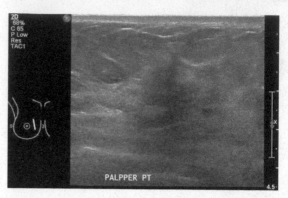

Ultrasound of right medial retroareolar breast demonstrates "hypoechoic mass" with "irregular" shape and "posterior acoustic shadowing."

4. Skin thickening can be related to mastitis and could be treated with antibiotics. However, it is important to follow the patient within a short time period of a few weeks to make sure that the treatment did work. If skin thickening persists and there are no other targets for biopsy on mammogram or ultrasound, patient needs to be transferred to surgeon for punch biopsy.

5. Further assessment and description of calcifications should be based on the magnification views. However, here the calcifications have a "segmental" or "regional" distribution and are not "scattered." This makes them more suspicious.

Pearls

- If feasible, ultrasound-guided biopsy is preferred over stereotactic biopsy due to better patient comfort.
- If there is need to prove that the calcifications have been sampled—which is not a crucial issue here—specimen radiograph of the tissue sampled by ultrasound-guided biopsy can be obtained.
- Please note that in this case, there was marked thickening of the skin in the inferior breast and periareolar breast as well as mild retraction of the right nipple.
- The histology did show intraductal invasive carcinoma and multifocal high-grade DCIS. The skin thickening did correlate to the presence of lymphovascular invasion of the tumor.

Suggested Reading

Soo MS, Baker JA, Rosen EL, et al. Sonographically guided biopsy of suspicious microcalcifications of the breast: a pilot study. *AJR Am J Roentgenol.* 2002;178(4):1007-1015.

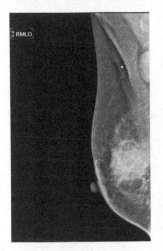 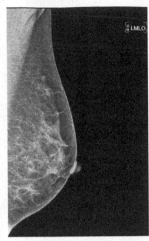 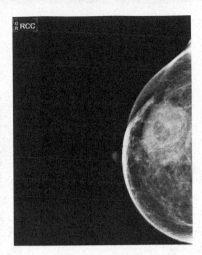 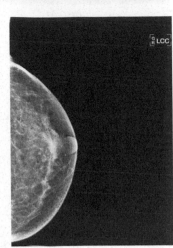

1. What BI-RADS classification should be used here?

2. What is the most likely pathology based on the imaging?

3. If there is no finding on mammography except lymphadenopathy, what is the imaging test that is recommended?

4. What stage is the tumor when it has metastasized to locoregional lymph nodes?

5. What are common sites for breast metastases?

Case ranking/difficulty: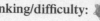

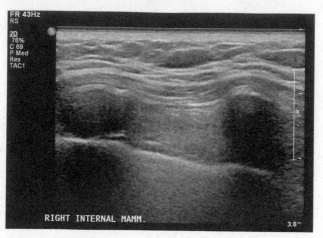

Looking for internal mammary nodes due to large central breast mass. An enlarged node in the internal mammary chain affects patient management when it comes to radiation treatment, as the field will be extended 1 cm across the sternum.

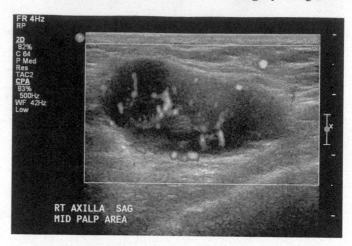

Vascular axillary node. Power Doppler often helps to distinguish a normal hilum, or, in this instance, may help direct the biopsy needle away from hitting one of these large vessels.

Answers

1. By the time a cancer has metastasized to axillary nodes, you should be able to give a BI-RADS 5 assessment without hesitation.

2. Fibroadenomas do not metastasize to axillary nodes. Primary breast lymphoma tends to present as a circumscribed mass in the breast. Hodgkin disease may present with bilateral axillary lymphadenopathy. The most common scenario with this type of imaging is a regular invasive ductal carcinoma with locoregional spread into the ipsilateral axillary nodes.

3. Whole breast ultrasound is not yet widely available, but may be helpful. MRI is the gold standard imaging procedure in this scenario, but is costly. PEM or BSGI may be of use, especially in dense breasts, and in patients unable to tolerate MRI. The downsides are the radiation dose.

4. Based on the size of the tumor, it is either a stage 2 or 3. It has metastasized to a lymph node and is therefore N1. Until formal staging is done, we do not know whether there are any metastases.

5. Bony and pulmonary metastases are common sites for metastases. Brain metastases may also occur frequently. Lobular cancer may metastasize to the peritoneum or a segment of bowel (beware the short segment stricture). Advanced disease can present with skin nodules.

Pearls

- Unilateral lymphadenopathy in the absence of known lymphoma should prompt a search for primary breast cancer.
- Mammography is frequently normal.
- MRI is the best imaging tool.

Suggested Readings

Ko EY, Han BK, Shin JH, Kang SS. Breast MRI for evaluating patients with metastatic axillary lymph node and initially negative mammography and sonography. *Korean J Radiol.* 2007;8(5):382-389.

Lanitis S, Behranwala KA, Al-Mufti R, Hadjiminas D. Axillary metastatic disease as presentation of occult or contralateral breast cancer. *Breast.* 2009;18(4):225-227.

Wang X, Zhao Y, Cao X. Clinical benefits of mastectomy on treatment of occult breast carcinoma presenting axillary metastases. *Breast J.* 2010;16(1):32-37.

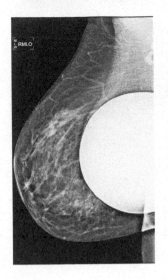
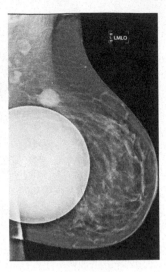
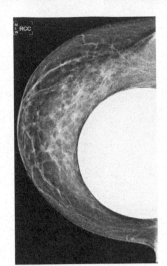
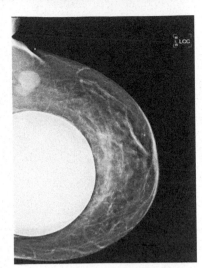

1. What is the BI-RADS category for this screening exam?

2. What other examinations do you normally do for patients with implants?

3. What is the most likely pathology?

4. What type and position of implant is present?

5. The mass is solid on ultrasound. What is your recommendation?

Case ranking/difficulty:

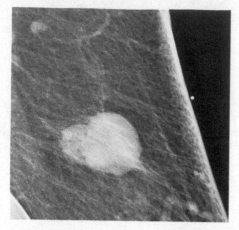

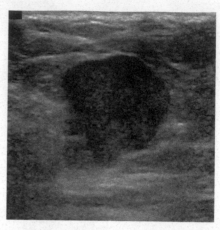

Left MLO spot compression. The question is: "Is this the index cancer or is this a metastatic lymph node, with unidentified primary?"

Mass identified on ultrasound. Margins are "circumscribed" in approximately 60% of its margin. The left lateral margins (often difficult to assess because of edge artifacts) show some "irregularity." As a result, the most suspicious descriptor wins out and prompts biopsy.

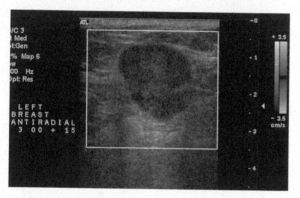

Doppler ultrasound—the mass is avascular. No vessels approaching the central part of the mass to indicate a hilum; therefore, more likely a primary breast mass. Only histology will be able to differentiate.

Answers

1. This is a screening exam with a positive finding. Recall for further views, including ultrasound examination. A physical examination by a trained professional could also be performed, especially if you have a multidisciplinary diagnostic breast clinic available for assessment of screen-detected abnormalities.

2. The additional views mean that some groups recommend known implant patients have diagnostic mammograms and get the implant displaced views routinely. MRI is the best test for implant complications. Ultrasound is the cheapest and quickest test for implant integrity, and lumps associated with an implant.

3. If you look at the margins of the mass, it is lobulated, but some parts of the margins are not clearly seen. Even a cancer-filled lymph node is a possibility in this site.

4. These implants are silicone and placed in a pocket BEHIND the pectoral muscle.

5. Parasitic infections are a rare cause of mass in the breast. You may see a calcified guinea worm on mammography, but in the western world, it does not cause presumed lymphadenopathy, or a mass in the breast. Ultrasound FNA may be used purely to establish a malignancy, but tissue is required for histology and for tissue biomarkers. Core biopsy is preferable. Surgical excisional biopsy has been replaced by percutaneous needle biopsy. MRI will be useful once malignancy has been confirmed.

Pearls

- In patients with implants, try to visualize as much glandular tissue as possible.
- Implant displaced views (EKLUND) have a major role in maximizing your chances of picking up a malignancy in patients with implants.
- Masses that look like intramammary nodes should still be fully worked up, especially if the presumed node is enlarged.

Suggested Readings

Grubstein A, Cohen M, Steinmetz A, Cohen D. Siliconomas mimicking cancer. *Clin Imaging*. 2011;35(3):228-231.

Nakaguro M, Suzuki Y, Ichihara S, Kobayashi TK, Ono K. Epithelial inclusion cyst arising in an intramammary lymph node: case report with cytologic findings. *Diagn Cytopathol*. 2009;37(3):199-202.

Tang SS, Gui GP. A review of the oncologic and surgical management of breast cancer in the augmented breast: diagnostic, surgical and surveillance challenges. *Ann Surg Oncol*. 2011;18(8):2173-2181.

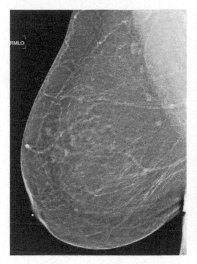
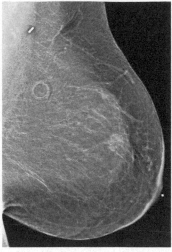
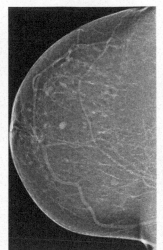
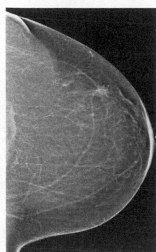

1. What BI-RADS classification should be used here?

2. What should be the next diagnostic imaging exam?

3. What type of biopsy would you consider with this lesion?

4. What mammographic surveillance would you recommend?

5. What signs are concerning for local recurrence in a scar?

Case ranking/difficulty: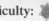

Category: Diagnostic

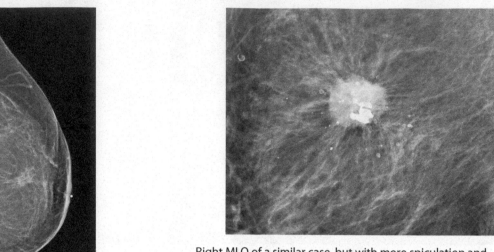

Right MLO of a similar case, but with more spiculation and calcifications—which was fat necrosis but even more concerning visually.

LM lateral view shows the relation of the soft density to the postsurgical distortion from the scar.

Answers

1. The postsurgical appearances can be described, and the finding is therefore benign. If this was a screening patient and you had no prior films and you may wish to do diagnostic views, you could give a BI-RADS 0 and then request diagnostic views.

2. If you have any doubt about the findings, you can perform diagnostic views. Tomosynthesis is an alternative to diagnostic views, as it can distinguish surgical scar from a mass. Ultrasound can be targeted to a palpable finding, but scanning a scar is not recommended, as you virtually always have suspicious findings, and may lock yourself into performing a biopsy. The features are diagnostic of a postsurgical scar, and so no further workup is required. Stability when compared with prior films is always useful.

3. The findings are normal postlumpectomy change. Therefore, no biopsy is indicated. If the scar gets denser over time, then that is usually a worrying sign, and ultrasound followed by core biopsy may be required. Cytology for scar recurrence is not recommended, as tumor markers will be required for treatment. MRI may sometimes help to distinguish a suspicious enhancing scar, from a normal postsurgical scar.

4. There are various approaches to the postoperative breast. If it is the first 5 years postsurgery, then your local lumpectomy protocol should be followed. After 5 years, many groups advocate for annual screening mammography. Others recommend diagnostic mammograms so that you can go direct to spot magnification plus or minus ultrasound if you detect any change. There is no evidence yet to warrant the addition of MRI screening surveillance to mammography in patients with a personal history of breast cancer.

5. There are several signs on mammography of possible scar recurrence. One is increasing density of the scar itself, following the maximal changes after radiation treatment (18 months). Scars usually soften over time. Developing microcalcifications in the scar, which are not characteristically dystrophic (fat necrosis) are suspicious and often provoke biopsy. Distortion related to the scar can be a normal reaction postop, with some patients having fat necrosis or exaggerated scarring causing these appearances. The only proviso is if the patient has had treatment for a lobular cancer, the finding is suspicious as lobular cancer recurrence may present in this type of manner.

Pearls

- Scars can be scary.
- Stability is good—look for prior films.

Suggested Readings

Cox CE, Greenberg H, Fleisher D, et al. Natural history and clinical evaluation of the lumpectomy scar. *Am Surg.* 1993;59(1):55-59.

Muir TM, Tresham J, Fritschi L, Wylie E. Screening for breast cancer post reduction mammoplasty. *Clin Radiol.* 2010;65(3):198-205.

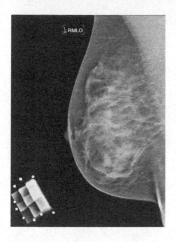
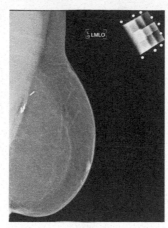
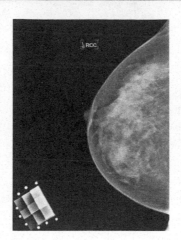
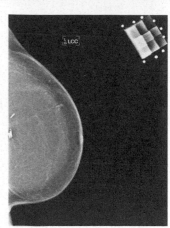

1. What BI-RADS should be used in this case?

2. What are the indications for a TRAM reconstruction?

3. What are the "breast" complications of TRAM flaps?

4. What is the best way to image TRAM reconstructions?

5. If a TRAM recurrence is suspected, what is the best way to biopsy the lesion?

Case ranking/difficulty:

Answers

1. This appearance is classic for a transverse rectus abdominis myocutaneous flap (TRAM). Mammograms may be performed, and may have this typical appearance. They are a benign finding, and therefore BI-RADS 2.

2. TRAM has been successfully used in patients having mastectomy for a variety of reasons, including risk reduction surgery for BRCA carriers. Poland syndrome affecting the breast has been successfully treated with TRAM augmentation.

   Patients who are likely to need postoperative radiation have in the past had their reconstruction delayed until they finished their radiation. However, this is no longer a contraindication. Patients do not need a mastectomy for ADH.

3. All forms of fat necrosis are very common following breast reconstruction, especially with TRAMs. Oil cysts and dystrophic calcifications are all part of the fat necrosis spectrum. There is no increased risk of malignancy, except for an increased risk of cancer due to having already had a primary breast cancer. Recurrence can occur in a TRAM flap, either in the lateral or in the medial margins.

4. MRI is the best tool in this scenario, with many papers documenting the imaging findings and complications.

5. Palpation-guided biopsy is less accurate than with image guidance, and ultrasound is usually the best method to guide a needle. Recurrence only needs a malignant diagnosis, and so many centers may feel that cytological diagnosis is enough. A core biopsy may provide additional information about histological type, grade, and receptor status.

Pearls

- TRAM reconstruction is common postmastectomy.
- Recognize the normal TRAM mammogram.
- Fat necrosis with calcifications is very common.

Suggested Readings

Glynn C, Litherland J. Imaging breast augmentation and Reconstruction. *Br J Radiol.* 2008;81(967):587-595.

Momoh AO, Colakoglu S, Westvik TS. Analysis of complications and patient satisfaction in pedicled transverse rectus abdominis myocutaneous and deep inferior epigastric perforator flap breast reconstruction. *Ann Plast Surg.* 2011;69(1):19-23.

Tan BK, Joethy J, Ong YS, Ho GH, Pribaz JJ. Preferred use of the ipsilateral pedicled TRAM flap for immediate breast reconstruction: an illustrated approach. *Aesthetic Plast Surg.* 2012;36(1):128-133.

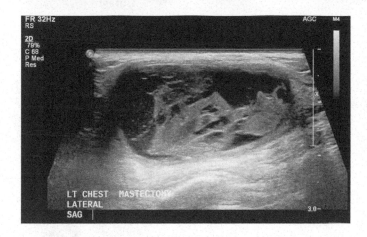
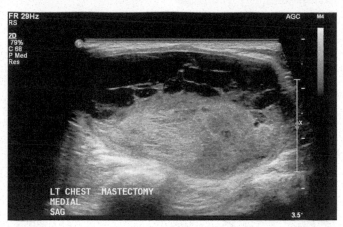

1. What is the BI-RADS category for this diagnostic exam?

2. What should be the next diagnostic imaging exam?

3. There is redness of the skin overlying this mass. What should I do next?

4. Now there is no skin redness, but the mass is visible under the skin. What further management recommendations do you want to make?

5. The mass has now settled. What imaging recommendations do you want to make?

Case ranking/difficulty:

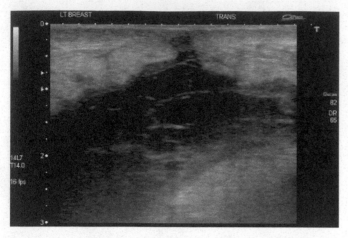

A patient with an abscess for comparison. There is thickening of the skin as well as a track for the infection up to the skin itself.

Answers

1. If this was a de novo case with no evidence of malignancy and no sign of infection, then this could be a complicated cyst that could be observed with short-term follow-up.

2. There is no residual breast tissue, and so diagnostic mammograms are unlikely to give important additional information. Tomosynthesis likewise is unlikely to help. If you are considering local recurrence, then MRI would be useful for staging and surgical planning. Positron emission mammography (PEM) is unlikely to give any useful information. No further diagnostic imaging is required at this stage. An intervention may be required.

3. Depending on whether you think there is minor inflammation present or a frank abscess, the intervention may be different. Redness of the overlying skin can be seen with masses that are not infected. Fat necrosis can do this, and even have evidence of local bruising. Observation with the use of oral antibiotics and short-term clinical follow-up is a reasonable management option. Percutaneous aspiration or drainage with installation of a catheter can be an option if you think there is an abscess, and the patient is symptomatic.

4. The features suggest some layered debris within this cystic space. Observation with short-term clinical examination and ultrasound follow-up is a good conservative plan. There is no evidence of an abscess, so emergent drainage is not required. Diagnostic aspiration may be attempted, but it is likely to show liquefied fat and blood products. If the mass does not settle, then core biopsy is reasonable. MRI is unlikely to add any further information at this stage.

5. Strictly, there is no reason to give any recommendations for annual mammograms, as the patient has bilateral mammograms. MRI has not been proven for the follow-up or surveillance of patients with bilateral mastectomies or of reconstructed breasts. However, in a young female, who already had multifocal breast cancer, she is at high risk of recurrence, and so some groups perform annual MRI in this setting. PEM and BSGI use isotopes for imaging and do not have a screening role.

Pearls

- Complications of mastectomy and reconstruction are more common following radiation treatment.
- Infection/inflammation through fat necrosis (which is more usually a delayed finding).
- Epidermal inclusion cysts are another finding.

Suggested Readings

Bittar SM, Sisto J, Gill K. Single-stage breast reconstruction with the anterior approach latissimus dorsi flap and permanent implants. *Plast Reconstr Surg.* 2012;129(5):1062-1070.

Sim YT, Litherland JC. The use of imaging in patients post breast reconstruction. *Clin Radiol.* 2012;67(2):128-133.

Tan BK, Joethy J, Ong YS, Ho GH, Pribaz JJ. Preferred use of the ipsilateral pedicled TRAM flap for immediate breast reconstruction: an illustrated approach. *Aesthetic Plast Surg.* 2012;36(1):128-133.

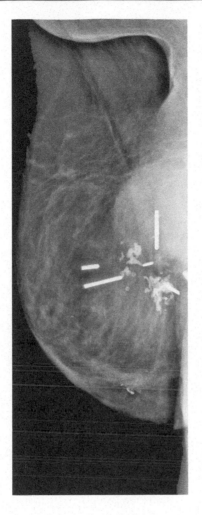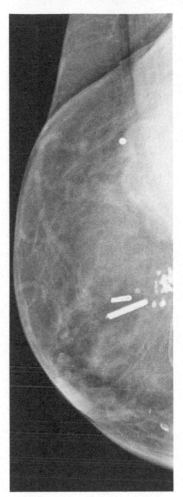

1. What BI-RADS classification is used for this entity?

2. What structure does the finding arise from?

3. What is the frequency of postradiation sarcoma, at 10 years?

4. What is the mainstay of treatment for this condition?

5. Which type of axial imaging is best to delineate the features of postradiation sarcoma?

Case ranking/difficulty:

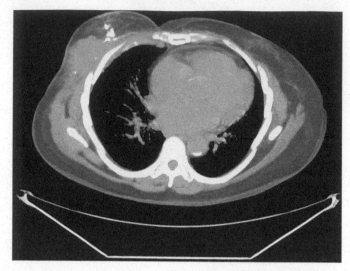

Non–contrast enhanced CT shows ill-defined soft tissue mass, which appears closely related to the chest wall. No destruction of ribs on bone window settings. No postradiation lung changes identified.

Answers

1. BI-RADS 0 is not appropriate in this setting, as it is not a screening exam. You could, however, give a BI-RADS 4 on this finding, as radiologically it is does not have characteristic descriptors of malignancy. In this particular setting, anything other than a malignancy is extremely unlikely, so BI-RADS 5 is the most appropriate assessment.

2. Secondary carcinomas usually arise from bone, connective tissue, or muscle as malignant fibrous histiocytomas or osteo/angio/fibro sarcomas. They are not related to breast cancer, and are not epithelial-based tumors.

3. OK it is rare, but not THAT RARE. Published data suggest a risk of postradiation sarcoma at 0.2%, but that is based on patients having radiation many years ago, and may not reflect current radiation treatment.

4. To have any chance of survival, the lesion needs to be widely excised. On the chest wall, this frequently includes removing ribs, as in this case. Chemotherapy has been used to varying effect. Radiation and hormone treatment have no place in the treatment of these sarcomas.

5. Plain radiographs are the best initial method of assessing coexistent bone involvement in patients with soft tissue sarcomas. MRI is the next step in imaging these lesions because of its superior soft tissue contrast, multiplanar imaging capability, and the absence of streak artifact. MRI is superior to CT in delineating tumor relationships to muscle, fat, fibrous tissue, and adjacent blood vessels. CT is superior to MRI only in the identification and evaluation of matrix/rim calcification and in the evaluation for pulmonary metastases.

Pearls

- Rare complication of radiation therapy.
- Mainly historic, but still occurs, and examiners often have one of these cases in their back pockets.
- When develops, prognosis is poor, but the mainstay of treatment is wide surgical excision.

Suggested Readings

Lagrange JL, Ramaioli A, Chateau MC, et al. Sarcoma after radiation therapy: retrospective multiinstitutional study of 80 histologically confirmed cases. Radiation Therapist and Pathologist Groups of the Fédération Nationale des Centres de Lutte Contre le Cancer. *Radiology.* 2000;216(1):197-205.

Pencavel T, Allan CP, Thomas JM, Hayes AJ. Treatment for breast sarcoma: a large, single-centre series. *Eur J Surg Oncol.* 2011;37(8):703-708.

Vojtísek R, Kinkor Z, Fínek J. Secondary angiosarcomas after conservation treatment for breast cancers [in Czech]. *Klin Onkol.* 2011;24(5):382-388.

Prior mastectomy for left breast cancer and prior lumpectomy for right breast cancer

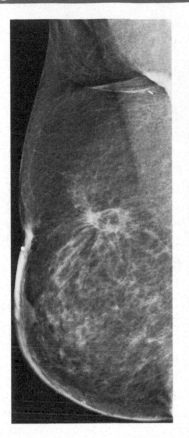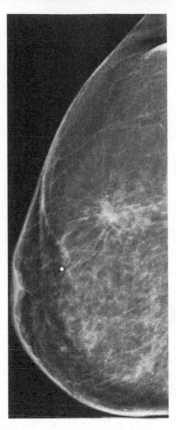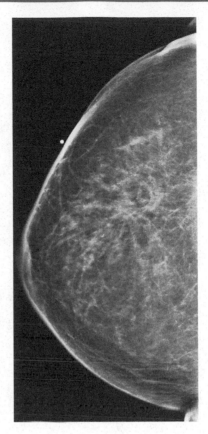

1. What BI-RADS classification should be used here?

2. What is the most likely pathology based on the imaging?

3. What is the frequency of fat necrosis following breast conservation surgery?

4. What type of biopsy should be performed?

5. What are the mammographic findings are signs of scar recurrence?

Case ranking/difficulty: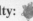

Category: Diagnostic

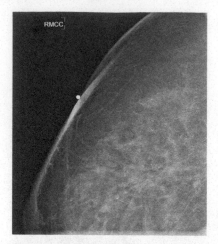

Right CC spot magnification view.

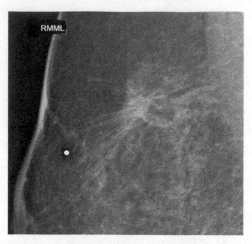

Right ML spot magnification view.

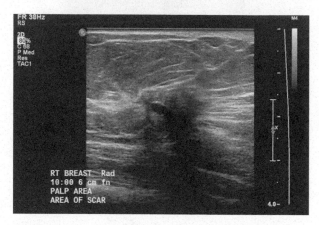

Ultrasound of scar—irregular mass with heterogeneous echo pattern and acoustic shadowing. There is no easy way around giving a BI-RADS 4 in this situation, which is why it is best to avoid scanning scars, unless you think there is a suspicious new finding on mammography.

Answers

1. This is a benign finding. Ignore the ultrasound image on the supplementary material, as ultrasound of scar is almost always "suspicious" in looks, and you can box yourself into doing an unnecessary biopsy. Despite the spiculation, the history of a lumpectomy at this site gives away the characteristic appearance of fat necrosis at the lumpectomy site.

2. The lucent fat-containing "cyst" at the center of the scar combined with dystrophic calcifications is characteristic of fat necrosis.

3. Fat necrosis is a common complication of breast conservation, seen more frequently in patients who have also had intraoperative radiation treatment (IORT). Radiotherapy terminology estimated 28% incidence.

4. The appearances are diagnostic, and biopsy is not required. If suspicious calcifications arise in the scar, and you cannot be certain of the location with ultrasound, a stereotactic core biopsy plus specimen x-ray may be required to establish the diagnosis.

5. Fine pleomorphic calcifications are always suspicious and require biopsy. They can, however, be found in a variation of fat necrosis, before the traditional coarse dystrophic calcification arises. A scar should soften over time, particularly after a (baseline) exam 2 years post–radiation therapy. Any increase in tissue density should raise concerns about scar recurrence.

Pearls

- A scar with a lucent center is characteristic of fat necrosis.
- Calcifications of fat necrosis occur in the wall of the inflammatory change.

Suggested Readings

Dershaw DD. Evaluation of the breast undergoing lumpectomy and radiation therapy. *Radiol Clin North Am*. 1995;33(6):1147-1160.

Rostom AY, el-Sayed ME. Fat necrosis of the breast: an unusual complication of lumpectomy and radiotherapy in breast cancer. *Clin Radiol*. 1987;38(1):31.

Wasser K, Schoeber C, Kraus-Tiefenbacher U, et al. Early mammographic and sonographic findings after intraoperative radiotherapy (IORT) as a boost in patients with breast cancer. *Eur Radiol*. 2007;17(7):1865-1874.

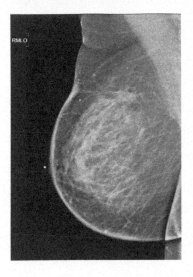 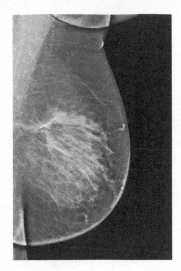 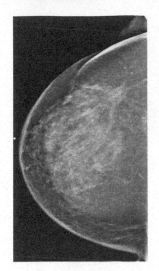 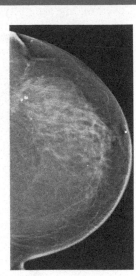

1. What BI-RADS classification should be used here?

2. What is the most likely cause for these findings on the left?

3. What is the percentage risk of associated malignancy with radial scars?

4. What radiographic factors may cause problems in postconservation breasts?

5. Which of the following are benign causes of calcifications following breast-conserving surgery?

Case ranking/difficulty: 🍁

Category: Diagnostic

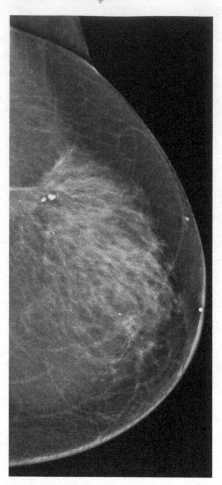

Left XCCL.

breast is frequently harder than normal for a number of years, and therefore less easily compressible. The biggest challenge technically is the positioning of the patient, to include as much breast tissue as possible and include the tumor bed. Additional view may need to be taken, such as XCCL. Fluid collections are normal postlumpectomy change, gradually being replaced by scar formation over a number of years. It assists with cosmesis, providing a corollary to the cavity from the surgery. Keloid may show up on a mammogram, but is not generally a technical factor in getting a good postconservation mammogram.

5. Dermal "calcifications" are frequently seen in the skin over the scar, and often are as a result of "trapping" of talcum powder or aluminum oxide in deodorant. An irregular scar may also cause the buildup of detritus that may be difficult for patients to clean off the skin. Fat necrosis calcifications are very common (approximately 25%) and also oil cysts. Suture calcifications may occur, and have characteristic appearances. Fine linear and branching calcifications are much more likely to be a high-grade DCIS recurrence and are a suspicious finding.

Pearls

- Post–breast conservation scars at first glance can look scary, especially if dense or are associated with calcifications.
- Take time to evaluate for stability (prior films are a must).
- Know what a normal scar looks like and the variants of calcifications that might occur.

Answers

1. BI-RADS 2—benign scar in both breasts. Look for prior films for stability. If NEW distortion, then perform a diagnostic exam and biopsy as necessary.

2. The appearances are much more of postsurgical scar, with dystrophic calcifications giving it away.

3. Most authorities quote a risk of associated DCIS of 20%. The issue of adequately sampling a radial scar to exclude associated DCIS is still controversial, as there are data for routine surveillance if enough biopsies are taken to surgical excision to completely exclude DCIS. This needs to be the subject of a clinical trial to inform future management.

4. There is not usually any difference in pain perception from a mammogram performed posttreatment, and a non–cancer patient. Following radiation therapy, the

Suggested Readings

Chansakul T, Lai KC, Slanetz PJ. The postconservation breast: part 1, Expected imaging findings. *AJR Am J Roentgenol.* 2012;198(2):321-330.

Chansakul T, Lai KC, Slanetz PJ. The postconservation breast: part 2, Imaging findings of tumor recurrence and other long-term sequelae. *AJR Am J Roentgenol.* 2012;198(2):331-343.

Dershaw DD, Shank B, Reisinger S. Mammographic findings after breast cancer treatment with local excision and definitive irradiation. *Radiology.* 1987;164(2):455-461.

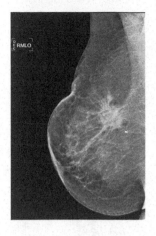
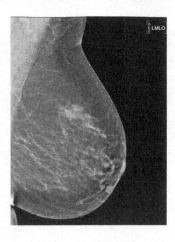
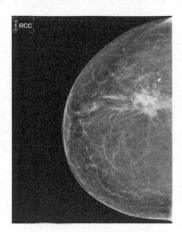
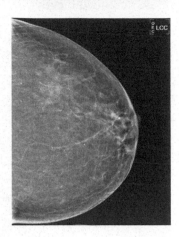

1. What is the BI-RADS category for this diagnostic exam?

2. What is the next best examination you recommend?

3. What is the most likely pathology?

4. What is the timescale you expect the maximal changes post–radiation therapy for breast cancer?

5. What is the most worrying feature of a surgical scar that would prompt you to biopsy?

Case ranking/difficulty: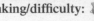

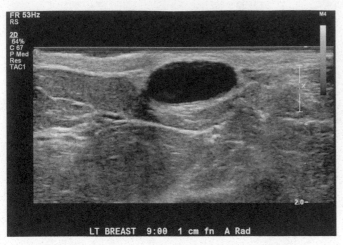

Ultrasound examination of palpable lump. Oval cystic mass identified, parallel to the skin. Some hyperechoic tissue around the wall, within the subdermal fat.

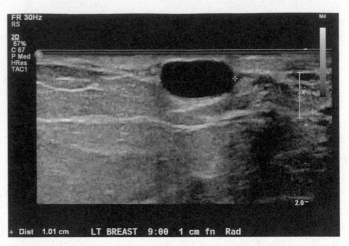

Compare with this exam: Ultrasound examination of palpable lump showing an oval intradermal mass with circumscribed margins and anechoic in nature, consistent with a subdermal cyst. The lower layer of the skin is stretched to include the mass.

Answers

1. (Stable) scar, postlumpectomy. No evidence of malignancy in either breast. There is a BB marker adjacent to the left nipple but no mass identified.

2. Further examination for a palpable lump using spot magnification views can be very helpful. In this case, it did not add anything, and we went directly to ultrasound.

3. A normal mammogram with a cystic lesion on ultrasound is a benign finding. The operative scar should not be mistaken for a cancer.

4. See BJR paper Buckley and Roebuck on time of maximal change. The skin thickening and parenchymal tissue edema should start to settle within 2 years following completion of radiation change. Any increase in edema following this should be regarded with suspicion.

5. Using first principles, any change that is not strictly benign (like obvious dystrophic calcifications) should prompt a biopsy for local recurrence.

Pearls

- Postoperative scars can look suspicious.
- Need prior films for stability.
- Watch for developing microcalcifications.

Suggested Readings

Buckley JH, Roebuck EJ. Mammographic changes following radiotherapy. *Br J Radiol*. 1986;59(700):337-344.

Ojeda-Fournier H, Olson LK, Rochelle M, Hodgens BD, Tong E, Yashar CM. Accelerated partial breast irradiation and posttreatment imaging evaluation. *Radiographics*. 2011;31(6):1701-1716.

Preda L, Villa G, Rizzo S, et al. Magnetic resonance mammography in the evaluation of recurrence at the prior lumpectomy site after conservative surgery and radiotherapy. *Breast Cancer Res*. 2006;8(5):R53.

Wong S, Kaur A, Back M, Lee KM, Baggarley S, Lu JJ. An ultrasonographic evaluation of skin thickness in breast cancer patients after postmastectomy radiation therapy. *Radiat Oncol*. 2011;6(6):9.

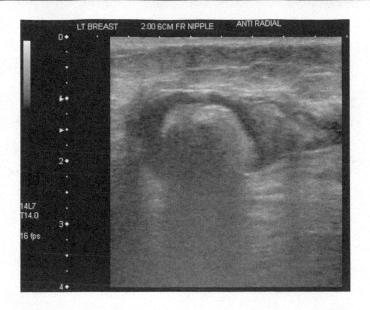

1. What BI-RADS classification should be used here?

2. In the setting of a postoperative patient, what should we be concerned about?

3. What is the next best imaging test?

4. What type of biopsy would you recommend?

5. What follow-up would you recommend?

Case ranking/difficulty: 🐾

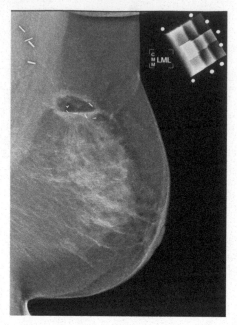

Fat/fluid level at lumpectomy site.

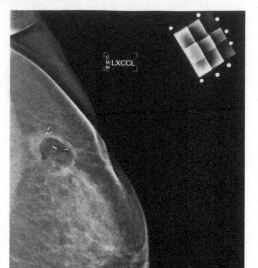

Lucency associated with surgical clips.

Answers

1. This is a benign finding in the presence of the mammographic findings, which will be made available on this page. The movable "debris" within the cystic cavity in a postoperative patient helps to make the diagnosis. Some people give a BI-RADS 0 until the mammographic workup is completed (which would be the normal way for this lesion to present). There is no finding, such as vascularity shown, which would make this finding suspicious of a possible intracystic papilloma.

2. The most common problems to occur postop in women with residual seromas are bleeding and hematoma formation, and infection. Fungus balls occur with aspergillus infection in lung cavities (aspergilloma). Patients are immunocompromised after having chemotherapy, but rarely get infection of the seroma.

3. Mammograms should have been performed before the ultrasound, so if they have not been done yet, now is the time. MRI in the postoperative breast is sometimes helpful in distinguishing clinical relevant problems from normal postoperative change, but there are many potential pitfalls. Tomosynthesis may be an answer for many of these findings, as it establishes its place in the workup of breast abnormalities.

4. This is a "normal" finding that can be followed, as no intervention is required.

5. Several answers are potentially correct, depending on the individual circumstances. Some groups advocate short-term physical examination and repeat ultrasound in atypical findings to ensure stability.

Pearls

- Fat necrosis common in later complication of breast conservation therapy.
- Contains fat.
- Hematoma can occur within the lipid cavity producing a fat/fluid level.
- No therapeutic or long-term sequelae from this complication unless the patient has a clotting disorder.

Suggested Readings

Drukteinis JS, Gombos EC, Raza S, Chikarmane SA, Swami A, Birdwell RL. MR imaging assessment of the breast after breast conservation therapy: distinguishing benign from malignant lesions. *Radiographics*. 2012;32(1):219-234.

Mendelson EB. Evaluation of the postoperative breast. *Radiol Clin North Am*. 1992;30(1):107-138.

Solomon B, Orel S, Reynolds C, Schnall M. Delayed development of enhancement in fat necrosis after breast conservation therapy: a potential pitfall of MR imaging of the breast. *AJR Am J Roentgenol*. 1998;170(4):966-968.

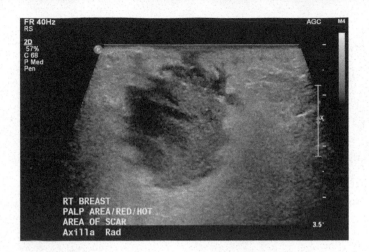

1. What BI-RADS classification should be used here?

2. What group of bacteria is likely to be found in an abscess?

3. A Doppler signal within an abscess means which of the following?

4. What are the possible management options for an abscess?

5. What are the ultrasound features of an abscess?

Case ranking/difficulty:

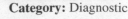

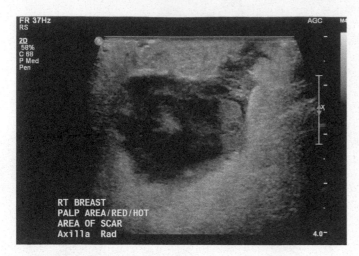

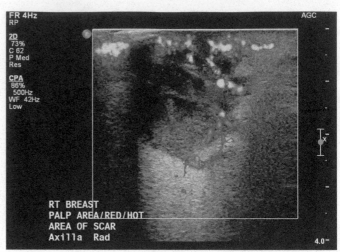

Another view shows the irregular mass and the extension superficially toward the skin.

Abscesses are inflamed and therefore vascular. There may be signal from movement of fluid within the abscess, so the gain needs to be turned down. It may be useful to identify vascular bands through the abscess, indicating that it is loculated, or is a phlegmon and might therefore need surgical intervention.

Answers

1. This is a special case situation, where the finding is of a benign lesion, but the BI-RADS descriptors are all suspicious. A summary phrase such as "a fluid collection with skin thickening and redness consistent with an abscess" would work well. BI-RADS 0 is not indicated as this is a diagnostic workup.

2. There is a low oxygen level within an abscess, and therefore anaerobic bacteria tend to colonize a surgical cavity and cause an abscess.

3. Increased Doppler signal throughout an abscess may occur when the abscess is loculated, but also at the stage where a phlegmon is present. A phlegmon is a confined focus of inflammatory tissue without liquefaction.

4. The management of an abscess depends on many factors, and it is important to work closely with the surgical team to ensure a correct treatment option for that patient. Treatment can be anything from watchful waiting during antibiotic treatment to diagnostic aspiration, drain placement, or surgery if there is a phlegmon that needs evacuating.

5. Abscesses may have myriad appearances, but, in general, they appear of mixed echogenicity, and you can observe movement of fluid within the cavity. There may be enhanced Doppler signals around or even within the abscess.

Pearls

- In the clinical setting of infection, think abscess until proven otherwise.

Suggested Readings

Boisserie-Lacroix M, Debled M, Tunon de Lara C, Hurtevent G, Asad-Syed M, Ferron S. The inflammatory breast: management, decision-making algorithms, therapeutic principles. *Diagn Interv Imaging*. 2012;93(2):126-136.

Leibman AJ, Misra M, Castaldi M. Breast abscess after nipple piercing: sonographic findings with clinical correlation. *J Ultrasound Med*. 2011;30(9):1303-1308.

Trop I, Dugas A, David J, et al. Breast abscesses: evidence-based algorithms for diagnosis, management, and follow-up. *Radiographics*. 2011;31(6):1683-1699.

Bloody nipple discharge—no nipple changes

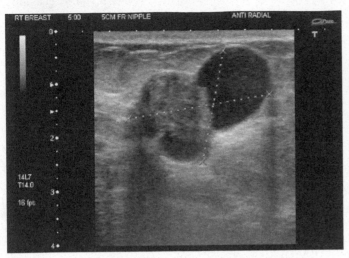 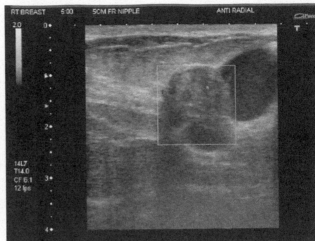

1. What BI-RADS classification should be used here?

2. What is the most likely pathology based on the imaging?

3. What is the next best imaging test?

4. Any other tests that you may consider?

5. What are common types of nipple discharge?

Case ranking/difficulty:

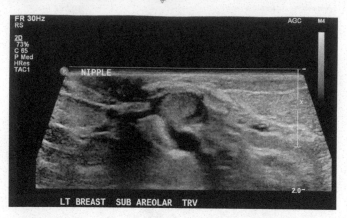

Ultrasound of another case of intraductal mass. It is possible to demonstrate the dilated duct extending from the nipple and the cystic space containing the solid mass.

Answers

1. This finding is suspicious, requiring biopsy, so a BI-RADS 4 is an appropriate classification. Until biopsy is performed, we cannot tell whether this is a simple papilloma, papillary lesion, or intracystic papillary carcinoma. In this case, the lesion appears to be possibly growing through the cyst wall and so a core biopsy showing papilloma was nonconcordant. Surgical excision was performed, confirming a simple papilloma.

2. Malignant cancers within the milk duct/cystic cavity are either invasive ductal or DCIS. Benign intraductal tumors are papillomas. A phyllodes tumor contains distorted ducts. Mucinous carcinoma can simulate a complicated cyst, with heterogeneous or low level echoes within the structure.

3. If older than 40 years, mammographic workup should really have been done first. If not, it is time to do it and decide what comes next. MRI can be performed but usually following a biopsy showing papillary DCIS (due to likely multifocality). These multifocal lesions can often be seen when you search for them with ultrasound.

4. A ductogram may help if there were no ultrasound finding, or you suspect multiple lesions early on. Some centers perform ductoscopy routinely. Ductal lavage can assist in deciding how hard you may wish to investigate a bloody nipple discharge.

5. If lactating or pregnant, milky discharge is normal physiology. Bloody nipple discharge is commonly due to duct ectasia or plasma cell mastitis, rather than cancer. Profuse watery nipple discharge is a potential symptom of DCIS. Brown, through yellow to light green and blue, is normal physiological nipple discharges.

Pearls

- When finding an intraductal mass, identify whether the echoes move (by toe/heel with the probe), suggesting proteinaceous plug or debris.
- Doppler ultrasound may help as papillomas have prominent vascular channels.
- Vessels entering perpendicular to the wall of the duct are highly suggestive of a papilloma.

Suggested Readings

Al Sarakbi W, Salhab M, Mokbel K. Does mammary ductoscopy have a role in clinical practice? *Int Semin Surg Oncol.* 2006;3(3):16.

Brookes MJ, Bourke AG. Radiological appearances of papillary breast lesions. *Clin Radiol.* 2008;63(11): 1265-1273.

Rizzo M, Linebarger J, Lowe MC, et al. Management of papillary breast lesions diagnosed on core-needle biopsy: clinical pathologic and radiologic analysis of 276 cases with surgical follow-up. *J Am Coll Surg.* 2012;214(3):280-287.

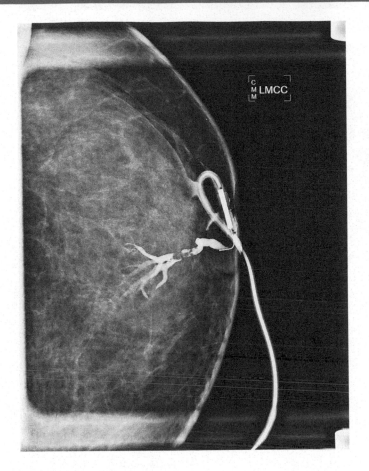

1. What are causes of bloody nipple discharge?

2. What are benign causes for bloody nipple discharge?

3. What volume of contrast is normally used in a ductogram?

4. What are contraindications to ductography?

5. What are the symptoms of extravasation of ductography contrast?

Case ranking/difficulty: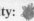

Category: Diagnostic

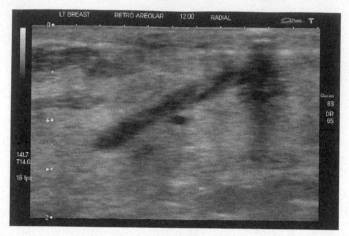

Ultrasound can be useful, but may just show a dilated duct, with possible proteinaceous debris.

Answers

1. Pagets disease is usually diagnosed on physical examination. Excoriation of the central milk ducts may cause bloody discharge. DCIS usually produces a profuse watery discharge. IDC may also cause a bloody nipple discharge (5–8% according to the literature). Eighty-five percent of bloody discharge is due to benign disease such as a papilloma.

2. Periductal mastitis and duct ectasia are the most common causes of bloody nipple discharge. Papillomatosis usually presents with watery nipple discharge like DCIS. Papilloma may present with bloody discharge.

3. Approximately 0.2 to 0.3 mL is all that is required to inject into a normal-caliber duct system. Occasionally, you may have to inject more. Use of a 1-mL syringe aids the injection of contrast, attached to the lacrimal catheter with connecting tubing.

4. Severe nipple retraction may physically prevent you from placing the cannula. Severe allergies to iodinated contrast are a relative contraindication (need to avoid intravenous puncture). If the patient says that she will not have surgery if something is found, there is no point in doing the procedure. A prior Hadfields procedure, where there has been a total duct excision, means that the ductogram is not technically possible, and a bloody nipple discharge should mean that one affected duct was not removed.

5. Extravasation is common in the first few ductograms, caused by injecting too much contrast. Patients do not get flushing, but may experience mild pain around the nipple. Most patients have no symptoms from extravasation.

Pearls

- Bloody nipple discharge is a rare cause of breast cancer.
- Periductal mastitis is the most common cause, and can be identified by periductal tiny lucencies from micro abscesses.
- A blocked duct is not pathognomonic of a papilloma, as proteinaceous plugs can cause the same effect.

Suggested Readings

Adepoju LJ, Chun J, El-Tamer M, Ditkoff BA, Schnabel F, Joseph KA. The value of clinical characteristics and breast-imaging studies in predicting a histopathologic diagnosis of cancer or high-risk lesion in patients with spontaneous nipple discharge. *Am J Surg.* 2005;190(4):644-646.

Dooley WC. Breast ductoscopy and the evolution of the intra-ductal approach to breast cancer. *Breast J.* 2009;15(Suppl 1):S90-S94.

Rissanen T, Reinikainen H, Apaja-Sarkkinen M. Breast sonography in localizing the cause of nipple discharge: comparison with galactography in 52 patients. *J Ultrasound Med.* 2007;26(8):1031-1039.

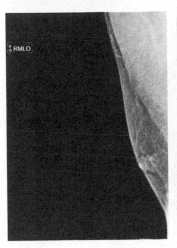
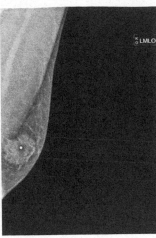
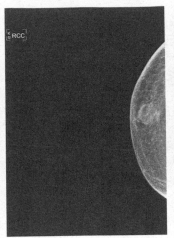
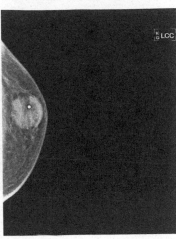

1. What is gynecomastia?

2. What is the etiology of gynecomastia?

3. What is the diagnostic algorithm for evaluation of palpable mass in males?

4. What is the role of ultrasound in the workup of palpable abnormality in males?

5. What is the epidemiology of male breast cancer?

Case ranking/difficulty:

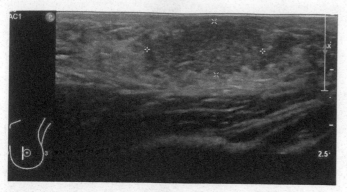

Category: Diagnostic

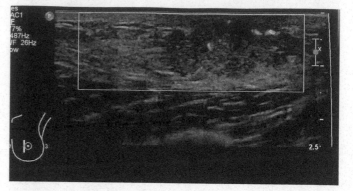

Ultrasound demonstrates lobulated hypoechoic nodular area corresponding to "lobulated" gynecomastia.

Ultrasound demonstrating lobulated hypoechoic nodular area with increased flow on duplex.

Answers

1. Gynecomastia is the most common benign finding in males with palpable breast abnormalities. It is best diagnosed on mammography—sometimes ultrasound can be helpful in addition. It might be symmetric but is often times asymmetric in appearance in both breasts. It has a peak in incidence in puberty and in higher age.

2. Any medication or medical condition that affects the balance between estrogen and testosterone in the body can result in proliferation of ducts and fibrotic tissue (gynecomastia) in the male breast—no connection to family history of breast cancer.

3. Mammography should always be the first choice, since it is diagnostic in most cases. Also calcifications can be best seen on mammogram. Gynecomastia can appear relatively concerning on ultrasound, since it might even show "posterior acoustic shadowing." In equivocal cases, ultrasound can be helpful to increase the specificity of mammography by searching for secondary signs for malignancy and lymphadenopathy. If suspicious abnormality is seen, ultrasound-guided biopsy is recommended.

4. See answer to question 3. Again, mammography is the first test of choice. Ultrasound can be helpful, but often times unnecessary.

   Increased flow on duplex or posterior echogenicity is not specific. More important are detection of secondary findings such as skin thickening, nipple retraction, or lymphadenopathy to increase specificity as seen on ultrasound.

5. Incidence is 1:100,000 and mean age of diagnosis is 67 years. Less than 6% occur in males younger than 40 years. Since gynecomastia is often seen in older patients, it can occur together with malignancy, although gynecomastia is not to be considered a precursor to breast cancer. Family history indeed is a significant risk factor as detailed above.

Pearls

- Bilateral standard mammography is the most important first test in the workup of palpable abnormalities in males—not ultrasound.
- Magnification views and or spot compression views may be useful in addition.
- Ultrasound can be helpful in case of equivocal mammogram findings.
- It is important not to miss lymphadenopathy, as secondary finding suggesting malignancy.
- Most common reason for breast lump in male is gynecomastia.

Suggested Readings

Chen L, Chantra PK, Larsen LH, et al. Imaging characteristics of malignant lesions of the male breast. *Radiographics*. 2006;26(4):993-1006.

Mathew J, Perkins GH, Stephens T, Middleton LP, Yang WT. Primary breast cancer in men: clinical, imaging, and pathologic findings in 57 patients. *AJR Am J Roentgenol*. 2008;191(6):1631-1639.

Prior prostate cancer—"lump" in the breast

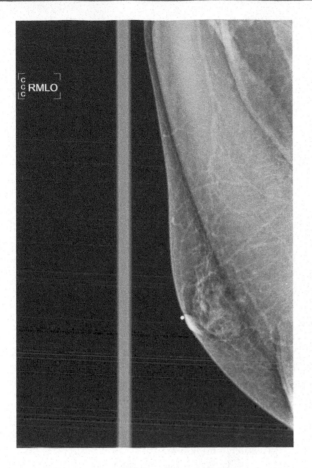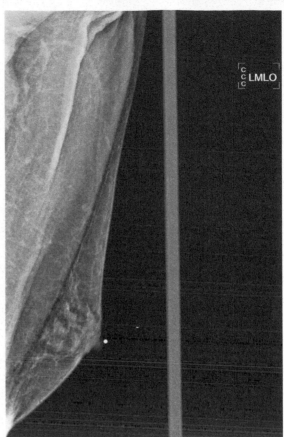

1. What is the most likely cause for these appearances?

2. Which drugs, or classes of drugs, cause these appearances?

3. What BI-RADS score is appropriate in this case?

4. What conditions are a cause of gynecomastia?

5. What treatment should be offered for this patient?

Case ranking/difficulty:

Category: Diagnostic

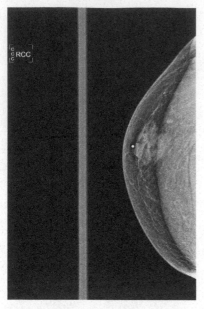

Right CC—BB marker on nipple.

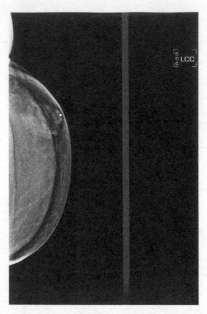

Left CC—BB marker on nipple. Note the large amount of pectoral muscle on the film, compared with a female. This male patient had little fat in the breast.

Answers

1. Usually medication related. In this case the estrogens used to treat prostate cancer.

2. The list of drugs known to cause gynecomastia is long and ever changing, because of the number of newer monoclonal antibody therapies for chronic conditions, which have similar side effects.

3. The finding is benign, with minor asymmetry only; therefore, BI-RADS 2. If there is truly a mass, it depends on your findings as to whether it becomes a BI-RADS 4. Remember that unless you get textbook pictures, an ultrasound of gynecomastia can look extremely worrying, and prompt biopsy.

4. Klinefelter syndrome is a reported cause of gynecomastia. Patients with chronic renal failure (end stage) often have reduced levels of testosterone and may have primary testicular failure. Amyloidosis and systemic lupus erythematosus do not cause gynecomastia. Hyperthyroidism may cause gynecomastia due to increased aromatase activity and increased levels of sex hormone binding globulin (SHBG). (SHBG binds androgens more avidly than estrogen, allowing for higher free levels to act on peripheral tissues such as the breast).

5. If gynecomastia is very mild and tolerable, then reassurance and observation may be appropriate. Tamoxifen is frequently given to males with gynecomastia to counter the estrogenic effect. It has its own list of side effects and may not be tolerated. Obviously, if possible, withdrawal of the offending drug would help, but the effects are not always reversible. Surgical excision is not recommended as primary treatment, especially if the underlying cause has not been removed.

Pearls

- Common complication of the use of a number of drugs.
- Need to remove the underlying cause, for example, change to a different drug within the same class.
- May not be reversible.

Suggested Readings

Fradet Y, Egerdie B, Andersen M, et al. Tamoxifen as prophylaxis for prevention of gynaecomastia and breast pain associated with bicalutamide 150 mg monotherapy in patients with prostate cancer: a randomised, placebo-controlled, dose-response study. *Eur Urol*. 2007;52(1): 106-114.

Grunfeld EA, Halliday A, Martin P, Drudge-Coates L. Andropause syndrome in men treated for metastatic prostate cancer: a qualitative study of the impact of symptoms. *Cancer Nurs*. 2011;35(1):63-69.

Thompson IM, Tangen CM, Goodman PJ, Lucia MS, Klein EA. Chemoprevention of prostate cancer. *J Urol*. 2009;182(2):499-507; discussion 508.

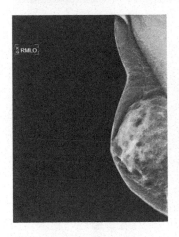
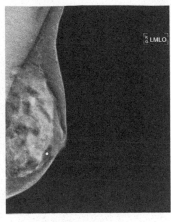
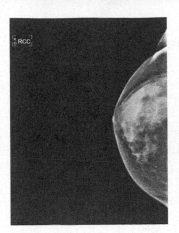
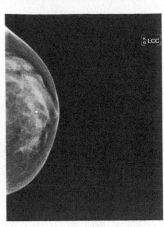

1. Why was the right as well as the left breast scanned?

2. What are the findings in regard to the symptomatic left side?

3. Is there a need for ultrasound?

4. What is the final diagnosis?

5. What would be the next step?

Case ranking/difficulty: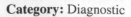

Category: Diagnostic

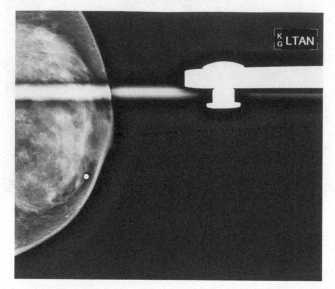

Spot compression left MLO view.

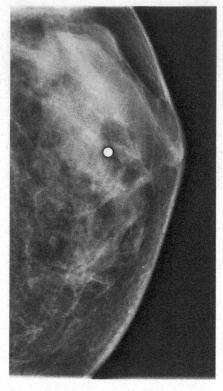

Spot compression left CC view.

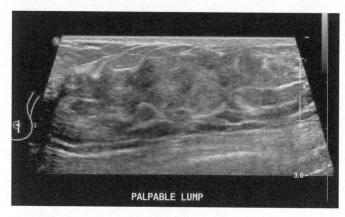

Ultrasound directed to the area of concern; left chest wall demonstrates normal fibroglandular tissue.

Answers

1. Patient is symptomatic on the left side. Nevertheless, patient received mammogram of both sides as a baseline to see if there is any focal asymmetry and also to assess the extent of the gynecomastia bilaterally.

2. Left side demonstrates normal fibroglandular tissue. No focal suspicious abnormality is identified.

3. Ultrasound is recommended for every palpable abnormality, in a male or female. In a male, mammogram, however, should be the first step.

4. The diagnosis is bilateral symmetric gynecomastia.

5. Patient with bilateral gynecomastia needs to be worked up clinically. There is no need for further imaging follow-up.

Pearls

- Example of extensive bilateral symmetric gynecomastia due to medication—in this case, spironolactone.

Suggested Readings

Cuculi F, Suter A, Erne P. Spironolactone-induced gynecomastia. *CMAJ*. 2007;176(5):620.

Haynes BA, Mookadam F. Male gynecomastia. *Mayo Clin Proc*. 2009;84(8):672.

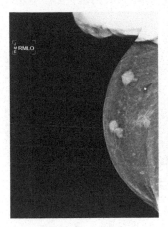

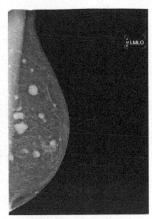

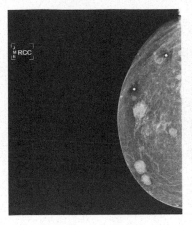

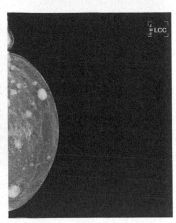

Right MLO.   Left MLO.   Right CC.   Left CC.

1. What is the first-line radiological examination in a patient with this history?

2. What will the ultrasound examination show?

3. What is the most likely pathology?

4. What is the cause of a vascular mass on the chest wall?

5. What should be the next radiological investigation?

Case ranking/difficulty: 🍁

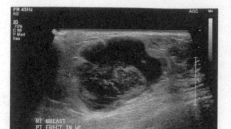

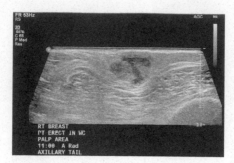

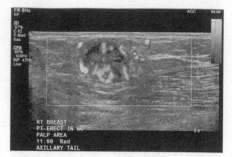

Ultrasound appears to be a complicated cystic structure.

Ultrasound—this view shows the mass to be "complex."

Power Doppler ultrasound shows a highly vascular solid lesion.

Answers

1. A quick noninvasive, nonionizing examination such as ultrasound is easy to perform and should give more information to inform you what should be the next step. In this case, the lumps were over the breast regions, so a mammogram would be a reasonable examination as well. If the patient already has a known malignancy, a PET/CT may be of assistance in staging the disease (although not in the choice of question 5 above). A chest x-ray has little place in the immediate workup of this patient. CT and MRI may be overkill.

2. They are predominantly "circumscribed masses," mainly "oval" in shape with "two or three gentle lobulations" (BI-RADS and Stavros).

3. Is there any evidence of multiple masses over the rest of the skin to suggest neurofibromatosis? Lipomas are typically HYPERECHOIC. Multiple hamartoma syndromes can look very similar to this. There are multiple different masses; therefore, unlikely to be multiple separate carcinomas. This patient had known multiple myeloma, and these were proven myeloma metastases (note the vascularity on Doppler).

4. Vascular malformations do not tend to present as breast masses. However, following a seat belt injury, it is possible to get fat necrosis mass formation that can be vascular (but not typically so). Hemangiomas of the breast tend to be smaller and circumscribed with fibrous septae. Angiosarcomas usually present like lobular cancer, in that they are infiltrative and permeative, rather than causing circumscribed masses. Metastases are often vascular, especially so with multiple myeloma.

5. Even with a known history of multiple myeloma, malignancy needs to be proven, and core biopsy is the next best investigation.

Pearls

- Metastases to the breast are most frequently found as round or oval masses with circumscribed margins on mammography.
- On ultrasound, they appear as hypoechoic masses with microlobulated or circumscribed margins and posterior acoustic enhancement.
- On MRI, mostly present as circumscribed masses with either marked or moderate homogenous enhancement.

Suggested Readings

Bartella L, Kaye J, Perry NM, et al. Metastases to the breast revisited: radiological-histopathological correlation. *Clin Radiol*. 2003;58(7):524-531.

Surov A, Fiedler E, Holzhausen HJ, Ruschke K, Schmoll HJ, Spielmann RP. Metastases to the breast from non-mammary malignancies: primary tumors, prevalence, clinical signs, and radiological features. *Acad Radiol*. 2011;18(5):565-574.

Yeh CN, Lin CH, Chen MF. Clinical and ultrasonographic characteristics of breast metastases from extramammary malignancies. *Am Surg*. 2004;70(4):287-290.

Routine follow-up post-breast reconstruction

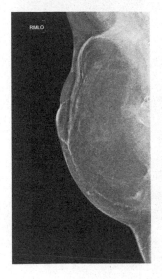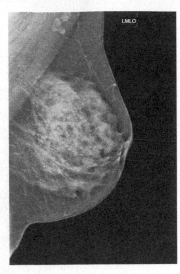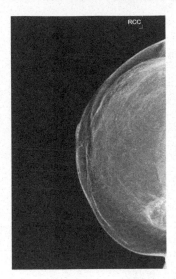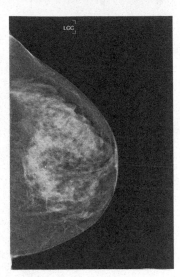

1. What BI-RADS classification should be used here?

2. What are the possible diagnostic imaging exams to work up this finding?

3. What type of biopsy would you recommend?

4. When you see microcalcification developing in a surgical scar, what is your differential?

5. What are the complications of breast reduction or reconstruction you should be looking for on surveillance?

Case ranking/difficulty:

Category: Diagnostic

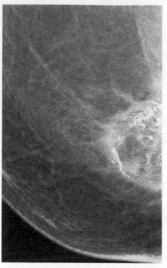

Close-up fat necrosis in TRAM reconstruction. Note that the calcifications make up a peripheral component to the mass.

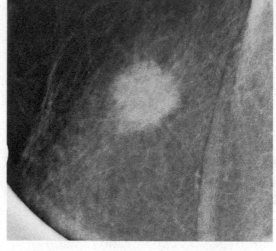

Close-up local recurrence in TRAM reconstruction.

Answers

1. BI-RADS 2 should be used, as this is a characteristically benign finding. BI-RADS 0 is not appropriate. If the patient was having a "tramogram," then it would be a diagnostic exam in the first place. Early fat necrosis can sometimes look suspicious, and therefore if this was one of those cases, a BI-RADS 4 may potentially be more appropriate.

2. All of the answers can be correct. If you have prior films and they are stable, no action need be taken. First visit, you may wish to work up with either spot (magnification) views or ultrasound. Ultrasound itself can appear suspicious when fat necrosis calcifies; therefore, it may not be a good exam in this instance. For reconstructed breasts, MRI is a good tool for surveillance. Tomosynthesis can be used in place of diagnostic special views.

3. This is a characteristic benign finding; therefore, no action other than follow-up is recommended.

4. Depends on what the lumpectomy was performed for. If there was ductal carcinoma in situ (DCIS) present in the surgical excision, then DCIS recurrence is always at the top of the list. "Dead DCIS" is said to be a recognized phenomenon in patients with lower-grade DCIS, who have undergone radiation therapy. Dystrophic calcifications commonly occur related to the development of fat necrosis. Dermal calcifications are usually seen only in the skin, but if there is marked posttreatment distortion, they may be projected over the surgical scar.

5. All of the answers can be true and can present as findings. However, in general practice, the common things you encounter are developing areas of fat necrosis that may be visible on both mammography and ultrasound. If they have had a breast reduction, they tend to have a characteristic pattern of parenchymal change with swirly lines, sometimes best seen on the CC and sometimes in the lower half on the MLO. Decreased breast volume related to lobular cancer is for global change over a time period, rather than just to the reduction surgery.

Pearls

- Benign condition relatively commonly seen in breast flap reconstructions.
- Characteristic appearance, and in typical locations, help make the diagnosis without the recourse to biopsy.

Suggested Reading

Eidelman Y, Liebling RW, Buchbinder S, Strauch B, Goldstein RD. Mammography in the evaluation of masses in breasts reconstructed with TRAM flaps. *Ann Plast Surg*. 1998;41(3):229-233.

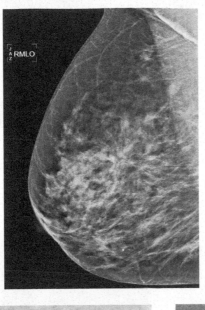
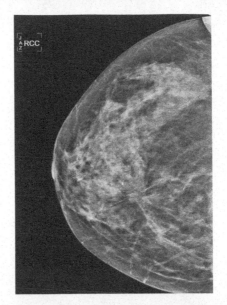
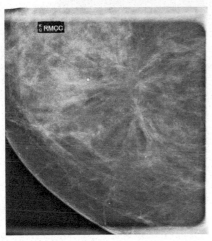
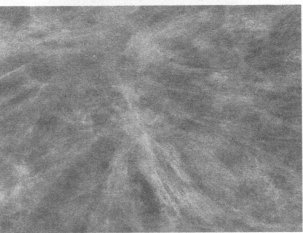

1. What are the pertinent findings on mammography?

2. What could be the etiology?

3. Which malignancy typically presents with distortion like this?

4. Are there any additional findings on the magnification view?

5. What is the consequence?

Case ranking/difficulty:

Category: Diagnostic

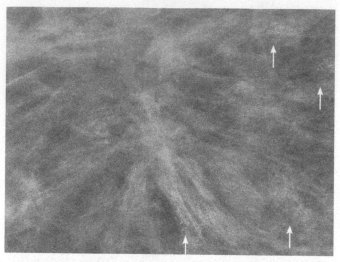

Diagnostic mammogram of right magnification CC view (additional electronically magnified) demonstrating several groups of "amorphous" calcifications.

Answers

1. Architectural distortion in the superior medial breast.

2. Differential diagnosis includes radial scar, malignancy, or prior surgery.

3. Any malignancy can result in the presence of distortion, but in general typical for this appearance would be tubular carcinoma. Tubular carcinoma is a malignancy with relatively good prognosis.

4. There are at least four groups of "amorphous" calcifications in proximity to the area of architectural distortion.

5. Given that all groups are similar in morphology, it would be reasonable to biopsy one group only as done in this case. Depending on the result, in case of positive for malignancy or atypia, all groups should be included into the excision. If the biopsy demonstrates benign, histology findings can be followed in 6 months.

Pearls

- "Architectural distortion" can be due to many different etiologies: prior lumpectomy, prior excisional biopsy, malignancy such as invasive ductal carcinoma, or radial scar.
- In this case, there is history of prior excisional biopsy, however; in addition, noted are several groups of indeterminate calcifications which, on additional magnification views, are "amorphous" and suspicious, and stereotactic biopsy was performed showing the presence of DCIS.

Suggested Reading

D'Orsi CJ, Bassett LW, Berg WA, et al. *Breast Imaging Reporting and Data System: ACR BI-RADS Mammography.* 4th ed. Reston, VA: American College of Radiology; 2003.

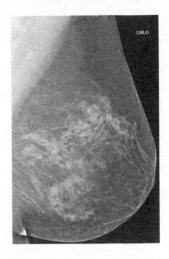
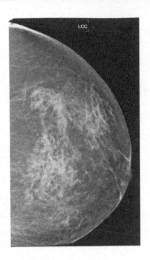
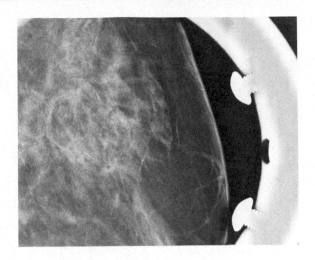

1. What BI-RADS classification should be used here?

2. What should be the next diagnostic imaging exam?

3. What are the causes of fat necrosis?

4. What calcification descriptor would you use in this case?

5. What type of biopsy would you recommend?

Case ranking/difficulty: **Category:** Diagnostic

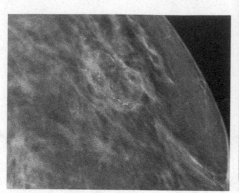

Left CC spot magnification view.

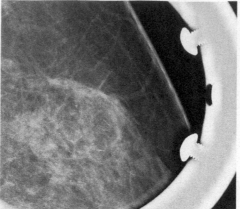

Left ML spot magnification view.

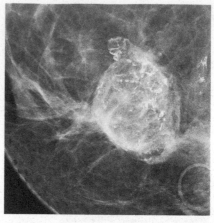

Different patient, similar mass but with much more calcifications.

Answers

1. These calcifications are mainly denser, rod like, and seen in orthogonal planes to lie around the periphery of the fat density mass. Fat density masses are characteristically benign. The appropriate assessment is therefore BI-RADS 2.

2. As there is calcification present, spot magnification views should be performed to characterize the calcific particles. Tomosynthesis may visualize an associated mass better. Ultrasound can be characteristic, with cystic changes and hyper-echogenicity. It can, however, be suspicious when there is calcification in the inflammatory wall of the necrosis. Non–fat-saturation MRI sequence would help to distinguish, if any remaining doubt.

3. Most of the above points may be a cause of fat necrosis. It is a response to injury, whether minor, as in grandchildren or pets climbing on to chest, or to a reaction to surgery and radiation treatment (can be marked in patients having intraoperative brachytherapy. Plastic surgery is a potent cause of fat necrosis.

4. Use of the "linear calcifications" descriptor is a suspicious term that you would use if you chose to biopsy this lesion. If this is stable and characteristically benign, then you should use a low-risk descriptor such as "curvilinear."

5. This patient has a palpable finding, and if you were concerned about the calcifications, stereotactic core biopsy could be performed. However, the calcifications are associated with the periphery of the fat necrosis mass, and therefore performing an ultrasound core biopsy of the margin of the mass and performing a specimen x-ray could be just as diagnostic.

Pearls

- Calcifications in fat necrosis start as fine or lacework like, and usually end up as classical dystrophic calcifications.
- In a patient with prior lumpectomy for DCIS, this may be a suspicious finding, prompting biopsy.

Suggested Readings

Bilgen IG, Ustun EE, Memis A. Fat necrosis of the breast: clinical, mammographic and sonographic features. *Eur J Radiol.* 2001;39(2):92-99.

DiPiro PJ, Meyer JE, Frenna TH, Denison CM. Seat belt injuries of the breast: findings on mammography and sonography. *AJR Am J Roentgenol.* 1995;164(2):317-320.

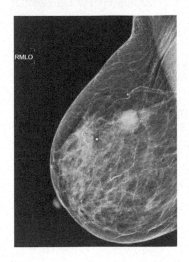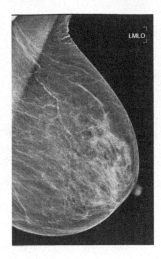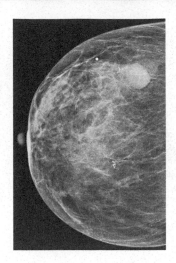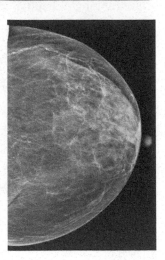

1. What BI-RADS classification should be used here?

2. What should be the next diagnostic imaging exam?

3. What is the likely pathology of a circumscribed mass?

4. What type of biopsy would you recommend?

5. If this is a malignancy, what would you expect to see on ultrasound?

Case ranking/difficulty:

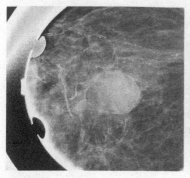

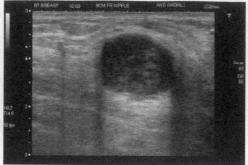

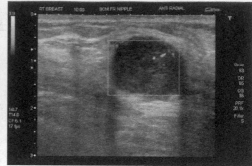

Right CC spot magnification views.   Targeted ultrasound.

Doppler ultrasound of mass.

Answers

1. In this context, this lesion does not fulfill the criteria for a benign mass; therefore, it should be treated with suspicion. See ultrasound images on page 2.

2. Tomosynthesis may not add anything extra in this lesion, but, in general, it is said to be equal to regular diagnostic projections for analyzing the margins of the mass. Ultrasound is the next most important exam to determine the nature of the lesion, and in this type of case, some would go directly to ultrasound from conventional mammography. MRI is not likely to add additional useful information. Core biopsy should not be performed before the diagnostic workup is complete.

3. In older patients who still have cysts, they may have stuck around for decades, and contain proteinaceous debris, such that there will never be a simple cyst, and likely to have appearances of a complicated cyst. *Note*: the term complex cyst was dropped in 2003 with the 4th edition of *BI-RADS*, as it was confusing. In the elderly and in the young, a malignancy may grow with circumscribed margins.

4. Ultrasound-guided core biopsy is appropriate here, as it is easy to find, cheap, and quick to perform. If the lesion was isoechoic and not easily visible, then stereotactic core biopsy would be appropriate.

5. The mass usually has some internal echoes (which may be difficult to appreciate if the patient has a mucus-secreting tumor). Vascularity within a mass is a suspicious ultrasound finding. The echo pattern is usually mixed echo (or heterogeneous) pattern.

Pearls

- "Circumscribed mass" can still be found in malignancies. Particularly,
  - Triple-negative cancers
  - Mucoid carcinomas
  - Colloid

Suggested Readings

Boisserie-Lacroix M, Mac Grogan G, Debled M, et al. Radiological features of triple-negative breast cancers (73 cases). *Diagn Interv Imaging*. 2012;93(3):183-190.

Gwak YJ, Kim HJ, Kwak JY, et al. Ultrasonographic detection and characterization of asymptomatic ductal carcinoma in situ with histopathologic correlation. *Acta Radiol*. 2011;52(4):364-371.

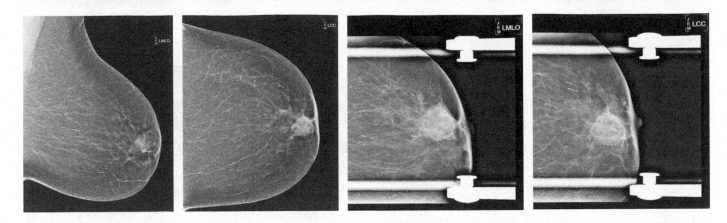

1. What is the best descriptor explaining the palpable abnormality?

2. What is the most likely reason for the palpable lump?

3. What are other typical findings of fat necrosis on mammography?

4. What are the features of fat necrosis on ultrasound?

5. What is an appropriate final assessment?

Case ranking/difficulty:

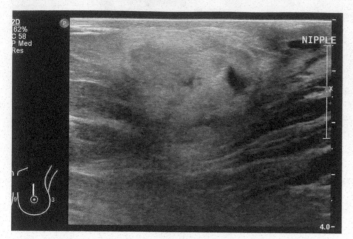

Diagnostic ultrasound demonstrates corresponding "complex mass" with mixed echogenicity and posterior shadowing.

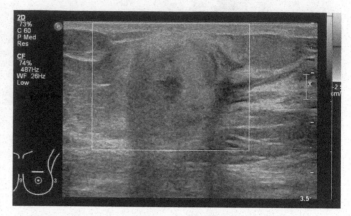

Diagnostic ultrasound demonstrates corresponding "complex mass" without increased flow on duplex.

Answers

1. Finding is consistent with round mass with "heterogeneous" density. It includes areas of low, fat-like density.

2. Given the history of recent infection, the finding most likely represents fat necrosis. The mammogram finding does correlate to fat necrosis given its heterogeneous density including areas of low fat density.

3. Fat necrosis can present in many different forms. Some findings are specific and can be classified as BI-RADS 2: benign, for example, fat-containing oil cysts, curvilinear calcifications associated with radiolucent mass. Some findings are more indeterminate such as "coarse" calcifications. Some findings cannot be differentiated from malignancy, and biopsy cannot be avoided, for example, in case of "spiculated" mass.

4. Fat necrosis again can show up in many different forms. Well-circumscribed mass may be classified as BI-RADS 2 or BI-RADS 3, while heterogeneous mass or ill-defined masses are unspecific and malignancy is difficult to exclude.

5. Given the presence of new palpable mass after infection, appropriate assessment is BI-RADS 3 (probably benign) and 6-month follow-up with mammogram.

Pearls

- Given the history of previous infection, which was treated with antibiotics, and the presence of a mass, which contains fat, the diagnosis of fat necrosis is most likely.

- Ultrasound does not help in regard to fat necrosis because it shows most likely a complex indeterminate mass.

- In this particular case, the finding was called BI-RADS 3 ("most likely" benign) and 6-month follow-up mammogram was recommended.

Suggested Reading

Taboada JL, Stephens TW, Krishnamurthy S, Brandt KR, Whitman GJ. The many faces of fat necrosis in the breast. *AJR Am J Roentgenol.* 2009;192(3):815-825.

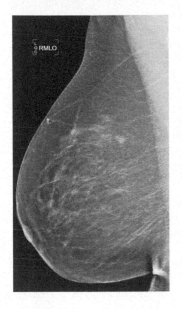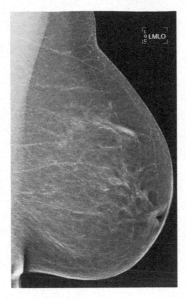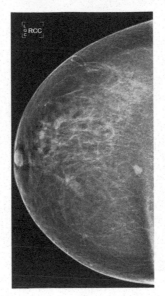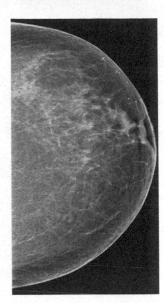

1. What is the correct BI-RADS classification in this case?

2. What is the next imaging test?

3. What are the features of a mass that distinguish a lymph node from another mass on mammography?

4. What are the features of a normal lymph node on ultrasound?

5. What ultrasound features are considered suspicious?

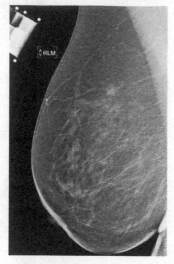

Right mediolateral.

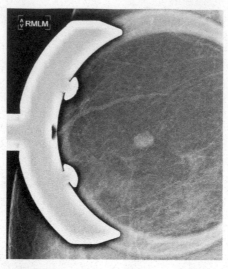

Right ML spot magnification.

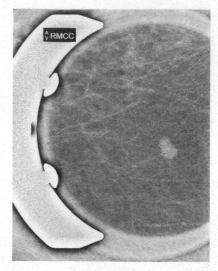

Right CC spot magnification shows "irregular" mass.

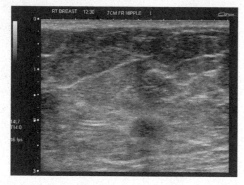

Targeted ultrasound.

be enlarged and therefore reactive following a diagnostic biopsy.

5. According to BI-RADS ultrasound, an "irregular mass" with "angular" or "microlobulated" margins are the descriptors of a suspicious lesion which should be biopsied. The "narrow zone of transition" is the opposite of the suspicious finding of a bright echogenic margin to a mass. The "parallel" orientation is the opposite of a taller-than-wide (or "non-parallel") mass that would be a suspicious finding.

Answers

1. This patient is a screening patient with a normal physical examination. The finding should therefore be given a BI-RADS 0 and further views plus ultrasound scanning recommended.

2. If you have tomosynthesis, then that test will replace the need for multiple examinations to determine the margins of the mass. Ultrasound will be required to determine the likely nature of the mass. There is no indication for an MRI at this stage.

3. The only features that help you make a diagnosis of lymph node from other type of mass is the presence of a hilum, either as a fatty lucency within the mass or as a radiological notch. Those are the pathognomonic features of a node. Supporting features include the typical position for an intramammary lymph node.

4. A vascular hilum and a thin smooth cortex are the features of a lymph node. Remember that the node can

Pearls

- Intramammary lymph nodes can occur in ectopic positions within the breast, not just in the axillary tail.
- The presence of a hilum/notch helps to clinch the diagnosis.

Suggested Readings

Hogan BV, Peter MB, Shenoy H, Horgan K, Shaaban A. Intramammary lymph node metastasis predicts poorer survival in breast cancer patients. *Surg Oncol.* 2010;19(1):11-16.

Pugliese MS, Stempel MM, Cody HS, Morrow M, Gemignani ML. Surgical management of the axilla: do intramammary nodes matter? *Am J Surg.* 2009;198(4):532-537.

Vijan SS, Hamilton S, Chen B, Reynolds C, Boughey JC, Degnim AC. Intramammary lymph nodes: patterns of discovery and clinical significance. *Surgery.* 2009;145(5):495-499.

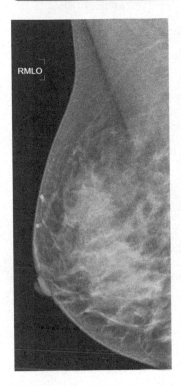 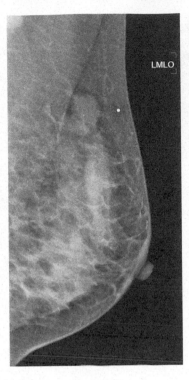 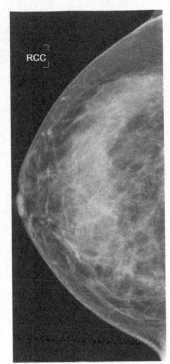 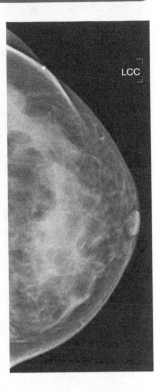

1. What BI-RADS classification should be used here?

2. What is the most likely pathology based on the imaging?

3. What mammographic views should you perform with these findings?

4. If you find abnormal nodes in the axilla, below the axillary vein, what levels are involved?

5. As a node is present, what staging tests would you perform?

Case ranking/difficulty:

Category: Diagnostic

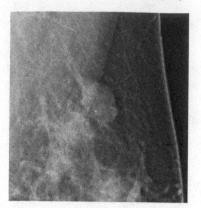

Left ML spot magnification view—in this plane, the masses are not easily seen.

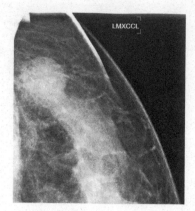

LXCCL spot magnification shows the lateral mass at the edge of the breast disc.

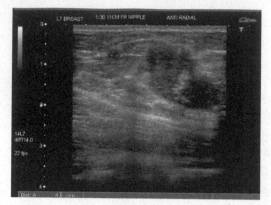

Left breast ultrasound shows not only the main lesion as an irregular mass containing calcification but also a second mass separate from the main mass consistent with a satellite lesion.

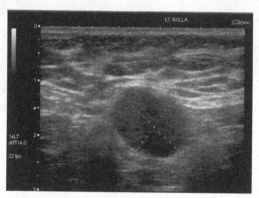

Left axillary ultrasound—here the enlarged solid node seen on mammography is demonstrated. Core biopsy confirmed metastatic adenocarcinoma.

Answers

1. BI-RADS 4 or 5 can be used here. The combination of features of an "irregular mass" containing highly suspicious microcalcification plus an abnormal lymph node allows BI-RADS 5 to be used.

2. The most common pathology with these findings is a high-grade IDC plus DCIS.

3. A lateral view is helpful for localization. However, the tumor is in the axillary tail in this instance, and if the mammo tech cannot get posterior enough, the tumor may not be visualized. An XCCL is helpful to determine the lateral extent of the disease. Spot magnification views are probably the best, as you get the maximum resolution to assess the margins of the mass, and to characterize the calcific particles. The Eklund technique is used to visualize breast tissue in front of the implants, known as the implant displaced view.

4. There is no such thing as level 0 or 4. Level 3 refers to disease superior to the boundary formed by the axillary vein. Levels 1 and 2 refer to the levels below the axillary vein.

5. Ultrasound staging of the locoregional nodes is important when you see a suspected malignancy with possible nodes on a mammogram. If the lesion is large, or is more likely to drain medially due to a central or medial position, then scanning longitudinally immediately alongside the sternum may identify involved internal mammary lymph nodes.

Pearls

- IDC with DCIS is usually high nuclear grade, and therefore more likely to metastasize.
- A focal asymmetry or mass associated with DCIS has a 50% risk of invasive cancer, and is a good target for biopsy, giving a higher yield of invasive disease.
- Watch for enlarged nodes on the mammogram, and consider adding axillary ultrasound staging to your routine ultrasound exam when you suspect a cancer.

Suggested Readings

Iakovlev VV, Arneson NC, Wong V, et al. Genomic differences between pure ductal carcinoma in situ of the breast and that associated with invasive disease: a calibrated aCGH study. *Clin Cancer Res.* 2008;14(14):4446-4454.

Meyerson AF, Lessing JN, Itakura K, et al. Outcome of long term active surveillance for estrogen receptor-positive ductal carcinoma in situ. *Breast.* 2011;20(6):529-533.

Diagnostic workup of group of indeterminate calcifications

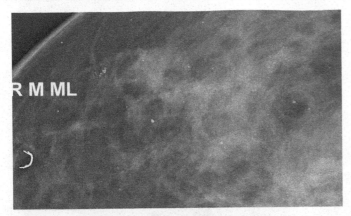
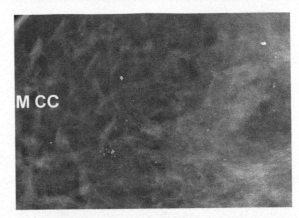
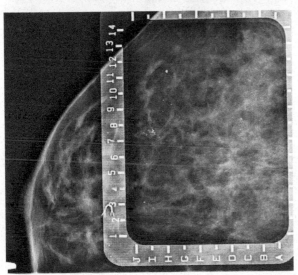
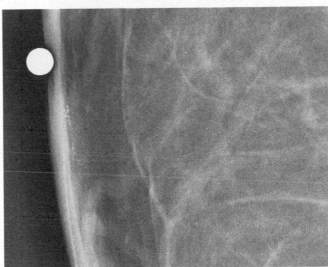

1. What is the best descriptor of this new group of calcification?

2. Why could that group of new calcifications be benign?

3. What is the next step after the standard ML and CC magnification view?

4. What is the appropriate technique to obtain tangential view?

5. What is the final assessment based on the tangential view?

Case ranking/difficulty: 🍂🍂

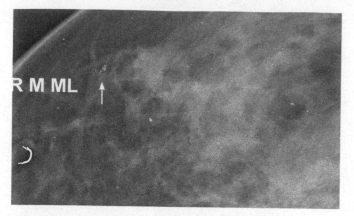

Diagnostic mammogram, right ML magnification view demonstrating group of indeterminate calcifications.

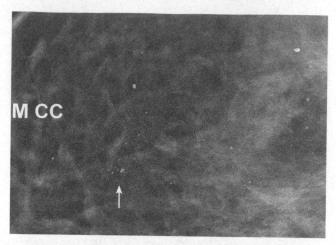

Diagnostic mammogram, right CC magnification view demonstrating group of indeterminate calcifications.

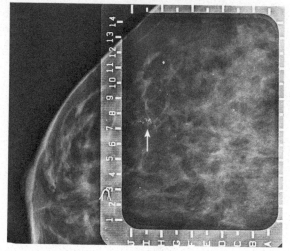

Diagnostic mammogram, right CC magnification view with grid demonstrating the group of indeterminate calcifications at the coordinates I—7.5.

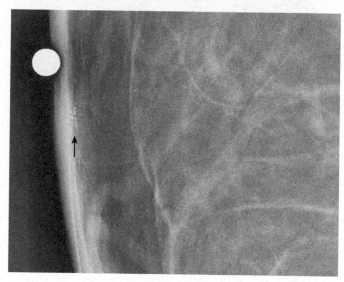

Diagnostic mammogram, tangential view with BB, demonstrates group of calcifications within the skin.

Answers

1. This is a group of "round and oval" calcifications, one or two of the calcifications demonstrate "lucent center."

2. Because one or two of the calcifications appear to have lucent center suspects that this could be skin calcifications.

3. Based on the standard ML and CC magnification views, the group of calcifications needs to be further worked up by obtaining a tangential view to prove their location within the skin.

4. The appropriate way is to have a paddle with grid to place a BB on the group of calcifications. An alternative could be to place the patient on the stereotactic biopsy table and place the BB. Next step is to obtain magnification view in second plane tangential to the BB—and thus tangential to the calcifications.

Stereotactic biopsy unit could also be used to calculate the Z value, which, in case of the presence of skin calcifications, had to be very small.

5. Calcifications are in the skin—BI-RADS 2 "benign" recommend patient to return for next screening mammogram in 1 year.

Pearls

- The appropriate workup of suspected skin calcifications requires to obtain tangential view with BB on the calcifications to prove if the group is close to the BB and therefore within the skin.

- If the presence of skin calcifications can be confirmed, the assessment is "benign" (BI-RADS 2) and the patient can return for next mammogram in 1 year.
- To obtain a tangential view, it is crucial to have a paddle with a grid, which in general is used to perform needle localizations. The same paddle can be used for the tangential view by putting a BB on the group of calcifications as seen within the grid—then, a second, tangential view can be obtained.
- An alternative to prove the presence of skin calcifications is to put the patient on the stereotactic biopsy table and prove that the calculated Z value is so small that the target has to be in the skin.

Suggested Readings

Berkowith JE, Gatewood OM, Donovan GB, et al. Dermal breast calcifications: localization with template-guided placement of skin marker. *Radiology.* 1987;163(1):282.

Linden SS, Sullivan DC. Breast skin calcifications: localization with a stereotactic device. *Radiology.* 1989;171(2):570-571.

Palpable finding in the right breast

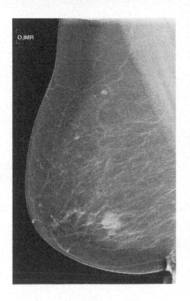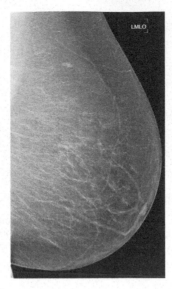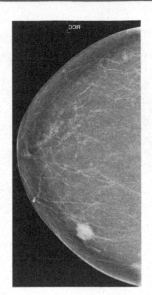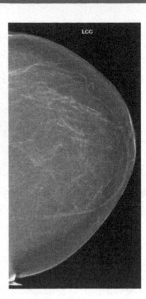

1. What BI-RADS classification should be used here?

2. What is the most likely pathology based on the imaging?

3. What is the next best imaging test?

4. What is the relevance of calcifications suspicious for DCIS outside of the tumor?

5. Do you have any recommendations for follow-up, other than normal mammography?

Case ranking/difficulty:

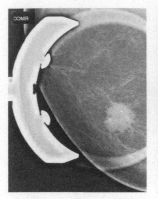

Right CC spot magnification view shows microcalcifications both within the tumor and outside extending anteriorly toward the nipple.

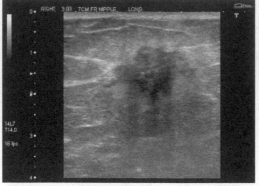

Ultrasound shows "irregular mass" with "angular margins," containing reflective echoes consistent with microcalcifications.

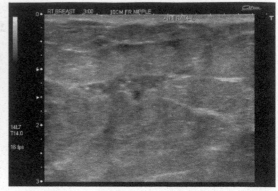

Ultrasound—another area closer to the nipple shows a "dilated duct" containing microcalcifications.

Answers

1. BI-RADS 4 or 5 can be given depending on your certainty. It is extremely unlikely to be a benign finding, so a BI-RADS 5 may be the best fit. This is not a screening exam; therefore, BI-RADS 0 should not be used. If it was a screening exam, then a BI-RADS 0 would be appropriate, along with recommendations for a diagnostic workup to include spot magnification views and targeted ultrasound.

2. DCIS masses can look like this, but are more likely to be noncalcified and circumscribed. Invasive lobular cancer can present like this, but it is extremely rare. This is much more of a typical situation where there is both DCIS and invasive cancer.

3. Ultrasound should be the first test to validate the presence of a mass, which can then be used to target for biopsy. For extent of DCIS, MRI is the best test, but expensive, and may over-estimate the disease, as it is often associated with proliferative change, especially in pre-menopausal women. There is currently no evidence that preoperative MRI improves the eventual outcome of the patient, but it may be helpful to map the disease for the surgeons.

4. DCIS is commonly found within tumors, but when seen outside it takes on a serious connotation. The disease outside of the index cancer is known as extensive intraductal component (EIC). This needs measuring and the distance from the primary tumor noting on the report. It has a significant impact on the local recurrence rate, even with a boost during radiation therapy. Some patients have a mastectomy to reduce this chance of recurrent disease.

5. Recurrent disease is likely to involve calcifications; therefore, ensure that all calcifications have been adequately removed at surgery. Some centers perform spot magnification views prior to radiation treatment to ensure there is no residual DCIS.

Pearls

- Calcifications outside a tumor are just as important to document.
- Extent of associated DCIS is best visualized by MRI.
- EIC has implications for the management of patients who are not able to have therapy with Intrabeam (intraoperative radiation treatment).
- May require completion mastectomy when found at surgery.

Suggested Readings

Schouten van der Velden AP, Boetes C, Bult P, Wobbes T. Magnetic resonance imaging in size assessment of invasive breast carcinoma with an extensive intraductal component. *BMC Med Imaging*. 2009;9(9):5.

Van Goethem M, Schelfout K, Kersschot E, et al. MR mammography is useful in the preoperative locoregional staging of breast carcinomas with extensive intraductal component. *Eur J Radiol*. 2007;62(2):273-282.

Yiu CC, Loo WT, Lam CK, Chow LW. Presence of extensive intraductal component in patients undergoing breast conservative surgery predicts presence of residual disease in subsequent completion mastectomy. *Chin Med J (Engl)*. 2009;122(8):900-905.

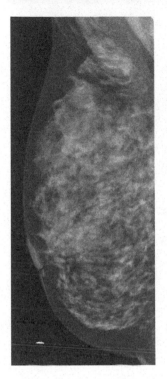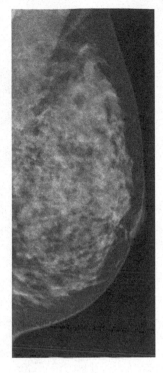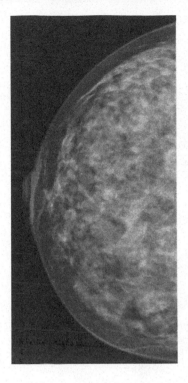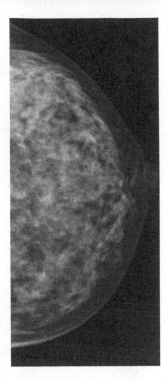

1. What could be the next step after a normal diagnostic mammogram in a high-risk patient?

2. If spot compression views and ultrasound are negative, what is the next step?

3. What is the appropriate scenario to order problem-solving MRI?

4. What is the finding of the breast MRI?

5. What is the consequence and next step after the MRI?

Case ranking/difficulty:

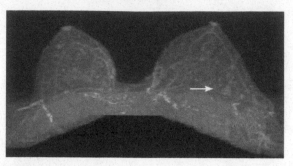

MRI post contrast Maximum Intensity Projection (MIP) demonstrates a small area of suspicious enhancement within the posterior left breast.

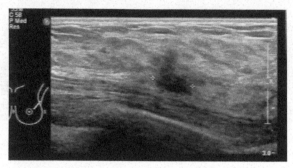

Second look gray-scale ultrasound image demonstrating corresponding "angular" mass.

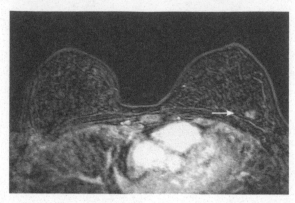

MRI after IV contrast with subtraction technique demonstrates focal area of enhancement left lateral posterior breast.

4. Noted is a mass in the left posterior superior breast, about 7 mm in diameter.

5. Since the lesion is very far back in the left breast near the chest wall, second look ultrasound is recommended as next step. MRI-guided biopsy would be technically very difficult, if not impossible. If ultrasound does not show corresponding lesion, MRI-guided biopsy or at least needle localization or marking of the lesion with clip is recommended to guide surgical excision.

Answers

1. Ultrasound, in general, would be the next step directed to the area of pain felt by the patient. However, if patient has a high-risk background, MRI as a problem-solving modality can also be considered.

2. This is a common scenario that patient feels a lump, or has some pain, and mammogram or ultrasound is unremarkable. It is not unreasonable to send patient with BI-RADS 1 (negative) assessment back to the referring physician and add a statement that "further assessment of the pain/lump should be based on clinical grounds." That basically means that if the pain/mass is highly suspicious to the clinician, it might still be necessary for the clinician to perform a non image guided biopsy based on palpation. MRI is also an option but should be used wisely. It cannot be used in every patient in that scenario.

3. Problem-solving MRI can be helpful but should be used wisely. In particular, it should not be used to characterize a lesion based on ultrasound, and/or mammographic morphological criterion is suspicious and needs biopsy. That means it would need biopsy, regardless of the finding on MRI. In this particular case, MRI was helpful, since it is a symptomatic high-risk patient with very dense tissue, and indeed abnormality was found.

Pearls

- This is a situation where MRI can be used as an additional "problem-solving" modality in patients with diffuse pain in the left breast and where mammogram is unremarkable.
- Despite initially normal targeted ultrasound, MRI did show, in this case, the presence of small suspicious lesion.
- Repeat second look ultrasound was performed and did show corresponding suspicious finding and ultrasound-guided biopsy confirms the presence of invasive ductal carcinoma.

Suggested Readings

Abe H, Schmidt RA, Shah RN, et al. MR-directed ("Second-Look") ultrasound examination for breast lesions detected initially on MRI: MR and sonographic findings. *AJR Am J Roentgenol.* 2010;194(2):370-377.

Moy L, Elias K, Patel V, et al. Is breast MRI helpful in the evaluation of inconclusive mammographic findings? *AJR Am J Roentgenol.* 2009;193(4):986-993.

Yau EJ, Gutierrez RL, DeMartini WB, Eby PR, Peacock S, Lehman CD. The utility of breast MRI as a problem-solving tool. *Breast J.* 2011;17(3):273-280.

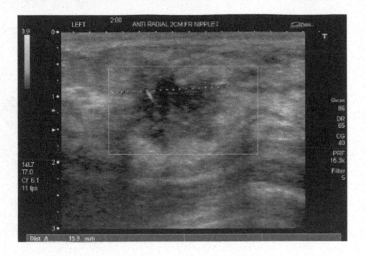 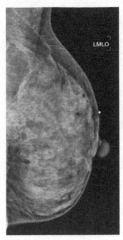 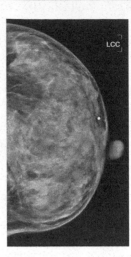

1. What BI-RADS classification should be used here?

2. In a lactating woman, what is the differential diagnosis?

3. If this patient was presenting to you for the first time, which imaging modality is your first choice?

4. What BI-RADS descriptors would you apply to this lesion?

5. What is the best staging test for this patient?

Case ranking/difficulty:

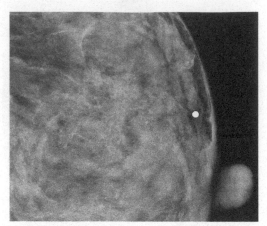

LCC spot magnification—minimal change seen. There is some distortion, but the mass is completely invisible because of lack of contrast. Some microcalcifications are also seen.

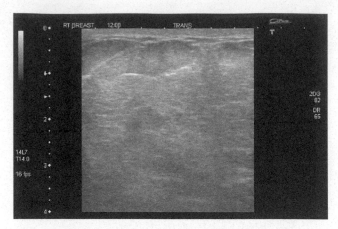

Another lactating patient showing what normal breast tissue can look like when lactating. Note the relatively bright glandular tissue with few features.

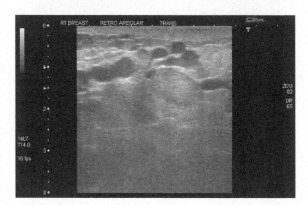

Another lactating patient showing prominent dilated milk filled ducts.

Answers

1. BI-RADS 4 or 5 can be used here based on the highly suspicious ultrasound. The mammogram is not particularly helpful, except from excluding associated DCIS microcalcifications.

2. All of the above are correct, as they can all present with a noncalcified mass in a lactating woman.

3. A nonionizing examination is the modality of choice in a young woman. This can be challenging in a woman who is lactating, but less so than in a pregnant patient, prepartum. If you see a suspicious abnormality, then mammography is warranted, as high-grade IDC can present first with microcalcifications in otherwise dense breasts. MRI can be reserved for challenging cases or for staging.

4. This is a suspicious lesion and suspicious BI-RADS descriptors should be used such as "irregular mass" and "angulated margins." It is taller than it is wide, which BI-RADS describes as "nonparallel" contrary to a benign lesion that is "parallel" to the skin.

5. MRI is the best (nonionizing radiation) exam. It may have decreased sensitivity because of the hormonal change related to postpartum. PEM and BSGI could be used to detect more than one lesion in the breast, but there is currently a significant radiation dose from the isotope used. PET/CT can be used if the lesion is large and there is evidence on nodal spread.

Pearls

• Palpable masses should always be taken seriously and explained, especially during pregnancy and lactation, even though the pretest probability for malignancy is low.

Suggested Readings

Espinosa LA, Daniel BL, Vidarsson L, Zakhour M, Ikeda DM, Herfkens RJ. The lactating breast: contrast-enhanced MR imaging of normal tissue and cancer. *Radiology*. 2005;237(2):429-436.

Sabate JM, Clotet M, Torrubia S, et al. Radiologic evaluation of breast disorders related to pregnancy and lactation. *Radiographics*. 2007;27(Suppl 1):S101-S124.

Saglam A, Can B. Coexistence of lactating adenoma and invasive ductal adenocarcinoma of the breast in a pregnant woman. *J Clin Pathol*. 2005;58(1):87-89.

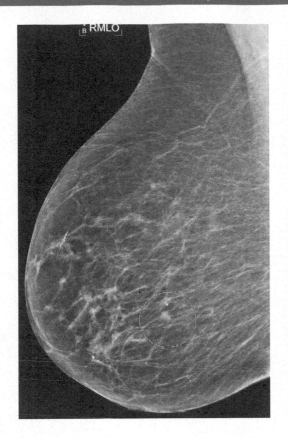 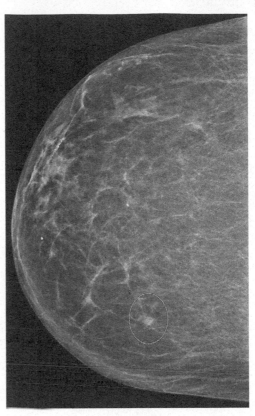

1. What is the next step?

2. What is the appropriate BI-RADS classification?

3. What is the appropriate description of the mammogram abnormality?

4. What is the differential diagnosis of this new mass based on mammogram?

5. If the finding is stable since several years on standard mammogram, what is the assessment?

Case ranking/difficulty:

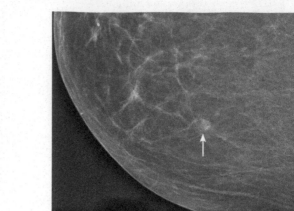

Diagnostic mammogram of right spot compression MLO view demonstrating small mass.

Diagnostic mammogram of right spot compression CC view demonstrating small mass.

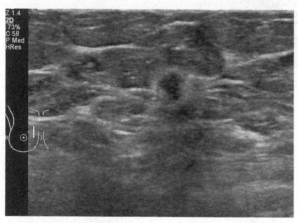

Gray-scale ultrasound demonstrating small corresponding "hypoechoic mass" with "irregular" shape with thick echogenic halo and "indistinct" margin.

Answers

1. Next step is diagnostic workup with spot compression views.

2. BI-RADS 0 incomplete exam—patient needs to be recalled.

3. This is a finding of a small mass with partially obscured margin and of equal density to the surrounding tissue and of "irregular" shape and "indistinct" margin.

4. The finding is indeterminate and could represent inflamed cyst, hematoma, or malignancy, which could include invasive ductal carcinoma, DCIS, and invasive lobular carcinoma.

5. If the finding is stable for more than 2 years on standard screening mammogram, it can be called BI-RADS 2. The finding is not specific and could also represent benign finding as discussed in question 4, for example, a complicated cyst. The presence of "irregular" shape and "indistinct" margin is not appreciated on standard views. In this particular case, the appearance on spot compression views and on the ultrasound makes a difference and raises concern.

Pearls

- The purpose of screening mammograms is to find abnormalities; however, detailed description should be spared for subsequent diagnostic mammogram that includes additional, more specific views, such as spot compression or magnification views.
- That is the reason why follow-up exams of "probably benign" findings should in general include the most specific images, such as spot compression or magnification views, since based on small changes in morphology, decision is made to further follow the finding or to biopsy the finding.

Suggested Reading

D'Orsi CJ, Bassett LW, Berg WA, et al. Breast Imaging Reporting and Data System: ACR BI-RADS–Mammography. 4th ed. Reston, VA: American College of Radiology; 2003.

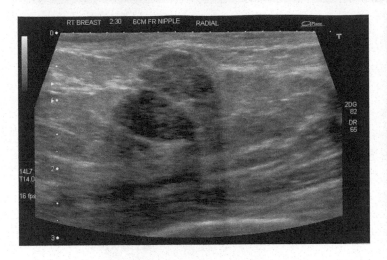
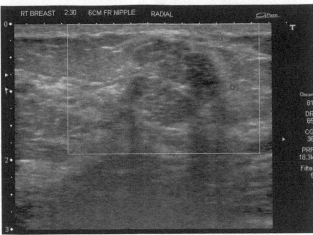

1. What BI-RADS classification should be used here?

2. What is the most likely pathology based on the imaging?

3. What is the next best imaging test?

4. What type of biopsy would you recommend?

5. If phyllodes tumor is found on biopsy, what is the appropriate management?

Case ranking/difficulty: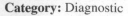

Category: Diagnostic

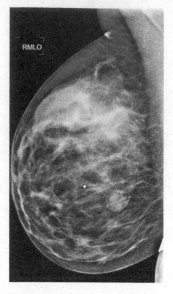

Right MLO.

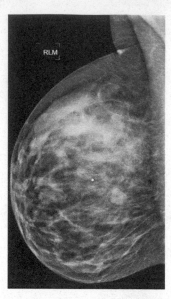

Right lateromedial exam. The mass was medial in the breast, so a LM exam is the preferred projection. "Lobulated circumscribed mass."

Answers

1. The ultrasound features are suspicious, in that it is an "irregular mass" with "microlobulated" margins, and a "heterogeneous echo pattern."

2. Strictly, all of the answers could be correct, as they all can appear with similar findings. The most likely finding in a 29-year-old woman is fibroadenoma or phyllodes tumor, and it is the concern about the latter that prompts biopsy.

3. All of the above have been performed before in this situation. MRI is expensive and likely to show an enhancing mass, which will not affect the outcome. Elastography may show some tissue stiffness, but in younger women, fibroadenomas often have a more cellular component and are therefore softer than fibroadenomas in older patients. In view of the suspicious imaging, biopsy needs to be performed. Mammography can be considered, especially with findings that are not definitely characteristic of a fibroadenoma.

4. If it is visible on ultrasound, then the best way to do is a biopsy. If the lesion is palpable, some surgeons may prefer to do the biopsy themselves, but ultrasound should be used to confirm that the biopsy is sampling the right parts of the mass.

5. Phyllodes tumors need to be excised with a good margin, as they have a high chance of local recurrence but do not metastasize. Fibroepithelial lesions are a type of fibroadenoma variant that has been recognized, which needs surgical excision, to ensure that the mass has been adequately sampled.

Pearls

• The most suspicious imaging modality usually trumps the least suspicious. This is not always the case; for example, a partially obscured mass on mammography may be an obvious simple cyst on ultrasound. A lesion that does not appear as a classical fibroadenoma should be regarded as suspicious and biopsy confirmed due to the risk of phyllodes tumor.

Suggested Readings

Chung A, Scharre K, Wilson M. Intraductal fibroadenomatosis: an unusual variant of fibroadenoma. *Breast J*. 2008;14(2):193-195.

Sklair-Levy M, Sella T, Alweiss T, Craciun I, Libson E, Mally B. Incidence and management of complex fibroadenomas. *AJR Am J Roentgenol*. 2008;190(1):214-218.

Thein KY, Trishna SR, Reynolds V. Benign and malignant breast lesions mimicking each other: imaging-histopathologic correlation. *Cancer Imaging*. 2011;11(Spec No A):S180.

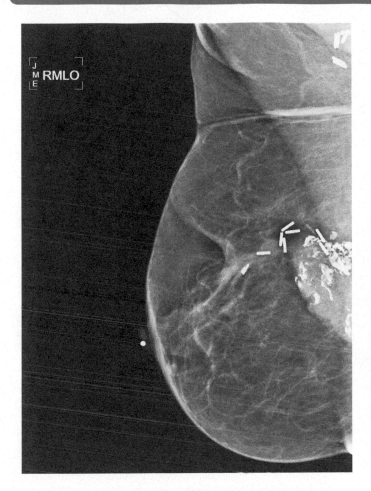
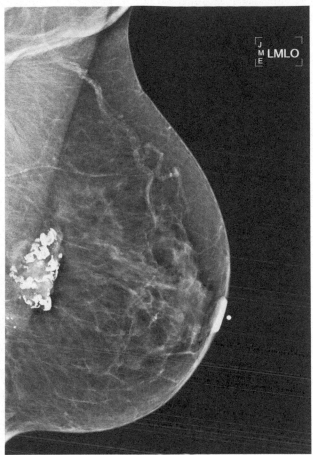

1. What BI-RADS classification should be used here?

2. What is the most likely pathology based on the imaging?

3. What type of implant causes calcified capsules?

4. What is the best examination for looking at implant integrity?

5. What is the name used for an intracapsular rupture of an implant on MRI?

Case ranking/difficulty:

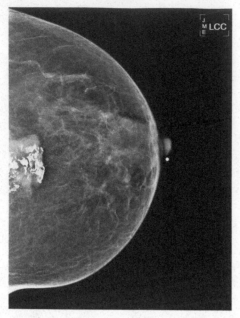

Right CC.

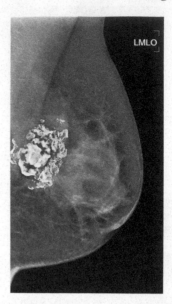

Another case—left MLO shows almost identical features. The calcification is coarse and "popcorn" like, but very extensive in the retro-pectoral space.

Answers

1. Whether screening or diagnostic, these findings are characteristically benign and therefore BI-RADS 2.

2. These are the appearances of collapsed calcified implant capsules following explantation of silicone pre-pectoral implants. Fat grafting gives changes similar to either lipomas or to fat necrosis, depending on how the body responds to the treatment. Injected silicone looks very dense and different to this type of density. Guinea worms look like irregular coils of calcium. Found when an adult dracunculus parasite dies, it is usually small in caliber, but can occasionally be very large. They do not tend to be seen bilaterally or symmetrically.

3. There is some evidence for calcified capsule formation with saline implants, but this is rare. Silicone leaking across the implant causes an intense inflammatory reaction, which is prone to calcifying. Capsular calcification is normally seen in the pre-pectoral type of implant, normally from a cosmetic surgery in the past. Saline implants are preferred for the retro-pectoral space, as they do not have any complications from rupture, unlike silicone gel. Trilucent implants were used in Europe for a time, before they were banned from use. They were relatively easy to see through, causing less obstruction of normal breast tissue.

4. MRI is the best exam for implant integrity, as you can see the whole of the implant and the capsule, as well as performing silicone dark and silicone bright sequences. Ultrasound is good for a palpable finding (usually on the anterior margin of the implant). Diagnostic mammograms can show complications of capsules, and contour abnormalities may suggest weakening of the implant wall, but is not the best test.

5. The term used is Linguine sign, of the collapsed inner capsule within the main capsule. Not to be confused with other delicious forms of Italian pasta.

Pearls

- The position of lesion and being bilateral and symmetrical gives you the diagnosis.
- Silicone implants, when they rupture, cause a marked inflammatory response, such that these calcified masses of the implant capsules may remain in the breast after surgical explantation.

Suggested Readings

Dershaw DD, Chaglassian TA. Mammography after prosthesis placement for augmentation or reconstructive mammoplasty. *Radiology*. 1989;170(1, Pt 1):69-74.

Peters W, Pritzker K, Smith D, et al. Capsular calcification associated with silicone breast implants: incidence, determinants, and characterization. *Ann Plast Surg*. 1998;41(4):348-360.

Peters W, Smith D, Fornasier V, Lugowski S, Ibanez D. An outcome analysis of 100 women after explantation of silicone gel breast implants. *Ann Plast Surg*. 1997;39(1): 9-19.

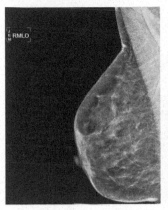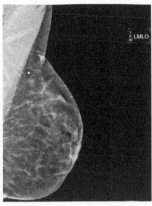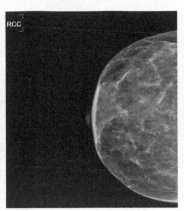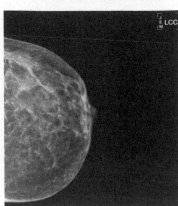

1. What is the first step of workup of palpable abnormality in a 73-year-old patient?

2. What would be the workup if patient had prior normal screening mammogram 7 months ago?

3. What would be the workup if there was a normal mammogram 3 months ago?

4. What is the most likely morphological appearance of low-grade DCIS?

5. What is the likelihood of the presence of malignancy in case of normal imaging despite the presence of palpable abnormality?

Case ranking/difficulty:

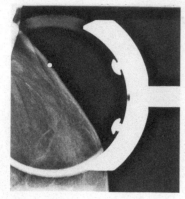

Spot compression left MLO view with BB marker on palpable abnormality demonstrating small mass.

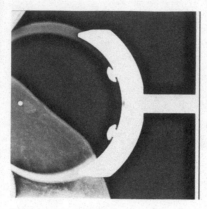

Spot compression left CC view with BB marker on palpable abnormality demonstrating small mass.

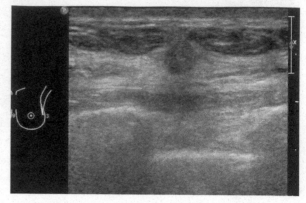

Gray-scale ultrasound image of palpable abnormality demonstrates small hypoechoic mass.

Answers

1. Workup of patients in that age group includes diagnostic mammogram with spot compression views with BB marker on the palpable finding and then ultrasound.

2. If patient had recent mammogram more than 6 months ago, in general, repeat mammogram is recommended. Remember, 6 months is the time frame used to follow BI-RADS 3 findings. There is no need to repeat mammogram at this point at the nonsymptomatic right side. This can be done when patient is due for next screening mammogram.

3. In general, if there is a normal mammogram available, performed less than 6 months ago, there is no need to repeat mammogram and it is not unreasonable to perform an ultrasound first. If the ultrasound is negative and the palpable abnormality is very questionable, it would be reasonable to stop here. However, this depends also on the confidence of the assessment of the last mammogram, performed less than 6 months ago. If breast parenchyma was very dense and therefore limits the assessment, it would not be unreasonable to repeat the mammogram, even if it was called BI-RADS 1 ("negative") less than 6 months ago. Remember at that time no spot compression views were obtained, since it was a screening mammogram.

4. In this case, a mass turned out to be low-grade DCIS, which is rather uncommon. In general, low-grade DCIS presents as a group of calcifications that are usually rather "amorphous" or "round and oval" and less likely "pleomorphic."

5. There are not many studies available looking at this issue. The study by Gumus et al. (2012) looked over a 12-year period of time at 251 patients with palpable abnormalities and normal imaging and found only

1.2% of the patients having malignancy (false-negative mammogram). However, the false-negative rate will also depend on the density of the breast parenchyma. It can be suspected that it will be even lower in "fatty replaced breast" versus in "extremely dense breast."

Pearls

- Any palpable abnormality is suspicious—the only finding that can be considered as definitely benign is a simple cyst.
- In this particular case, the finding is not a simple cyst and remains indeterminate and has even suspicious features such as "taller-than-wide" (Stavros) shape and the mass was subsequently biopsied under ultrasound guidance and did show the presence of low-grade DCIS.
- If there is no abnormality seen on imaging, including ultrasound, "further management of palpable abnormality should be based on clinical grounds" and the exam can be called "negative" BI-RADS 1 and patient can return to screening.
- In very rare situations, biopsy of palpable findings based on the palpation and without imaging guidance, performed by breast surgeon, can show malignancy.

Suggested Readings

DiPiro PJ, Meyer JE, Denison CM, Frenna TH, Harvey SC, Smith DN. Image-guided core breast biopsy of ductal carcinoma in situ presenting as a non-calcified abnormality. *Eur J Radiol.* 1999;30(3):231-236.

Gumus H, Gumus M, Mills P, et al. Clinically palpable breast abnormalities with normal imaging: is clinically guided biopsy still required? *Clin Radiol.* 2012;67(5):437-440.

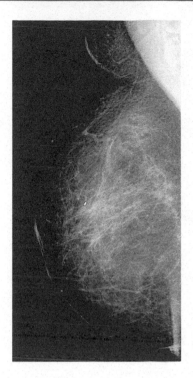 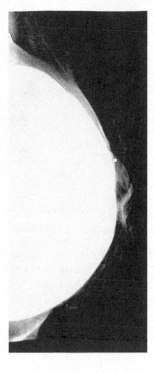 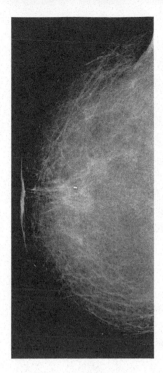 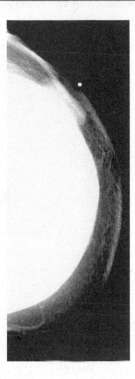

1. What BI-RADS classification should be used here?

2. Which is the best modality to assess implants?

3. Which is the best modality to assess a palpable finding associated with an implant?

4. What further tests do you recommend at this stage?

5. If a patient has an implant reconstruction as part of a mastectomy, what is the initial implant used?

Case ranking/difficulty: **Category:** Diagnostic

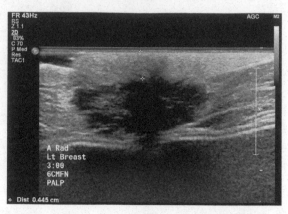

Ultrasound—relationship with implant and skin—technique using gentle pressure with standoff gel.

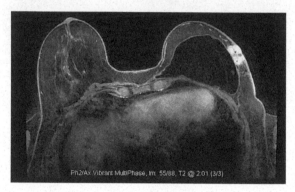

MRI—T1 postcontrast, unsubtracted exam.

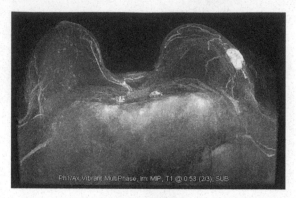

Subtracted MIP image in axial plane.

however, some centers have these tests as local protocol for any patient with a breast cancer recurrence. MRI is the most helpful initial test to determine the extent of the recurrence and check on skin coverage for surgical planning, which is usually a completion mastectomy in a patient who has had breast conservation. This patient, however, has already had a mastectomy with tissue expanders and followed by implant reconstruction.

5. The patient has a special type of implant inserted, which is a tissue expander. This type of implant has a saline bag and tubing with a valve, which is gradually expanded over a period of weeks to stretch the skin. Once the skin has reached the required volume, the expander is switched out for a conventional implant.

Answers

1. You can either use BI-RADS 4 straight off or wait until you have done the ultrasound and give a combined BI-RADS assessment. There is a vague density seen on the left ML, but best seen in this instance on the CC view. Implant-displaced views cannot be performed because there is no "breast tissue," as this implant was placed following a tissue expander.

2. MRI is the only modality that allows for full assessment of implants. Using silicone suppression sequences allows for distinguishing between cysts and silicone granulomas. MRI can see the posterior aspect of the implant, no accessible with ultrasound.

3. Ultrasound should be the first modality to use, as no ionizing radiation, and can be targeted easily, and correlated with the physical findings. MRI overall is the best modality for assessing implants themselves.

4. If there is no biochemical evidence of metastatic deposits, then PET or bone scans may not be needed;

Pearls

- Any new mass in a patient who has had a mastectomy and reconstruction for breast cancer should be treated expeditiously.
- High yield for breast cancer.
- If originally presented with a mass, a recurrence with a further mass is more common.

Suggested Readings

Destounis S, Morgan R, Arieno A, Seifert P, Somerville P, Murphy P. A review of breast imaging following mastectomy with or without reconstruction in an outpatient community center. *Breast Cancer*. 2011;18(4):259-267.

Patterson SG, Teller P, Iyengar R, et al. Locoregional recurrence after mastectomy with immediate transverse rectus abdominis myocutaneous (TRAM) flap reconstruction. *Ann Surg Oncol*. 2012;19(8):2679-2684.

Sim YT, Litherland JC. The use of imaging in patients post breast reconstruction. *Clin Radiol*. 2012;67(2):128-133.

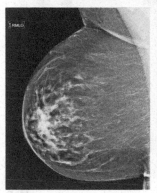
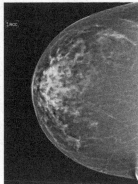
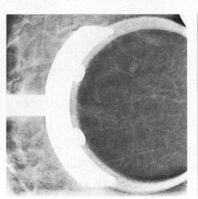
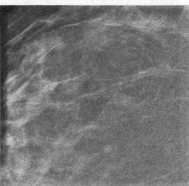

1. What is the difference between an asymmetry and a mass?

2. What is the workup of an asymmetry on a first screening mammogram?

3. If there is a finding on ultrasound—which correlates to the mammogram—what is the next step?

4. What is the next step in regard to the "focal asymmetry" if it is new?

5. What would be a way to correlate an ultrasound with a mammogram finding, if in doubt?

Case ranking/difficulty:

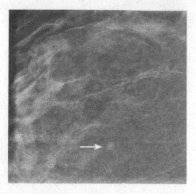

Mammogram of right spot compression CC view confirming small 3–4 mm mass on the right lateral breast.

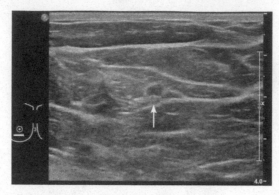

Ultrasound directed to the right breast demonstrating small hypoechoic mass of corresponding size in the central breast.

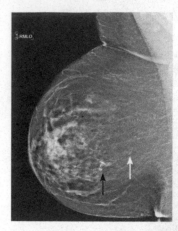

Diagnostic mammogram, right MLO view demonstrates iodine contrast (*black arrow*) and mass (*white arrow*).

Answers

1. BI-RADS differentiates between "mass" and "asymmetry." Mass is always seen in two projections and has a clear border and conspicuity which is visible on both projections. An asymmetry is sometimes seen only in one projection, but can be seen on two projections as well and is less defined. A "focal asymmetry" is differentiated from a larger "global asymmetry" by size alone. A global asymmetry can involve an entire quadrant and is in general more likely to represent normal tissue.

2. The patient needs to be recalled for a diagnostic work up including spot compression views CC and MLO. Then ultrasound should be performed. It is also important to confirm that there is no palpable abnormality in that area. In the absence of an underlying palpable abnormality, the finding can be followed in 6 months and classified as "probably benign" if ultrasound is normal.

3. The ultrasound finding has to be a simple cyst to justify calling this a benign finding and return the patient to screening. Any other finding should be biopsied, since this is a new mass on mammogram. An exception could be cluster of small cysts and follow-up in 6 months could be performed. However, if there is any doubt, biopsy would be preferred in case of a new mass on mammogram.

4. If the finding is a new asymmetry and has not any corresponding finding on ultrasound, it has to be biopsied or excised—BI-RADS 4 (suspicious). First step would be to attempt stereotactic biopsy. If finding is not visible on the stereotactic biopsy table, needle localization and subsequent surgical excision can be performed.

5. One way is to place a BB on the ultrasound finding and perform a tangential view to see if it correlates. Other methods would be to aspirate the finding, in case it is a

cyst, and repeat mammogram to see if the mammogram finding is gone. Other options could be to place a Homer needle (removable needle localization) and repeat mammogram, or to inject small trace of air or iodine contrast and repeat mammogram. This can be helpful if there are multiple small findings or if the findings are so small that cyst aspiration is technically difficult.

Pearls

- To correlate ultrasound finding to mammogram finding of small mass can be challenging, in particular if the mass is very small or because of the presence of multiple lesions.
- Correlation can be achieved by placing BB on the skin next to the ultrasound finding and repeat mammogram and even sometimes tangential views.
- Placement of a Homer needle can be used to mark the ultrasound finding and then perform mammogram.
- It might be sometimes helpful to inject small amount of air or iodine contrast (1-mL tuberculin syringe) adjacent to the ultrasound finding and then repeat mammogram for more definite correlation.
- If the ultrasound finding does not correlate to a new mass seen on mammogram, stereotactic biopsy is recommended.

Suggested Readings

Ellis RL. Sonographic confirmation of a mammographically detected breast lesion. *AJR Am J Roentgenol.* 2011;196(1):225-256.

Sickles EA. The spectrum of breast asymmetries: imaging features, work-up, management. *Radiol Clin North Am.* 2007;45(5):765-771, v.

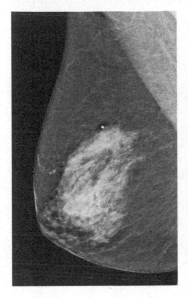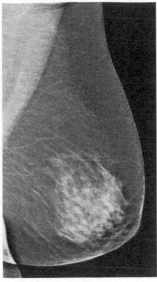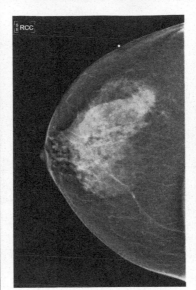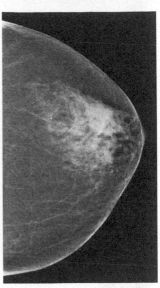

1. What BI-RADS classification should be used here?

2. What is the next imaging test?

3. If calcification is seen with this finding, what is the likely pathology?

4. This lesion is palpable. What type of biopsy should be performed?

5. Based on the imaging, what is the likely pathology on core biopsy?

Case ranking/difficulty:

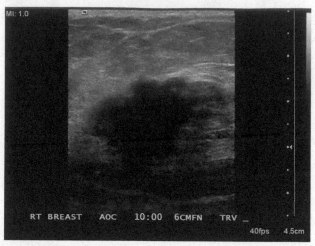

Ultrasound showing an "irregular" mass with "microlobulated" superior "margins."

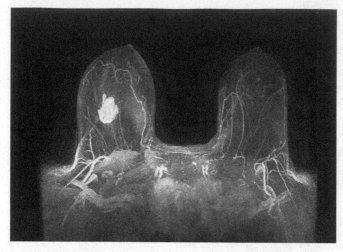

Axial subtracted MIP showing 4.3-cm solitary enhancing mass.

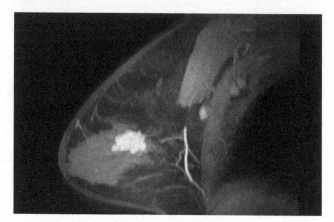

Right breast sagittal subtracted thin MIP.

Answers

1. Either BI-RADS 4 or 5 is a valid answer. Even though you are not supplied with spot or spot magnification views, you get the impression that this is quite a large lesion.

2. Ideally, you want to maximize the information you can get from mammography before proceeding to other tests. Lateral projection and spot or spot magnification films should be used to get a better idea of the extent of this lesion. If available, tomosynthesis may help to evaluate the mass margins. Ultrasound is the next examination when this is done. In some patients with very dense breasts, it is not possible to adequately measure the extent of disease, and MRI may be the more accurate modality.

3. In the setting of a "spiculate mass," there are several possibilities, which include benign conditions such as fat necrosis (where the calcification is usually easier to distinguish as appears dystrophic), radial scar, or complex sclerosing lesion, which can be associated with DCIS in 20%. Lobular cancer may be associated with amorphous calcifications. A classic "spiculate mass" with "fine linear pleomorphic" calcifications is usually a high-grade invasive ductal cancer with high-grade DCIS.

4. Although palpation guidance can be used, ultrasound guidance allows you to confirm that the needle passes through different areas of the mass, and gets the most representative samples of the tumor. If the lesion is not clearly seen on ultrasound, or there are confounding appearances on ultrasound, such that your confidence for sampling the mass accurately is low, then consider stereotactic core biopsy.

5. The appearances of a mass with distortion are more likely to be a feature of invasive ductal carcinoma. Invasive lobular cancer may present as a mass (better seen on the CC) but is more common as subtle distortion, a slowly shrinking breast, or even with no mammographic findings, but obvious palpation abnormalities or ultrasound changes.

Pearls

- Dense breasts represent a challenge to the reader.
- Tomosynthesis holds promise in this area.
- Look for disruption of normal lines/structures in the breast.
- Comparison with opposite side is important.

Suggested Reading

Huynh PT, Jarolimek AM, Daye S. The false-negative mammogram. *Radiographics*. 2006;18(5):1137-1154; quiz 1243-1244.

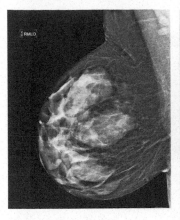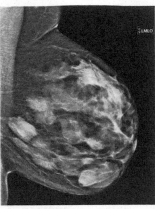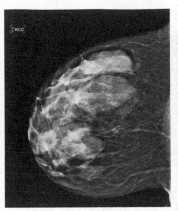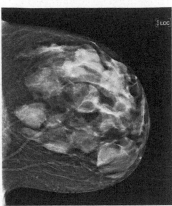

1. What are the findings on the screening mammogram?

2. What is the most likely etiology?

3. What is the next step after screening mammogram of asymptomatic patient?

4. What is the appropriate BI-RADS assessment?

5. What is the likelihood of malignancy in this case? (best answer)

Case ranking/difficulty: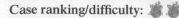

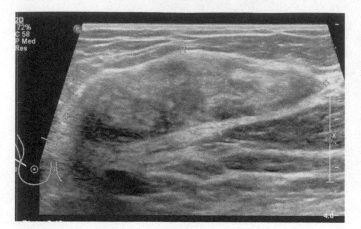

On B-mode ultrasound, there are scattered benign-appearing, well-circumscribed masses noted in the right breast.

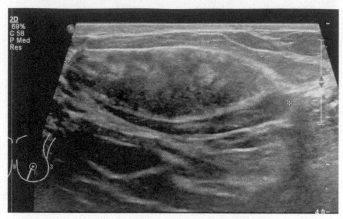

On B-mode ultrasound, there are scattered benign-appearing, well-circumscribed masses noted in the left breast.

Answers

1. Noted are bilateral scattered benign-appearing masses.

2. Most likely bilateral masses will be due to the presence of bilateral fibrocystic changes (cysts) or less likely due to bilateral fibroadenomas.

3. In general, there is no need for further workup, since it has been shown that the likelihood of malignancy is not higher than in normal screening population. In this particular case, the patient felt multiple lumps and therefore ultrasound was performed.

4. The appropriate classification is BI-RADS 2 (benign) and next screening exam is due in 1 year.

5. Among 1440 patients with bilateral scattered masses, only 2 interval cancers were found based on a study by Leung and Sickles (2000), which results in an incidence rate of malignancy of 0.14% that is lower than the age-matched ultrasound incident cancer rate of 0.24%.

Pearls

- In the absence of palpable abnormality, multiple benign-appearing masses on a screening mammogram can be classified as "benign" and there is no need for recall.
- Based on the study by Leung and Sickles (2000), the incidence of breast cancer in a mammogram with bilateral "benign"-appearing masses is not higher than in the absence of bilateral "benign masses" and there is no need for workup, unless there is significant change, new abnormal morphology, or new clinical symptoms.

Suggested Reading

Leung JW, Sickles EA. Multiple bilateral masses detected on screening mammography: assessment of need for recall imaging. *AJR Am J Roentgenol.* 2000;175(1):23-29.

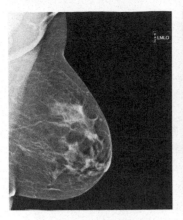 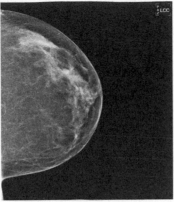 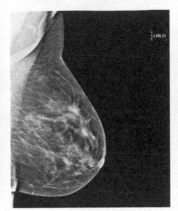 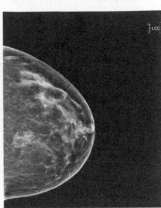

1. What is the pertinent finding?

2. What malignancy can present in that way?

3. Would MRI, in this case, help to eliminate biopsy?

4. Does it make a difference if there were no old images available?

5. Why is ultrasound necessary for workup in this case?

Case ranking/difficulty:

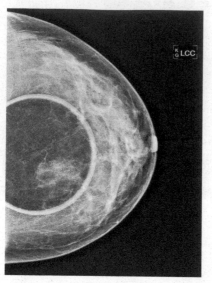

Diagnostic mammogram, left CC spot compression view, demonstrating "focal asymmetry."

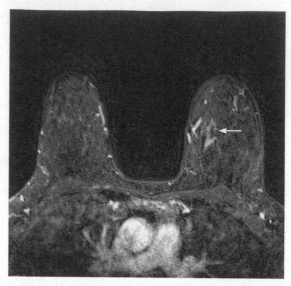

MRI, T1-weighted sequence after IV contrast with subtraction technique, demonstrating "non–mass-like" area of enhancement.

Answers

1. Noted is the development of subtle "focal asymmetry" in the left superior breast, posterior depth.

2. All malignancies can present as "focal asymmetry." Pseudoangiomatous stromal hyperplasia (PASH) is not a malignant lesion but can present as focal asymmetry.

3. In general, the negative predictive value of breast MRI is high, close to 100% but not exactly 100%. Therefore, the mainstream opinion is to biopsy any suspicious abnormality seen on mammogram—including developing "focal asymmetry." However, there is a recent shift and there are more publications suggesting that negative MRI might eliminate the need for biopsy. The article from Europe in 2011, for example, suggests that this is feasible.

4. If this was a "focal asymmetry" on a baseline mammogram, the workup would be the same. But if there was no underlying suspicious morphology, the finding could be classified as BI-RADS 3 and could be followed in 6 months, and again 6 months later and then 1 year later to have a monitoring period of 2 years in total.

5. In case of a new asymmetric density, it is necessary to determine if there is any corresponding abnormality that could be biopsied under ultrasound guidance. In case of an asymmetric density on a baseline mammogram, ultrasound is necessary to further exclude corresponding abnormality. If ultrasound is normal, it can be followed in 6 months.

Pearls

- Any developing density that persists on spot compression views is suspicious (BI-RADS 4), and despite of lack of ultrasound finding, stereotactic biopsy should be performed.
- In this case, MRI was performed before the biopsy. It demonstrates corresponding "non–mass-like" area of enhancement—subsequently performed stereotactic biopsy demonstrates findings consistent with PASH, which is concordant.
- If this patient had no prior screening study, the finding would be BI-RADS 3 based on the mammogram and negative ultrasound, and could be followed in 6 months.

Suggested Readings

Dorrius MD, Pijnappel RM, Sijens PE, van der Weide MC, Oudkerk M. The negative predictive value of breast magnetic resonance imaging in noncalcified BI-RADS 3 lesions. *Eur J Radiol.* 2012;81(2):209-213.

Leung JW, Sickles EA. Developing asymmetry identified on mammography: correlation with imaging outcome and pathologic findings. *AJR Am J Roentgenol.* 2007;188(3):667-675.

Piccoli CW, Feig SA, Palazzo JP. Developing asymmetric breast tissue. *Radiology.* 1999;211(1):111-117.

Bilateral calcifications on first screening exam

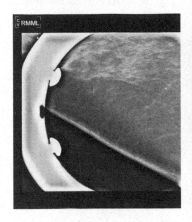 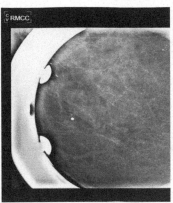 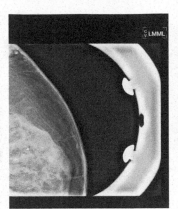 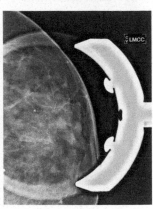

1. What would be the description of these calcifications on a screening exam?

2. What is the consequence these descriptors?

3. What other benign proliferative changes can cause pleomorphic calcifications?

4. What is the consequence of the presence of pleomorphic calcifications on diagnostic exam?

5. Pathology showed fibrocystic changes and sclerosing adenosis on the right side (calcifications seen in specimen) and DCIS on the left side. What is the management?

Case ranking/difficulty:

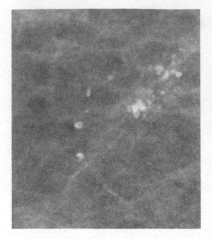

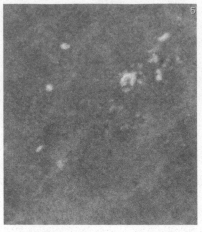

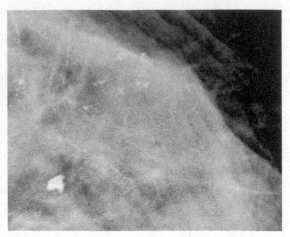

Right ML magnification view with additional electronic magnification demonstrating group of "pleomorphic" calcifications.

Right CC magnification view with additional electronic magnification demonstrating group of "pleomorphic" calcifications.

Left ML magnification view with additional electronic magnification demonstrating group of "pleomorphic" calcifications.

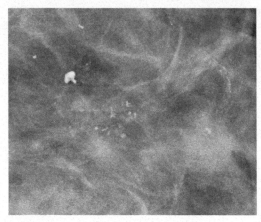

Left CC magnification view with additional electronic magnification demonstrating group of "pleomorphic" calcifications.

Answers

1. Screening mammogram demonstrates bilateral scattered benign calcifications and also group of indeterminate calcifications in the right inferior medial breast and left superior lateral breast. On screening mammogram, calcifications should not be further characterized. All indeterminate calcifications need to be magnified and then can be further described with appropriate BI-RADS descriptors.

2. Patient needs to be recalled for additional magnification views bilaterally.

3. Sclerosing adenosis and early calcifications in a fibroadenoma can present as "pleomorphic" calcifications.

4. "Pleomorphic" calcifications indicate the need for biopsy.

5. Both findings are concordant. Patient needs lumpectomy of left breast and 6-month follow-up mammogram of right side with magnification views. A preoperative MRI would also be helpful. Any benign biopsy in general will be followed in 6 months. Any follow-up of calcifications has, by definition, to include magnification ML and CC views. The same principle applies to follow-up of "focal asymmetries" or "masses"; it should always include spot compression views. You want to have the best information to follow something that is considered BI-RADS 3 or was recently biopsied to look for change.

Pearls

- There is a large overlap between benign proliferative changes and associated calcifications related to DCIS.
- For example, sclerosing adenosis as a form of benign proliferative change of breast parenchyma can cause "pleomorphic" calcifications indistinguishable from "pleomorphic" calcifications as a result of high-grade DCIS.
- That explains why about 70% of biopsies will not show malignancy—the benchmark (true positive rate) is to have malignancy, including DCIS, in about 30% to 40% of biopsies performed (PPV).

Suggested Reading

Burnside ES, Ochsner JE, Fowler KJ, et al. Use of microcalcification descriptors in BI-RADS 4th edition to stratify risk of malignancy. *Radiology*. 2007;242(2):388-395.

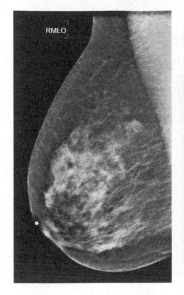 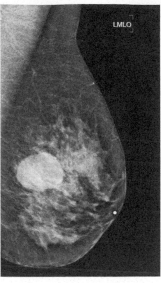 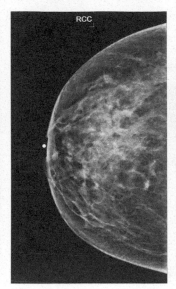 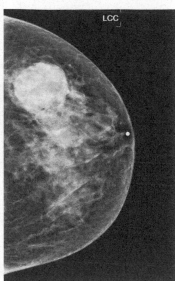

1. What BI-RADS classification should be used here?

2. What is the most likely pathology based on the imaging?

3. What is the next best imaging test?

4. A biopsy shows DCIS with papillary features. What is your next step?

5. What type of biopsy would you recommend?

Case ranking/difficulty: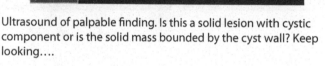

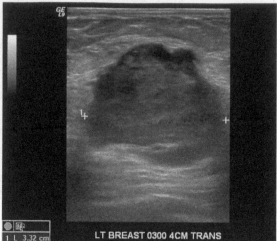

Ultrasound of palpable finding. Is this a solid lesion with cystic component or is the solid mass bounded by the cyst wall? Keep looking....

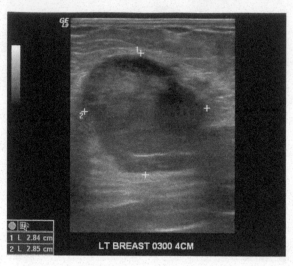

Ultrasound shows an intracystic mass that has irregular margins. There is no sign of the mass extending beyond the cyst wall.

Answers

1. The mammographic findings are suspicious. As the patient has a palpable finding, this is a diagnostic exam, and therefore a BI-RADS 0 should not be given. A BI-RADS 4 (suspicious) is the most appropriate assessment in this case.

2. The mammographic appearances could be due to any of the above findings. The ultrasound appearances are what clinch the diagnosis. If you chose any of the answers, you could be correct.

3. There are two approaches to this finding. If you think that further diagnostic workup will assist you in seeing the margins of the mass more clearly, or if you suspect calcifications being present, then diagnostic views are recommended. Many groups go direct to ultrasound when you have a mass, as if you can diagnose a simple cyst on ultrasound; you can prevent further unnecessary workup and radiation.

4. While working in multidisciplinary teams, surgeons like to know early about a patient in case they wish to do further clinical evaluation. If this is a mass like this, you may be so suspicious of invasive disease and you may want to sample more of the lesion to show potential invasion. DCIS rarely has spread into the axilla. Papillary DCIS is far from an indolent lesion, and can be very aggressive in expanding throughout the breast. Further workup is needed to determine whether it is possible to perform breast-conserving surgery. Papillary DCIS has a tendency to be rapidly multifocal and may spread to different segments, making it multicentric.

5. Fine needle aspiration can give suspicious findings with papillary carcinoma, and tissue is better. Smaller core biopsies may just give fragments of a papillary lesion, and then surgical diagnostic excision may be required. Pathologists like to see a relatively intact or larger specimen so that they can understand the architecture, which is why some authors recommend wide-bore vacuum-assisted biopsy in this situation.

Pearls

- If the lesion is vascular on Doppler ultrasound, with vessels entering perpendicular to the wall of the cyst/duct, then it is more likely to be a papillary lesion.
- If you see more than one lesion, it could be simple papillomatosis or papillary DCIS.

Suggested Readings

Bhargava R, Esposito NN, Dabbs DJ. Intracystic papillary carcinomas of the breast are more similar to in situ carcinomas than to invasive carcinoma. *Am J Surg Pathol.* 2011;35(5):778-779; author reply 779-781.

Kitada M, Hayashi S, Matsuda Y, Sato K, Miyokawa N, Sasajima T. Surgical treatment of intracystic carcinoma of the breast. *World J Surg Oncol.* 2011;9(9):116.

Wang H, Li F, Luo B. Breast intracystic papillary carcinoma. *Breast J.* 17(6):676-677.

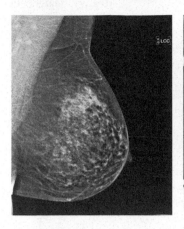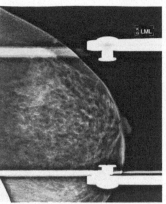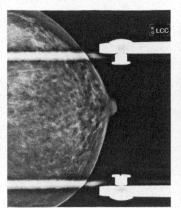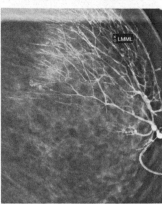

1. What are the findings on the mammogram and ductogram?

2. What other exam should be included in the workup?

3. What is the next step after MRI is normal?

4. What would be the last resort the breast surgeon could offer?

5. What is the most suspicious form of nipple discharge?

Case ranking/difficulty:

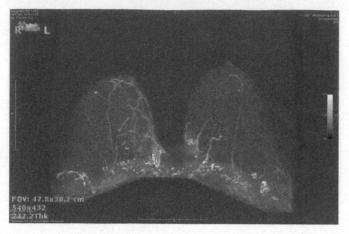

Demonstrates no abnormality in the left breast.

Answers

1. Mammogram and ductogram are unremarkable.

2. Ultrasound should also be performed. If there are still no findings, MRI might be considered.

3. The next step would be to send patient to breast surgeon for clinical evaluation.

4. The gold standard would be to perform selective duct excision. That is the reason why, in some institutions, no ductogram is done, because it could be argued that the ultimate step (duct excision) should be done anyway, even in the presence of normal imaging, if the discharge is clinically worrisome enough.

5. Spontaneous unilateral bloody or clear discharge is of most concern. During pregnancy, spontaneous bloody discharge bilaterally can be physiologic.

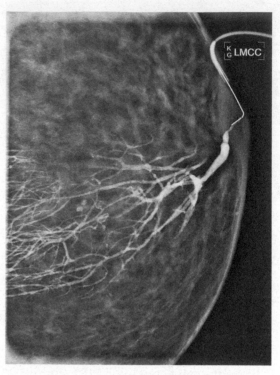

Ductogram of left breast, CC spot compression view is unremarkable.

- Although negative predictive value of additional MRI is very high, there are no data currently available supporting negative MRI eliminating the need for further action in the situation of high clinical concern, such as patients with new spontaneous, bloody nipple discharge.

Pearls

- Negative predictive value of normal mammogram, ultrasound, and ductogram is very high in the presence of nipple discharge.
- However, in selected cases, surgical excision of the duct might still be considered, which is still considered the gold standard.

Suggested Readings

Montroni I, Santini D, Zucchini G, et al. Nipple discharge: is its significance as a risk factor for breast cancer fully understood? Observational study including 915 consecutive patients who underwent selective duct excision. *Breast Cancer Res Treat*. 2010;123(3):895-900.

Nelson RS, Hoehn JL. Twenty-year outcome following central duct resection for bloody nipple discharge. *Ann Surg*. 2006;243(4):522-524.

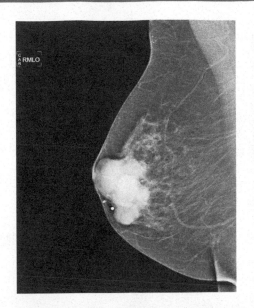
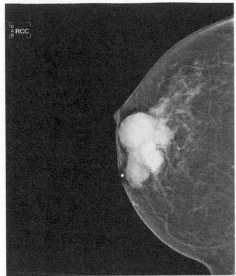
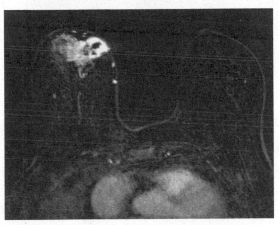
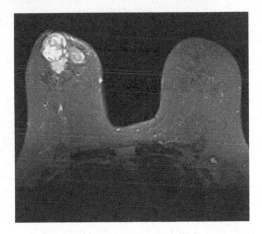

1. What would make you suspicious that this could be a phyllodes tumor?

2. What are the typical clinical features of a phyllodes tumor?

3. How frequent is the finding of phyllodes tumor?

4. How can we differentiate benign from malignant phyllodes tumor?

5. What is the appearance of phyllodes tumor on MRI?

Case ranking/difficulty:

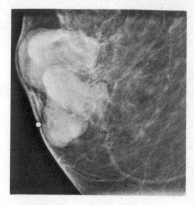

Diagnostic mammogram, right spot compression MLO view, demonstrating large mass with "lobular" shape.

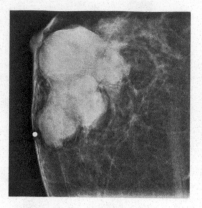

Diagnostic mammogram, right spot compression CC view, demonstrating large mass of "high density" and "circumscribed" margin.

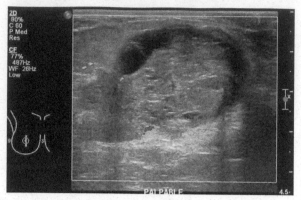

Ultrasound of right breast demonstrating large mass with cystic component.

Answers

1. Phyllodes tumors, oftentimes, cannot be distinguished from fibroadenoma. Fast growing masses with relatively benign morphological features raise the question of the presence of phyllodes tumors. Phyllodes tumors often occur in older patients than in typical patients with fibroadenomas.

2. Phyllodes tumors have local recurrence rates of up to 46% and sometimes metastasize most likely to the lung. The likelihood of metastasis depends on the histology. It is extremely rare in young patients but is described in up to 12% in case of the presence of sarcomatous elements.

3. 0.3% to 1% of breast neoplasm are phyllodes tumors.

4. Histology is the only way to differentiate benign from malignant phyllodes tumors by showing polymorphia of stromal cells and the presence of sarcomatous elements.

5. Phyllodes tumors in general show smooth margins, the presence of internal cysts, septations, and hemorrhage. Differentiation between phyllodes tumor and fibroadenoma is not possible. Both fibroadenoma and phyllodes tumor show unspecific contrast enhancement pattern.

- In general, they occur in the age group of mid-40 years. Secondary signs of malignancy such as perifocal edema, skin thickening, or nipple retraction are absent.
- On ultrasound, phyllodes tumors are well-defined masses with heterogeneous echogenicity; some tumors show posterior enhancement; most tumors show cystic parts within the tumor.
- On histology, the presence of nuclear polymorphia of the stromal cells is characteristic of malignant phyllodes tumors.
- Epithelial cells are not helpful to differentiate benign from malignant phyllodes tumor—that is one reason fine needle aspiration (FNA) is not appropriate to distinguish benign from malignant phyllodes tumor, since FNA oftentimes does not include stromal and epithelial cells.
- The recurrence rate of malignant phyllodes tumors is up to 46%. Distant metastasis by vascular spread is being described in about 3% to 12%.

Pearls

- On mammography, phyllodes tumors are often well defined, round, and lobulated, and belong to the fastest growing breast masses.

Suggested Readings

Buchberger W, Strasser K, Heim K, Müller E, Schröcksnadel H. Phyllodes tumor: findings on mammography, sonography, and aspiration cytology in 10 cases. *AJR Am J Roentgenol.* 1991;157(4):715-719.

Grebe P, Wilhelm K, Brunier A, Mitze M. MR tomography of cystosarcoma phyllodes. A case report [in German]. *Aktuelle Radiol.* 1992;2(6):376-378.

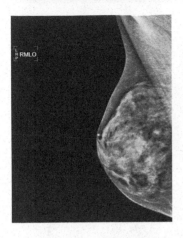 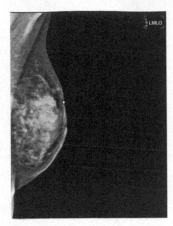 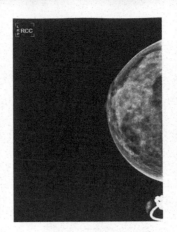 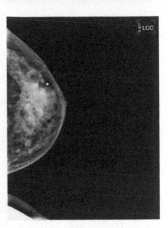

1. What BI-RADS classification should be used here?

2. Which ethnic groups of young women are at increased risk of triple-negative breast cancer?

3. What is the next best imaging test?

4. This patient turned out to have a triple-negative cancer with a basal subtype. What are the tissue biomarker findings?

5. What type of biopsy would you recommend?

Case ranking/difficulty: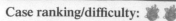

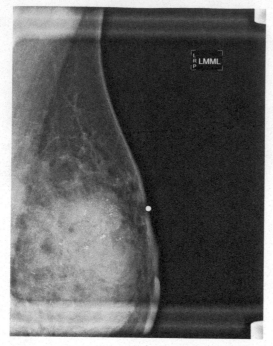

Left lateral spot magnification confirms an "ill-defined mass" or "focal asymmetry" containing "segmental pleomorphic" calcifications.

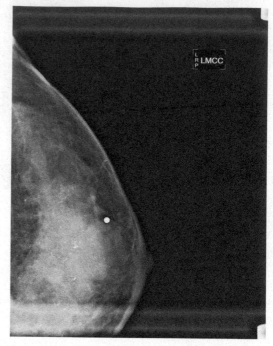

Left CC spot magnification.

Answers

1. Diffuse increased density associated with "pleomorphic" microcalcifications indicates aggressive disease.

2. Young black women. TN breast cancer affects younger women in general than regular invasive carcinoma.

3. Depends on your approach, as strictly a full mammographic workup should be completed before performing an ultrasound exam. However, this patient is unlikely to be having breast conservation, and may be having neoadjuvant chemotherapy. Ultrasound can then be the initial diagnostic exam, with axillary and internal mammary node staging, prior to biopsy. MRI will then also need to be performed prior to neoadjuvant chemotherapy or surgery for staging purposes. PEM may be of assistance in a patient with a palpable lump and suspicious ultrasound but not in a patient with dense breasts.

4. Triple-negative breast cancer refers to the negative status of ER, PR, and c-ERB receptor (HER2). As more subtypes are being found, future terms may include quadruple-negative breast cancer, and so on.

5. A good-quality core biopsy is needed with larger cores, as the HER2 overexpression will need to be redone on the surgical specimen (which may be after neoadjuvant chemotherapy).

Pearls

- Triple-negative breast cancer is more common in younger females.
- ER-, PR-, HER2-.
- Metastasizes early (at a small size).
- May present as circumscribed or partially obscured masses.

Suggested Readings

Kojima Y, Tsunoda H, Honda S, et al. Radiographic features for triple negative ductal carcinoma in situ of the breast. *Breast Cancer*. 2011;18(3):213-220.

Kojima Y, Tsunoda H. Mammography and ultrasound features of triple-negative breast cancer. *Breast Cancer*. 2011;18(3):146-151.

Uematsu T. MR imaging of triple-negative breast cancer. *Breast Cancer*. 2011;18(3):161-164.

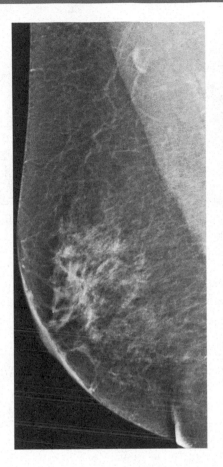 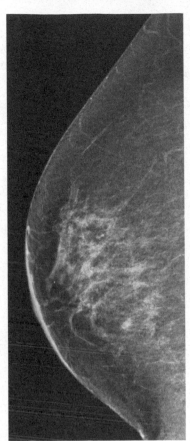 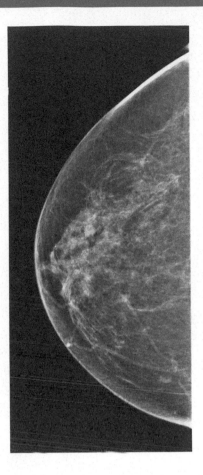

1. What is the finding on the mammogram?

2. Why is mammogram workup warranted before ultrasound?

3. What is the best ultrasound method for assessment of a small hypoechoic mass?

4. Why would it be inappropriate to classify the ultrasound lesion as BI-RADS 3?

5. What is the next step after the imaging?

Case ranking/difficulty:

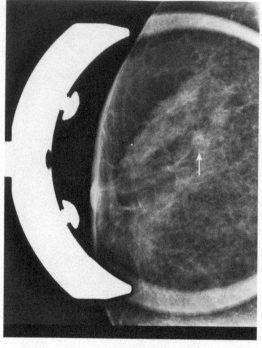

Diagnostic mammogram of right spot compression CC view.

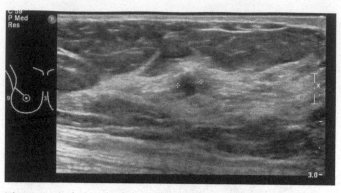

Ultrasound of right breast demonstrating small "mass" with "irregular" shape.

Answers

1. Noted is a small mass right 11–12:00.

2. Mammography workup with spot compression views is still warranted to further assess if the finding on the screening exam is real and also to better localize the lesion, and also to assess shape, margin, and density. This is, in particular, important if the finding is not seen on ultrasound.

3. A combination of B-mode imaging duplex and possibly elastography will have the highest specificity to determine the need for biopsy and the appropriate classification as BI-RADS 3 or BI-RADS 4. However, in most practices, the B-mode images alone will be used to characterize the mass.

4. Because of the "irregular" shape and "indistinct" margin on B-mode images.

5. Ultrasound-guided biopsy would be the next step to assess the suspicious finding.

Pearls

- This is an example where a hypoechoic nodule can be difficult to be classified, in part due to small size. The differential diagnosis could be "complicated cyst" versus solid "mass."
- Other methods that could help to differentiate cystic from solid lesion are elastography and the use of Doppler ultrasound in particular in the presence of extensive fibrocystic changes with multiple cysts.
- Elastography is used to semiquantitatively measure stiffness of tissue by calculating the displacement of each pixel relatively to the surrounding pixels in real time. A solid mass would be stiffer than a cyst and elastography would subsequently result in different signal.
- Ultrasound Doppler, on the other side, can help to show the presence of vessels which would prove the presence of solid mass and raises concern for the presence of malignancy and biopsy is warranted.

Suggested Reading

Cho N, Jang M, Lyou CY, Park JS, Choi HY, Moon WK. Distinguishing benign from malignant masses at breast US: combined US elastography and color Doppler US—influence on radiologist accuracy. *Radiology.* 2012;262(1):80-90.

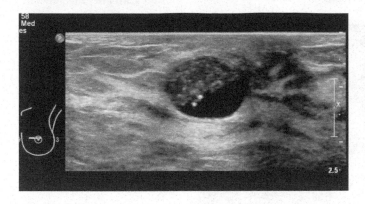 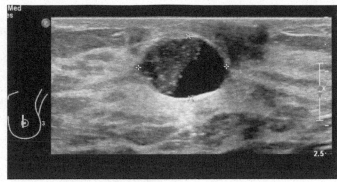

1. What are the criteria to call a lesion a simple cyst?

2. What additional test would be helpful to characterize the finding?

3. What is the appropriate classification of the cystic mass?

4. What is the next step?

5. What is the final BI-RADS classification?

Case ranking/difficulty: 🍁🍁

Category: Diagnostic

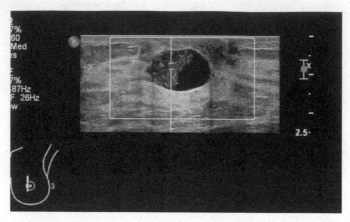

Ultrasound with duplex demonstrating "complicated cyst" in the left breast corresponding to palpable abnormality.

Answers

1. Simple cyst has to be "well circumscribed" and "oval or round," "anechoic" with "posterior acoustic shadowing."

2. If layering can be shown, this is proof that it is not a mass but debris. Positive duplex does prove the presence of intracystic mass and biopsy is recommended.

3. This is the typical presentation of a "complicated cyst." All other terms are not BI-RADS descriptors.

4. The options here would be cyst aspiration or 6-month follow-up.

5. BI-RADS 3 ("probably benign") would be an appropriate assessment.

Pearls

• Cysts can be divided into "simple cysts" and "complicated cysts."
• Simple cysts are "round," "well circumscribed," and "anechoic" with "posterior acoustic enhancement" and are BI-RADS 2 ("benign") finding.
• All other cysts are called "complicated cysts" and the option is cyst aspiration; or if there are no signs of intracystic mass, follow up in 6 months—BI-RADS 3.
• If there is a definite mass seen within a cyst, it should be called "complex mass" and biopsy should be performed.

Suggested Reading

Berg WA, Campassi CI, Ioffe OB. Cystic lesions of the breast: sonographic-pathologic correlation. *Radiology.* 2003;227(1):183-191.

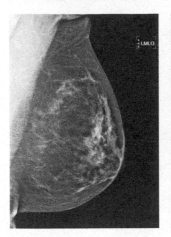 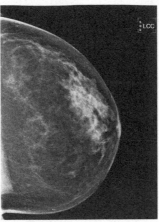 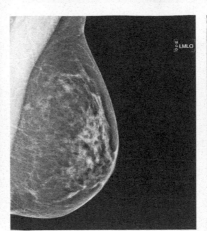 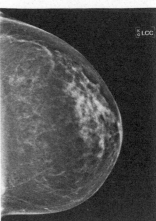

1. What is the pertinent finding?

2. What is the appropriate BI-RADS assessment for the screening mammogram?

3. What are the possible consequences if ultrasound does not show simple cyst?

4. What would you do if the aspiration fluid is bloody and the cyst has collapsed?

5. Where is the mass located?

Case ranking/difficulty:

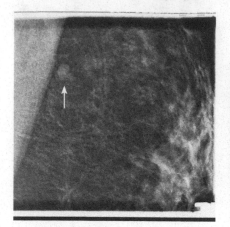

Diagnostic mammogram, left MLO spot compression view.

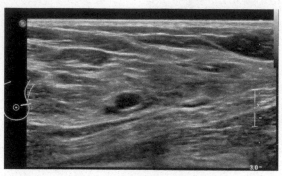

Ultrasound, left lateral breast demonstrates corresponding cluster of relatively simple cysts.

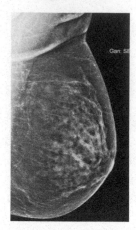

Mammogram, left MLO view after cyst aspiration demonstrates resolution of the small mass.

Answers

1. Noted is the interval development of a small mass in the left upper outer quadrant projecting on MLO view close to the pectoralis muscle and on the CC view posterior depth laterally.

2. Any new mass like in this case requires diagnostic workup and the assessment of the screening mammogram is BI-RADS 0, incomplete exam. Patient needs to be recalled for additional workup. On the screening mammogram, there is no need to describe shape and margin of the mass—this should be done based on the spot compression views at the time of diagnostic workup. To call the mass "indeterminate" is appropriate on screening mammogram.

3. If the finding is not a simple cyst, cyst aspiration or biopsy is recommended. Since, in this case, it was most likely a cluster of two cysts, cyst aspiration was performed first—cyst did collapse and subsequently the mass was not seen any more on repeat, post-aspiration mammogram.

4. Typical cyst-like fluid can be discarded—yellow and brownish fluid. Any bloody fluid, unless iatrogenic, should cause some concern. The pitfall is that if the cyst is aspirated, the lesion cannot be found in the future. Therefore, it is essential to leave a clip in that case.

5. The mass is located in the upper breast on the MLO view and in the lateral breast on the CC view—based on the rule of L it would be L(!)ower on the ML view because it is L(!)ateral on the CC view and therefore 3:00 is the best location as confirmed on ultrasound.

Pearls

- In case of new mass on mammogram, if corresponding ultrasound shows simple cyst—and the level of confidence is high that it correlates to the mammogram finding—finding is BI-RADS 2 ("benign") and patient can return to screening mammography.
- If the cyst is more complicated on the ultrasound, or if it is more uncertain and corresponding to the mammogram finding, cyst aspiration or short-term follow-up (BI-RADS 3) is recommended—depending on the situation.
- Simple cyst is defined by a well-circumscribed, homogeneous, and anechoic mass with posterior acoustic enhancement.
- Repeat mammogram after cyst aspiration should be performed to prove resolution of the new mass as seen on mammogram.

Suggested Reading

Kopans DB, Meyer JE, Lindfors KK, Bucchianeri SS. Breast sonography to guide cyst aspiration and wire localization of occult solid lesions. *AJR Am J Roentgenol.* 1984;143(3):489-492.

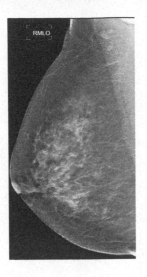 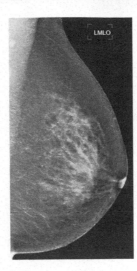 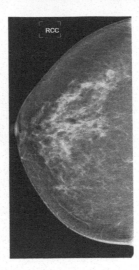 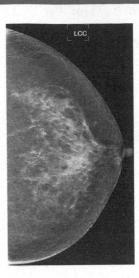

1. What is the BI-RADS category for this screening exam?

2. What further mammographic views do you wish to do?

3. What is the differential diagnosis of this lesion?

4. If this lesion is NOT visible on ultrasound, what would be your recommendations?

5. Given the mammographic appearances, what risk of malignancy would you estimate this lesion to have?

Case ranking/difficulty: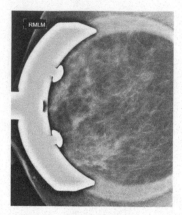

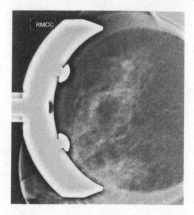

Right CC spot magnification view.

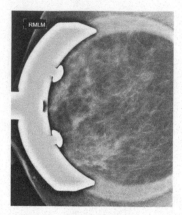

Right lateral spot magnification views. Even with the improved resolution of the spot magnification view, the mass remains irregular and the margins of the mass remain indistinct.

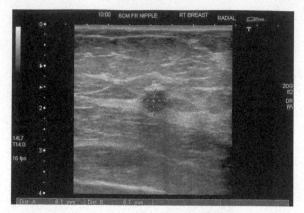

Ultrasound of mass shows that the mass is "irregular" with "ill-defined" margins, and containing low-level echoes.

Answers

1. This is an abnormal screening examination so that a BI-RADS assessment of 0 should be rendered, and further workup ordered. At this stage, there is no clear evidence of malignancy, and the outcome could still be a simple cyst or fibroadenoma. If you know that the prior mammogram was normal, this is a developing focal asymmetry (or mass), which automatically raises your concern about a developing malignancy.

2. The reason for doing a mediolateral rather than a lateromedial mammogram is that the abnormality is in the lateral breast. Spot compression films are required to further define the lesion from the surrounding glandular tissue. Many centers use spot magnification to increase the resolution of the examination. If this was a soft call, and you thought that the finding is likely superimposition, then repeating the CC and MLO would confirm or refute your hypothesis. However, it would not help to further characterize the lesion margins.

3. The lesion is so difficult to characterize, but appears to be more of a mass than a distortion, so more likely an intraductal origin. Lobular cancers tend to present as a vague asymmetry or distortion.

4. If the lesion is round and circumscribed on further mammograms and you think the patient has either a cyst or fibroadenoma, and the patient has no prior exams, then a 6-month follow-up may be appropriate. If prior films show no abnormality, this is a developing focal asymmetry or a mass and should be further worked up. You could do a problem-solving MRI or even positron emission mammography (PEM) or similar nuclear medicine scan. However, given the developing mass, this

is likely to require biopsy, and a stereotactic biopsy is the quickest and most accurate way to establish a diagnosis in a focal asymmetry that is not seen on ultrasound.

5. Based on the limited imaging so far, this lesion could be benign or malignant and therefore lies in a wide range from 10% to <95% (BI-RADS 4B–4C)—BI-RADS 5th edition ACR.

Pearls

- This can be a challenging malignancy to diagnose because of its benign-appearing features on mammography and ultrasound.
- It is very slow growing and may never metastasize in the patient's lifetime, according to molecular subprofiling.
- Look for indistinct margins of a benign lesion in an elderly patient.

Suggested Readings

Bode MK, Rissanen T. Imaging findings and accuracy of core needle biopsy in mucinous carcinoma of the breast. *Acta Radiol*. 2011;52(2):128-133.

Laucirica R, Bentz JS, Khalbuss WE, Clayton AC, Souers RJ, Moriarty AT. Performance characteristics of mucinous (colloid) carcinoma of the breast in fine-needle aspirates: observations from the College of American Pathologists Interlaboratory Comparison Program in Nongynecologic Cytopathology. *Arch Pathol Lab Med*. 2011;135(12):1533-1538.

Le-Petross H, Lane D. Challenges and potential pitfalls in magnetic resonance imaging of more elusive breast carcinomas. *Semin Ultrasound CT MR*. 2011;32(4):342-350.

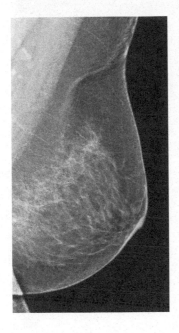 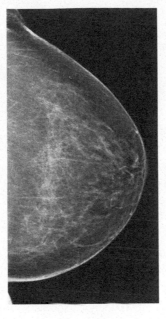 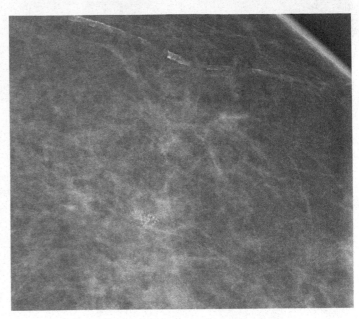

1. Are there any additional findings seen on the screening mammogram except small group of calcifications in the left upper outer quadrant?

2. What is the workup of a group of calcifications?

3. Is the pathology of lobular carcinoma in situ (LCIS) concordant with a group of calcifications?

4. What is the relationship between LCIS and invasive breast cancer?

5. What are potential consequences after diagnosis of LCIS?

Case ranking/difficulty:

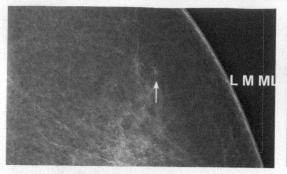

Diagnostic mammogram, left ML magnification view.

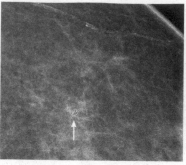

Diagnostic mammogram, left CC magnification view.

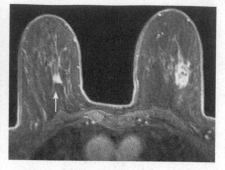

MRI T1-weighted sequence after IV contrast with index lesion in the left breast and additional 8-mm mass in the right central breast.

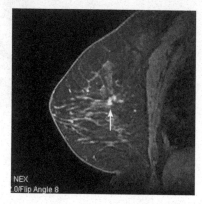

MRI T1-weighted sequence, sagittal image, postcontrast, demonstrating the mass in the right central breast.

Answers

1. Noted is the group of indeterminate calcifications in the left upper outer quadrant—otherwise no focal lesions.

2. The most appropriate workup is to perform a ML standard view to better localize the calcifications within the breast and for better planning of the subsequent stereotactic biopsy. ML and CC magnification views are standard for workup of calcifications. There is no indication for a MLO magnification view at all. An exception could be that in ML projection it is impossible to cover the calcifications due to location in the very posterior breast. ML and CC plane for magnification views is standard, since this is the best way to demonstrate "milk of calcium" as a typical form of benign calcifications—which would not require biopsy.

3. Yes—LCIS can present as group of calcifications. Although, in this case, MRI was performed, it is not standard of care at this time.

4. LCIS was initially thought to be a precursor for lobular invasive carcinoma. However, it was shown that this is false and that lobular carcinoma is now considered a risk factor for future development of malignancy in both breasts. Malignancy in the future can be lobular or ductal.

5. In general, most patients return to screening. In the face of the higher risk of malignancy, additional MRI screening is recommended. Other option could be bilateral mastectomy. If there is concern that there is additional suspicious morphology, then excisional biopsy is recommended.

Pearls

- Atypical lobular hyperplasia (ALH) and LCIS are associated with increased risk of breast cancer in the future in both breasts, including invasive ductal and lobular carcinomas—by 3- to 4-fold with ALH and 8- to 10-fold increase with LCIS.
- Both lesions are not considered a precursor to invasive lobular carcinoma.
- Management options include (1) lifetime surveillance with MRI added to mammography, (2) local excision of the lesion, and (3) bilateral prophylactic mastectomy.
- In this particular case, breast MRI was performed immediately after the diagnosis of LCIS was made, which showed an additional contralateral 8 mm highly suspicious mass in the right breast, which on subsequent MRI-guided biopsy was consistent with invasive ductal carcinoma.
- This case shows that mammogram with scattered fibroglandular tissue failed to show an 8-mm invasive ductal carcinoma, despite comparison with several old mammograms (not submitted for the book).

Suggested Readings

Oppong BA, King TA. Recommendations for women with lobular carcinoma in situ (LCIS). *Oncology (Williston Park)*. 2011;25(11):1051-6, 058.

Sung JS, Malak SF, Bajaj P, Alis R, Dershaw DD, Morris EA. Screening breast MR imaging in women with a history of lobular carcinoma in situ. *Radiology*. 2011;261(2):414-420.

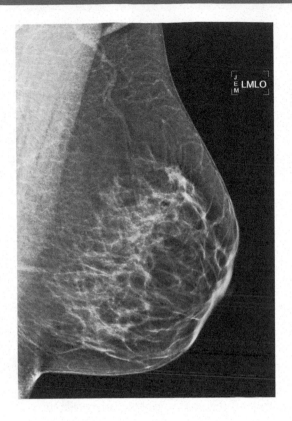
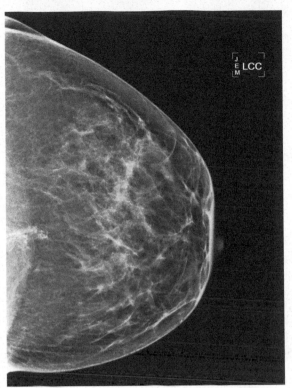

1. What is the abnormality seen on the mammogram?

2. If you see most likely artifact on a screening mammogram, what would you do?

3. What other patient-related artifacts are seen on mammograms?

4. What artifact could the abnormality be?

5. What would be an option if patient is still in the office?

Case ranking/difficulty:

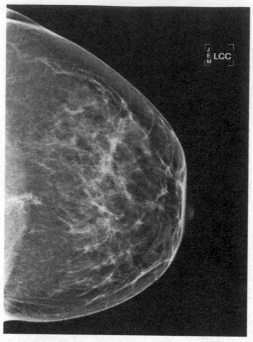

Screening mammogram, left CC view, demonstrating linear density in the posterior central breast.

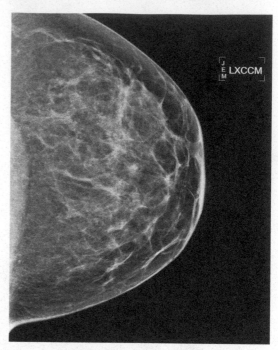

Repeat left CC view, with medially exaggerated scan field (LXCCM), demonstrates resolution of the density.

Answers

1. Noted is the linear density of left posterior breast—near chest wall.

2. Mammogram should be classified as BI-RADS 0 (incomplete exam) and patient should be called back for "technical repeat." That means the projection should be repeated showing the artifact. Anything suspected of causing the artifact, such as deodorant, powder, or hair should be removed before the film is taken.

3. All these are related to the patient. However, artifacts due to underexposure are more related to the setup of the machine (not enough mAs or kV) and not directly related to the patient.

4. The linear area could represent hair artifact from overlying hair.

5. If patient is still in office, there is no need to turn the exam into a diagnostic study. The images can be repeated and if the abnormality disappears and was due to artifact, this is a "technical repeat" and the study can remain screening exam.

Pearls

- When artifact, in this case hair artifact is suspected, patient needs to be recalled for "technical repeat."
- If the technologist does recognize the finding at the time the patient is still there, the issue can be addressed immediately.

Suggested Reading

Hogge JP, Palmer CH, Muller CC, et al. Quality assurance in mammography: artifact analysis. *Radiographics*. 1999;19(2):503-522.

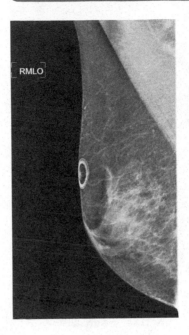
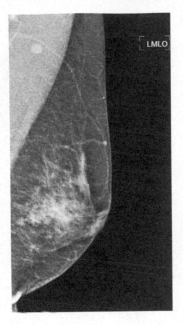
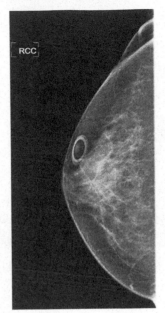
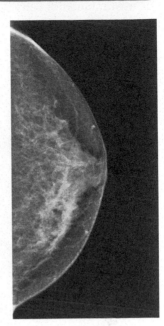

1. What is the BI-RADS category for this screening exam?

2. What is the next best examination you recommend?

3. What is the best description for the distribution of calcifications?

4. What is the most likely pathology in this case?

5. This case is a type of "developing" focal asymmetry. What is the likely risk of malignancy?

Case ranking/difficulty:

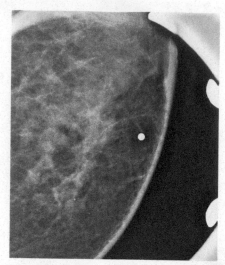

Left CC spot magnification views. The finding was palpable, and so a BB marker is seen over the palpable mass.

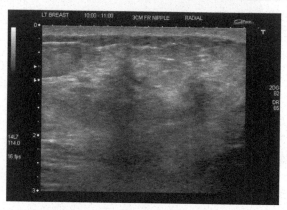

Left breast targeted ultrasound to palpable thickening shows vague decreased echogenicity within the glandular tissue and also some complex acoustic shadowing.

Answers

1. There is a subtle asymmetry in the left breast with possible distortion. There are possible calcifications associated with this asymmetry that are hard to evaluate on these films.

2. Further mammographic workup is indicated with an orthogonal mammogram in the lateral plane, plus spot magnification views to further characterize the calcific particles. Ultrasound is a good adjunct examination, but best performed when the mammographic workup is complete.

3. If you think these calcifications are likely malignant, then a more suspicious descriptor modifier such as "segmental" should be used. If you think these calcifications are likely benign, but associated with

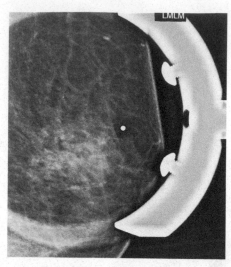

Left lateral spot magnification views show the asymmetry to be palpable. Some amorphous calcifications are also seen to be associated with this asymmetry. These are usually the reason biopsy is prompted.

a different process, then "regional" may be a better description.

4. Both lobular and tubular cancers present with asymmetries associated with distortion.

5. Based on the "developing focal asymmetry" alone, there is a risk of malignancy of approximately 20%, but may be up to 50% or more when there are new calcifications with it. This is the case in this particular example. These findings should prompt you to recommend biopsy.

Pearls

- Lobular cancer is difficult to diagnose on a mammogram.
- Findings are often very subtle.
- Distortion (especially in one view) is a common presentation.
- Beware of the "shrinking breast."

Suggested Readings

Choi BB, Kim SH, Park CS, Cha ES, Lee AW. Radiologic findings of lobular carcinoma in situ: mammography and ultrasonography. *J Clin Ultrasound*. 2011;39(2):59-63.

Heil J, Buehler A, Golatta M, et al. Do patients with invasive lobular breast cancer benefit in terms of adequate change in surgical therapy from a supplementary preoperative breast MRI? *Ann Oncol*. 2012;23(1):98-104.

Kim SH, Cha ES, Park CS, et al. Imaging features of invasive lobular carcinoma: comparison with invasive ductal carcinoma. *Jpn J Radiol*. 2011;29(7):475-482.

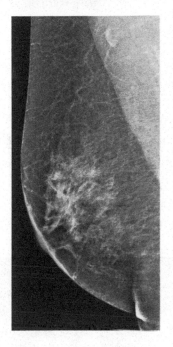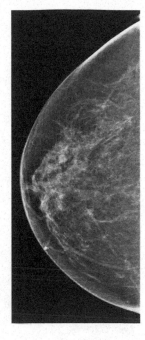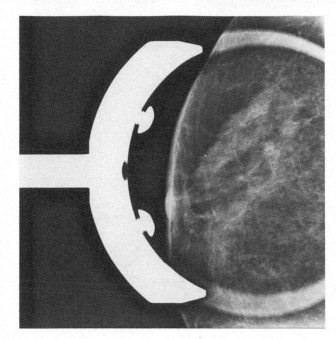

1. What is the finding on the mammogram?

2. How can the mass be described on spot compression view?

3. Where is the mass located?

4. What is the description of the ultrasound finding?

5. What are the descriptors on ultrasound that are suggestive or malignancy?

Case ranking/difficulty:

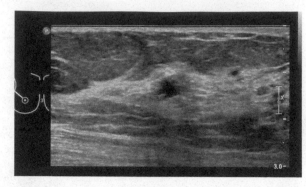

Ultrasound directed to the mass shows suspicious hypoechoic mass as best seen on tissue harmonic imaging.

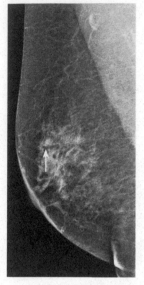

Screening mammogram, right MLO view.

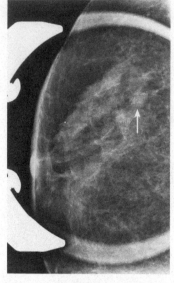

Spot compression right CC view confirms mass right lateral breast, anterior depth close to the nipple.

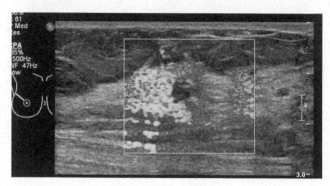

On power Doppler with vocal fremitus images, there is lack of color artifact within the area of concern.

Answers

1. There is a subtle mass seen on the right upper outer quadrant, which can be confirmed with spot compression views. Nodule is not a BI-RADS term.

2. The mass is irregular in shape, has "partially obscured and indistinct margins," and is of "equal density" to the surrounding fibroglandular tissue.

3. Mass is located superior to the MLO view and lateral to the CC view, which results in 10:00. It is also located in the anterior depth.

4. The mass is "irregular" in shape with "spiculated" margin and "hypoechoic" in comparison with the fat tissue. There is only minimal posterior acoustic shadowing.

5. All descriptors that are not round or oval in shape are suspicious, including "irregular"; all margin descriptors including "indistinct" or "angular," "microlobulated," or "spiculated" are of concern. Stavros et al. uses the term "taller than wide"; BI-RADS uses the terms "parallel" and "not parallel."

- If lesion is near isointense on ultrasound on B-mode images, harmonic imaging improves lesions conspicuity with higher image contrast and the surrounding fatty tissue appears less dark than the targeted lesion.
- Second ultrasound technique to differentiate lesion from surrounding fat is called "vocal fremitus technique," which uses acoustic vibrations from the chest wall to create color artifacts in normal tissue but not within the tumor on power Doppler ultrasound.

Suggested Readings

Kim MJ, Kim JY, Yoon JH, et al. How to find an isoechoic lesion with breast US. *Radiographics*. 2011;31(3):663-676.

Stavros AT, Thickman D, Rapp CL, Dennis MA, Parker SH, Sisney GA. Solid breast nodules: use of sonography to distinguish between benign and malignant lesions. *Radiology*. 1995;196(1):123-134.

Pearls

- Any developing density is potentially suspicious—if the density is seen in two plains and has convex margin, it is called "mass."

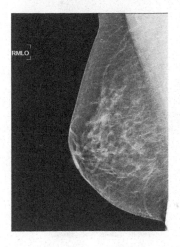 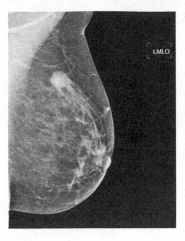 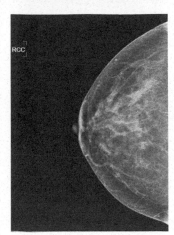 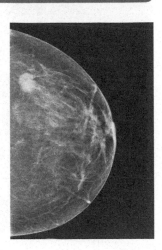

1. What is the BI-RADS category for this screening exam?

2. What is the background breast density?

3. If you want to recall this patient, what are your recommendations?

4. What type of biopsy should be performed?

5. Pathology shows florid inflammatory change around a hematoma. There is no history of trauma. What do you do next?

Case ranking/difficulty: **Category:** Screening

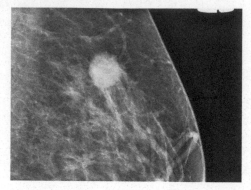

Left mediolateral spot magnification view for characterization of margins of mass—soft "spiculation" is seen, particularly in the plane toward the nipple.

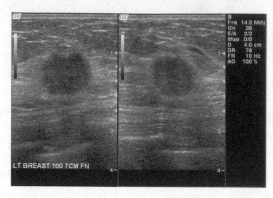

Orthogonal view of the mass seen on the mammogram. The mass appears relatively circumscribed in one plane. Take the ultrasound appearances in context with the mammogram to come to your final assessment.

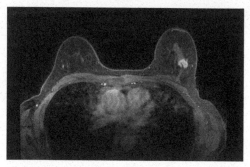

MRI for extent. Note signal void from recent biopsy within the enhancing mass.

Answers

1. This is a screening exam and thus should be 0; needs additional workup, negative, or benign. Although you are most likely to be correct to think that this is a malignant neoplasm, BI-RADS recommends that you fully work up this lesion mammographically, and possibly sonographically, before you come to a final assessment, and make a recommendation about management. Some benign lesions, including fat necrosis and prior lumpectomy, can mimic these appearances.

2. Some readers would classify this breast density as almost entirely fat, and some scattered fibroglandular densities. There is marked disagreement between readers when it comes to breast density. The assessment of breast density is currently subjective, until we have a reliable and reproducible automated way of defining breast density.

3. For most questions these days, tomosynthesis needs to be included. If you have tomosynthesis at screening, you likely have all the information you are going to get about the mass margins, but if there are calcifications, currently spot magnification views cannot be beaten. Ultrasound is the next modality to interrogate the mass. Whole breast

ultrasound can be performed looking for second lesions, but there is a significant false-positive rate that will need to be addressed.

4. Even if palpable, ultrasound-guided biopsy is more accurate giving a better chance of accurately sampling a mass. Sometimes, the lesion is not easily visible on ultrasound, and then you have to resort to stereotactic core biopsy.

5. In this case, it is possible that the imaging findings are due to fat necrosis, but with the spiculation I would give it a BI-RADS 5 lesion, as I will not accept a benign result. The pathology is of a hematoma and inflammatory change. The imaging does not fit with this. Therefore, the lesion has been under-sampled, and a larger-core biopsy could be performed. The finding is palpable and so needle localization should not be required.

Pearls

- Spot magnification views are useful to assess the margins of a mass, as well as for calcifications.
- Ensure that imaging findings correlate with pathology at biopsy.

Suggested Readings

Brenner RJ, Bassett LW, Fajardo LL, et al. Stereotactic core-needle breast biopsy: a multi-institutional prospective trial. *Radiology*. 2001;218(3):866-872.

Flowers CI. Breast biopsy: anesthesia, representative sampling and rad/path concordance. *Applied Radiol*. 2012;41(1):9-14.

Richter-Ehrenstein C, Müller S, Noske A, Schneider A. Diagnostic accuracy and prognostic value of core biopsy in the management of breast cancer: a series of 542 patients. *Int J Surg Pathol*. 2009;17(4):323-326.

Palpable lump in the right breast

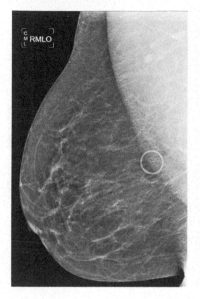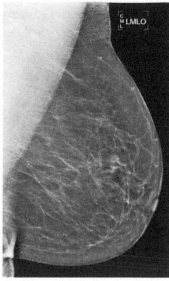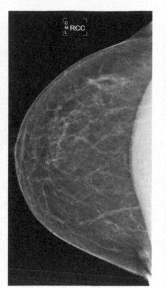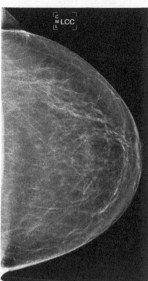

1. What is the BI-RADS category for this diagnostic exam?

2. What should be the next diagnostic imaging exam?

3. What are the clinical features of a sebaceous cyst?

4. What type of intervention would you recommend?

5. What is the malignant transformation rate of sebaceous cysts over 10 years?

Case ranking/difficulty: **Category:** Diagnostic

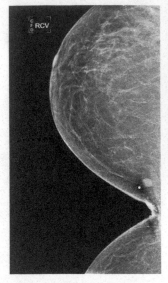

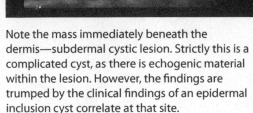

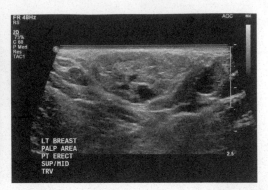

Right cleavage view shows position of mass more clearly.

Note the mass immediately beneath the dermis—subdermal cystic lesion. Strictly this is a complicated cyst, as there is echogenic material within the lesion. However, the findings are trumped by the clinical findings of an epidermal inclusion cyst correlate at that site.

Similar mass in a young woman who is breast-feeding. In this case, it appears as a complex mass BETWEEN the layers of skin, and therefore of dermal origin. The second "layer" of skin being displaced backward by the increasing intradermal mass. This is a sebaceous cyst.

Answers

1. This is a diagnostic examination and you should not give a BI-RADS 0 assessment, even if you are awaiting to do the ultrasound. As the findings are of a benign lump and the patient was shown to have a sebaceous cyst on clinical examination, you could even stop here and not do an ultrasound.

2. Tomosynthesis may include the lesion, but special views are needed when the lesion in the lower inner quadrant is so close to the sternum, and cleavage views are the best way of demonstrating this type of lesion. Once worked up, targeted ultrasound can be performed if there is no clinical evidence of sebaceous cyst. MRI and PEM are overkill for a skin lesion.

3. A sebaceous cyst is easily picked up on physical examination, and if your patient is still in the examination room, then a quick physical exam may obviate the requirement of further workup. A lump is usually fixed to the skin, but can become variably deep. If the lump is not attached to the skin, think of a different differential diagnosis. Redness can occur if a sebaceous cyst becomes infected, but is not a normal finding. A rash in a dermatome distribution is characteristic of herpes zoster infection.

4. No intervention is required apart from reassuring the patient that there is no evidence of malignancy.

5. They have a very low risk of malignant transformation. Development of a squamous cell malignancy within an epidermal inclusion cyst is very rare.

Pearls

- Sebaceous cysts can simulate a cancer occurring in the inferior mammary fold or in the medial breast on the CC view.
- They are harmless.
- Physical examination with the finding of a skin mass with a punctum is diagnostic of a sebaceous cyst.
- Ultrasound may be required for an epidermal inclusion cyst.

Suggested Readings

Giess CS, Raza S, Birdwell RL. Distinguishing breast skin lesions from superficial breast parenchymal lesions: diagnostic criteria, imaging characteristics, and pitfalls. *Radiographics*. 2011;31(7):1959-1972.

Kalli S, Freer PE, Rafferty EA. Lesions of the skin and superficial tissue at breast MR imaging. *Radiographics*. 2010;30(7):1891-1913.

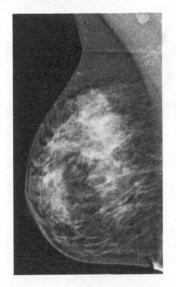
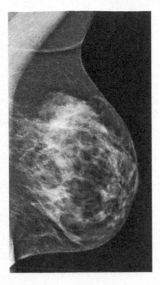
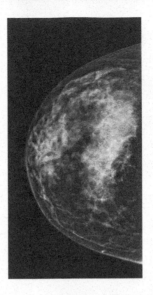
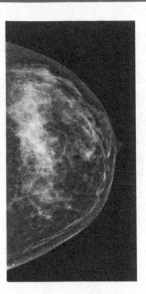

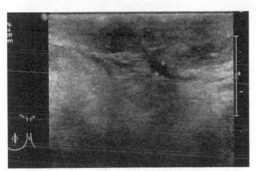
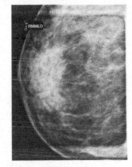
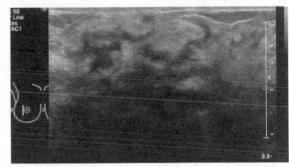

Diagnostic mammogram, right spot compression MLO view.

Ultrasound, B-mode image demonstrating prominent ducts and a large area of shadowing posterior depth.

1. What is the appropriate workup for bloody nipple discharge?

2. Would the ductogram have been helpful in this case?

3. What are the technical reasons for an insufficient ultrasound?

4. What is the most suspicious form of nipple discharge?

5. Ultrasound image was submitted by technologist as prominent ducts—anything else?

Case ranking/difficulty:

Category: Diagnostic

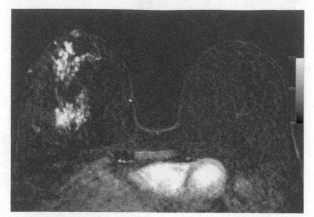

MRI axial T1-weighted image after IV contrast after subtraction demonstrates large area of "non–mass-like enhancement" retroareolar and also posterior right breast.

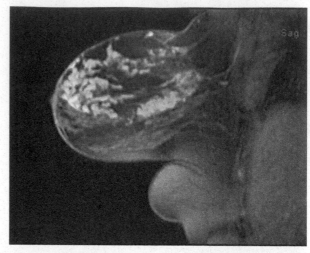

MRI sagittal T1-weighted image after IV contrast demonstrates large area of enhancement retroareolar and also posterior breast.

Answers

1. The first step is standard MLO and CC views of the symptomatic side and then additional SC views of the retroareolar tissue. Next standard routine step is an ultrasound directed to the right retroareolar breast—however, this case also demonstrates the remainder of the right breast if nothing is found. MRI could be an additional test if the patient is symptomatic and imaging does not find any abnormality. Ductogram can be helpful, but it is in general performed if the discharge is from one or two ducts and might show intraductal filling defect.

2. The nipple discharge in this case is due to large invasive ductal carcinoma that erodes the ductal system. An intraductal filling defect like seen with papilloma is unlikely here. Thus, the ductogram would likely not have helped to solve the situation.

3. An imperfect ultrasound can be due to incorrect gain, positioned focal zone or depth

4. The most suspicious form of discharge is clear or bloody discharge, spontaneously from one duct in one breast. Typical discharge due to proliferative fibrocystic changes is milky, greenish, or brownish bilateral discharge on pressure. Bloody nipple discharge during pregnancy or lactation is less of a concern because of increased blood flow to the parenchyma.

5. This is a case of a large mass not well appreciated on the images. Focus of the exam was directed to the retroareolar breast and the more deeper parts were not well examined and the large mass was missed in the deeper tissue.

Pearls

- This case demonstrates how easy it is to misjudge even the presence of a large invasive ductal carcinoma in dense fibroglandular tissue.
- It is crucial to set the focal zone of the ultrasound machine deep enough to be able to assess the breast parenchyma deep to the level of the chest wall.
- Ultrasound was originally misjudged as "presence of dominant ducts."
- Patient received MRI due to discrepancy between ultrasound and mammogram and clinical concern based on bloody nipple discharge and palpable mass, which did show the malignancy.

Suggested Reading

Baker JA, Soo MS, Rosen EL. Artifacts and pitfalls in sonographic imaging of the breast. *AJR Am J Roentgenol.* 2001;176(5):1261-1266.

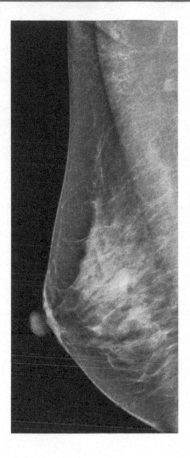
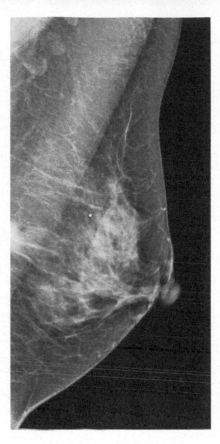
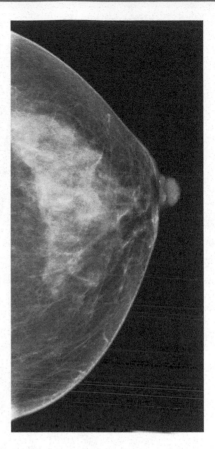

1. What is the BI-RADS category for this screening exam?

2. What structures are at risk in a patient with a possible posterior placed malignancy?

3. What are the appropriate tests during diagnostic workup in this patient?

4. What is the likely position of this mass based on the distribution of malignant lesions in the breast?

5. How do the majority of posterior located malignancies present?

Case ranking/difficulty: 🏵️ 🏵️

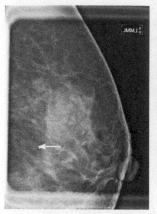

LML spot view at diagnostic workup—patient now states she can feel something in the left breast.

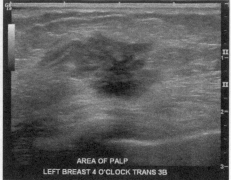

"Ill-defined mass" with (fine) "ductal extension."

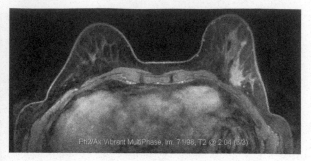

MRI was performed as the lesion was close to the chest wall. The extent is much greater than originally appreciated on mammography or ultrasound.

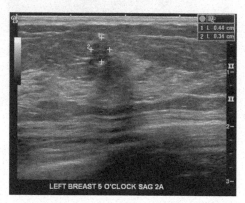

Second-look ultrasound showed multiple other masses, which were also biopsied and confirmed malignancy.

Answers

1. This is a screening examination, which should generate a BI-RADS 0, 1, or 2 assessment. As there is a finding, which is not typically benign, it should be classified as BI-RADS 0 and recalled for further workup.

2. With a lesion being so far posterior, it has potential for pectoral muscle involvement. Surgery to breast cancer includes cutting away the pectoral fascia when the mass is posterior. However, that is more likely to cause a poorer cosmetic outcome, with skin tethering. MRI is useful to see if there is muscle involvement, manifested as enhancement of the muscle.

3. Sometimes, it is not possible to find the lesion on orthogonal mammographic projections, and therefore difficult to find on ultrasound, and MRI could be useful to determine the location of the mass.

4. The distribution of both benign and malignant lesions are similar in frequency in the different areas, as follows:

   a. Upper outer quadrant, 45%
   b. Subareolar, 25%
   c. Upper inner quadrant, 15%
   d. Lower inner, 10%
   e. Lower outer, 5%

   Quadrant location does not predict benign versus malignant pathology (data and quotation used with permission from E. A. Sickles, MD).

5. Posterior lesions are not infrequently found by the woman when bathing. These are easily missed because of their position at mammography.

Pearls

- Watch edges of films when otherwise appears normal.
- Watch danger areas.
- Be prepared to recommend additional diagnostic views to work up this apparent finding.
- Computer-aided detection (CAD) can assist the radiologist pointing out an area to second look.

Suggested Readings

Brem RF, Baum J, Lechner M, et al. Improvement in sensitivity of screening mammography with computer-aided detection: a multi-institutional trial. *AJR Am J Roentgenol.* 2003;181(3):687-693.

Skaane P, Kshirsagar A, Hofvind S, Jahr G, Castellino RA. Mammography screening using independent double reading with consensus: is there a potential benefit for computer-aided detection? *Acta Radiol.* 2012;53(3):241-248.

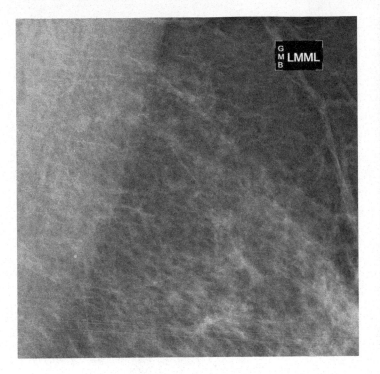 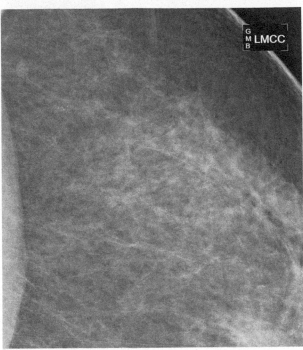

1. What is the definition of DCIS?

2. What is the prevalence of DCIS in a screening population?

3. What are the characteristics of high-grade DCIS?

4. What is the typical appearance of DCIS on MRI?

5. What is the value of MRI in regard to DCIS?

Case ranking/difficulty:

Category: Diagnostic

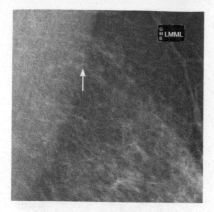

Diagnostic mammogram of left ML magnification view demonstrating group of "round and oval" calcifications.

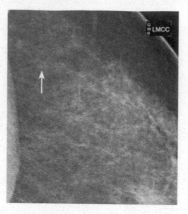

Diagnostic mammogram of left CC magnification view demonstrating group of "round and oval" calcifications.

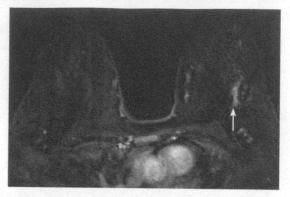

MRI after IV contrast demonstrating linear area of increased enhancement in the lateral superior breast. It exceeds the extent of the small group seen on the mammogram.

Answers

1. Ductal carcinoma in situ (DCIS; synonyms: intraductal carcinoma, noninvasive carcinoma) is a form of malignant transformation of epithelial cells lining the mammary ducts and lobules. The proliferating cells are confined by an intact basement membrane.

2. The overall prevalence is 32.5 per 100,000 women; the rate is as high as 88 per 100,000 women between the ages of 50 and 54.

3. High-grade DCIS on mammography most likely demonstrates calcifications as well, although there is a higher likelihood of the presence of "asymmetry" or "mass," in comparison with low-grade DCIS. On MRI, high-grade DCIS will more likely represent with vascular neogenesis and therefore will show contrast enhancement and is well seen.

4. Most frequently, DCIS appears on MRI as "non–mass-like clumped" enhancement. The kinetics of contrast enhancement varies between "early enhancement and washout kinetics" and also "mild early enhancement with increasing kinetics" over time.

5. MRI is helpful to reduce the chance to obtain positive margins after surgery and also to detect multifocal disease (as seen in retrospect in 23% of patients).

Pearls

- MRI has gained reputation over the past years for excellence in the detection of DCIS (sensitivity near 90%).
- Low-grade DCIS might be missed because of lack of vascular neogenesis; however, clinical significance of low-grade DCIS is controversial.
- MRI, however, shows often better the extent of DCIS than mammography and therefore is helpful for presurgical planning.
- Most common MRI finding in DCIS is "clumped, non–mass-like enhancement" in ductal or "linear" distribution.
- Enhancement kinetics vary and can include early enhancement, as well as delayed enhancement.

Suggested Readings

Kuhl C. Why do purely intraductal cancers enhance on breast MRI images? *Radiology*. 2009;253:281-283.

Mossa-Basha M, Fundaro GM, Shah BA, et al. Ductal carcinoma in situ of the breast: MRI imaging findings with histopathologic correlation. *Radiographics*. 2010;30:1673-1687.

Vag T, Baltzer PA, Renz DM, et al. Diagnosis of ductal carcinoma in situ using contrast-enhanced magnetic resonance mammography compared with conventional mammography. *Clin Imaging*. 2008;32(6):438-442.

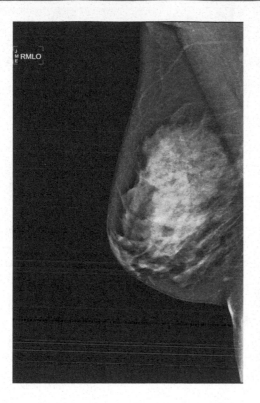 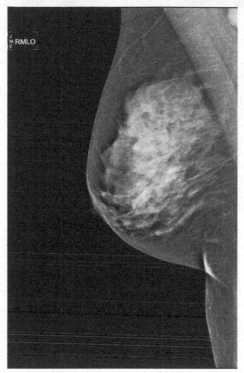

1. Given that the breasts appear normal, what is the most appropriate BI-RADS category to use?

2. What is the next best imaging test?

3. The ultrasound shows a solid node. What is the next imaging test?

4. The node shows metastatic adenocarcinoma on FNA. What is the next imaging test?

5. What is the differential for lymphadenopathy on mammography?

Case ranking/difficulty:

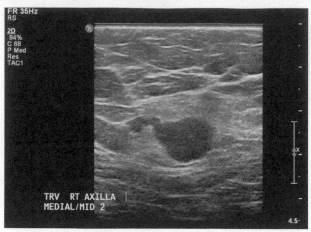

Ultrasound of the right axilla shows a nodule arising in the cortex of the lymph node. The lymph node has an irregular margin. The nodule is the most suspicious part of the lymph node, and the best place to target your biopsy.

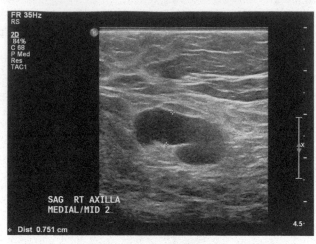

Ultrasound of the right axilla. In this view, the cortex appears smooth but thickened—beyond the 3-mm threshold for biopsy.

Answers

1. As this is a diagnostic exam and you are going to recommend a biopsy, a BI-RADS 4 is the best category to use, as it gives the message of a suspicious finding. Some people use BI-RADS 0 in the situation of a diagnostic exam, which requires an ultrasound scan that cannot be done at the same time. The downside to this is that the degree of suspicion or urgency is not conveyed in the same way. Some people also argue that you should use BI-RADS 1 as the breasts are negative for malignancy, but there is a coincidental finding in the axilla, which requires action.

2. There is nothing to be seen in the breast to indicate an axillary recurrence, so diagnostic films or tomosynthesis is unlikely to give any extra information at this point. MRI may be required later following interrogation of the axillary node. As yet we have no proof that this is an axillary recurrence—need cytology or histology. PET/CT may be required later if this is proven to be breast cancer recurrence, but not at this stage.

3. Establishment of recurrent malignancy needs to be made before we recommend additional expensive tests. FNA cytology is sufficient to detect recurrent malignancy; however, if possible, a small-gauge core biopsy will give tissue for biomarkers as well and guide any further treatment. If cancer is proven in the nodes, and the breasts are dense, PEM is an alternative way to determine lesions in breasts.

4. This is where MRI is probably the best test, just as in patients who present with metastatic axillary lymph nodes

of unknown origin. MRI is likely to show any recurrent focus within the breast. If the breasts are very dense and enhancing, or if the patient is unable to have an MRI, then PEM or BSGI may assist in finding the primary.

5. After metastatic cancer, lymphoma is the most obvious cause for lymphadenopathy. Localized rupture of silicone implants can also cause enlarged nodes. Sarcoid is normally picked up incidentally on a chest radiograph. Infections are a cause, including "cat-scratch" disease. Brucellosis is a known cause.

Pearls

- Don't forget to notice change in axilla.
- Not all breast cancer recurrence is visible within the breast.
- Workup for a suspicious node with no mammographic finding.

Suggested Readings

Barton SR, Smith IE, Kirby AM, Ashley S, Walsh G, Parton M. The role of ipsilateral breast radiotherapy in management of occult primary breast cancer presenting as axillary lymphadenopathy. *Eur J Cancer.* 2011;47(14):2099-2106.

Ho A, Morrow M. The evolution of the locoregional therapy of breast cancer. *Oncologist.* 2011;16(10):1367-1379.

Ruano Pérez R. Incidence of axillary recurrence after a negative sentinel lymph node result in early stages of breast cancer: a 5-year follow-up. *Rev Esp Med Nucl Imagen Mol.* 2012;31(4):173-177.

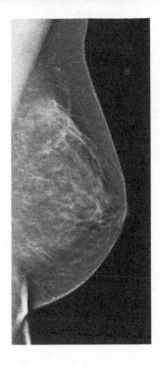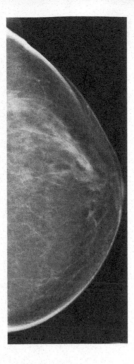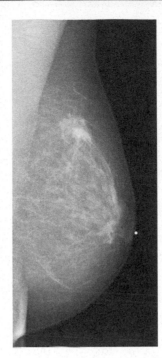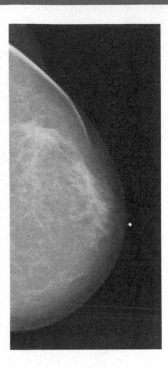

1. What is the finding on the current screening mammogram?

2. In case the density is not palpable and not visible on ultrasound, what is the next step?

3. If stereotactic biopsy is not technically feasible, what is the next step?

4. Where is the abnormality located?

5. What would be the correct description of the likely finding on ultrasound?

Case ranking/difficulty:

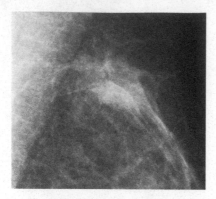

Diagnostic mammogram, left spot compression MLO view demonstrates development of "focal asymmetry" with subtle "architectural distortion."

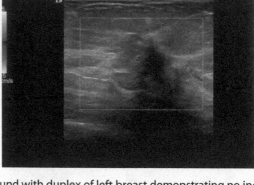

Ultrasound with duplex of left breast demonstrating no increased flow in the mass.

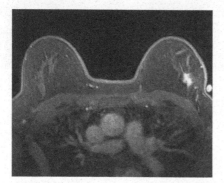

MRI, T1-weighted postcontrast image, demonstrates spiculated mass in the left upper outer quadrant.

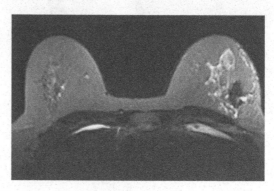

MRI, T2-weighted image, demonstrates corresponding low-signal mass in the left upper outer quadrant.

Answers

1. Noted is the development of subtle "focal asymmetry" and "architectural distortion" in the left upper outer quadrant best seen on the MLO view.

2. In this case, finding can be classified as BI-RADS 4 and stereotactic biopsy should be attempted. Since the mass that has developed in the interval is "spiculated," it could be even argued that it could be classified as "highly suspicious," BI-RADS 5. The consequence would be that any benign pathology, for example "focal fibrosis," would be considered as being not concordant and patient had to go to surgery.

3. Any finding seen on two mammogram projections can be excised, since finding can be marked with needle localization.

4. Since it is lateral on the CC view and superior on the MLO, it would be slightly lower on an ML view; therefore, while located in the upper outer quadrant, its more precise location is about 2:00 then 12:00 to 1:00. Take home point: anything L(!)ateral on CC view is L(!)ower on ML in comparison with MLO view.

5. The BI-RADS lexicon has also descriptors for ultrasound findings—in this case, this is a "hypoechoic mass" with "irregular" shape and "spiculated" margin and "posterior acoustic shadowing."

Pearls

- If mammogram raises concern for the presence of architectural distortion, workup should include spot compression views and ultrasound.
- If ultrasound cannot demonstrate corresponding abnormality, stereotactic biopsy should be performed.
- Remember that prior surgery, or even large-bore core biopsies, may also explain the presence of architectural distortion.

Suggested Reading

Piccoli CW, Feig SA, Palazzo JP. Developing asymmetric breast tissue. *Radiology.* 1999;211(1):111-117.

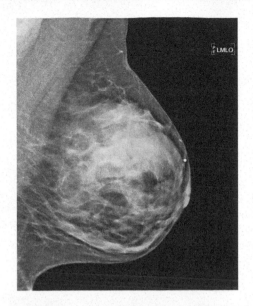
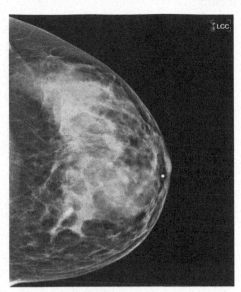
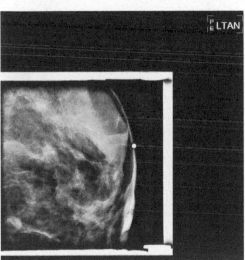
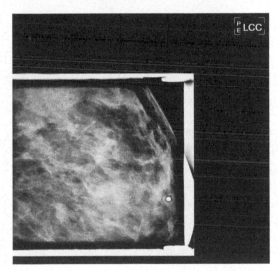

1. What does PASH stand for?

2. What is the typical appearance of PASH on mammography?

3. What is the typical appearance of PASH on sonography?

4. What is the consequence of a biopsy showing PASH?

5. What can PASH be confused with by the pathologist?

Case ranking/difficulty:

Category: Diagnostic

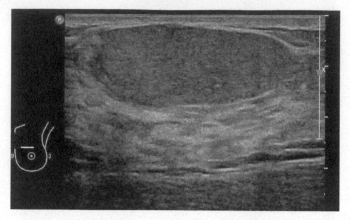

Ultrasound directed to the area of concern demonstrates well-circumscribed mass.

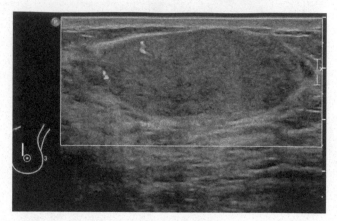

Ultrasound directed to the area of concern demonstrates well-circumscribed mass with some increased flow.

Answers

1. Pseudoangiomatous stromal hyperplasia.

2. PASH presents, in general, as a benign-appearing mass or as a focal asymmetry.

3. PASH has no specific morphological features and is found in up to 25% as incidental finding on breast biopsies. However, it appears most frequently on ultrasound as a benign mass with the appearance of a fibroadenoma or a hypoechoic area.

4. If the imaging is concordant with the benign diagnosis of PASH, patient can return back to screening mammogram. For example, if PASH is the diagnosis after stereotactic biopsy of "pleomorphic," "highly suspicious calcifications" (BI-RADS 5), excisional biopsy is recommended because PASH might be only an incidental finding.

5. Angiosarcoma can be confused histologically with PASH. While PASH is not a high-risk lesion and not being related to subsequent development of malignancy, angiosarcoma is considered malignant tumor and requires wide excision and chemotherapy.

Pearls

- PASH is benign proliferative change and can appear on mammograms as "focal asymmetry," "architectural distortion," calcifications, or without any abnormality at all.
- Patient with sonographic finding consistent with well-circumscribed oval hypoechoic mass, like in this particular case, can also be concordant with PASH.
- PASH is identified as an incidental finding in as many as 25% of breast biopsies.
- If the imaging findings are concordant with the diagnosis of PASH, then it is appropriate to return the patient back to screening.
- It is important to remember that if there are suspicious features seen on imaging, excision of the lesion is warranted.
- Angiosarcoma can be confused with PASH at histology. Angiosarcoma requires surgical treatment +/− chemotherapy.

Suggested Reading

Hargaden GC, Yeh ED, Georgian-Smith D, et al. Analysis of the mammographic and sonographic features of pseudoangiomatous stromal hyperplasia. *AJR Am J Roentgenol.* 2008;191(2):359-363.

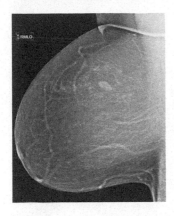 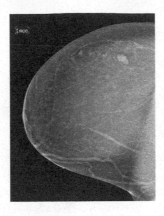 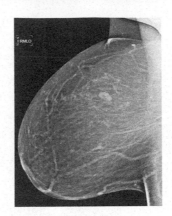 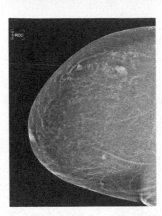

1. What is the pertinent finding?

2. Which should be the most important comparison year reading screening mammogram?

3. What is the other reason and why comparison with 2-year prior mammogram is essential?

4. Where is the suspicious mass located?

5. If you believe the ultrasound is a "complicated cyst," what could you do?

Case ranking/difficulty: 🍁🍁

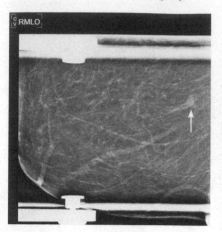

Diagnostic mammogram, right MLO spot compression view demonstrating new mass.

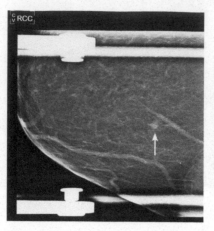

Diagnostic mammogram, right CC spot compression view demonstrating new mass.

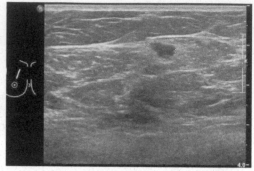

Gray-scale ultrasound demonstrating corresponding "hypoechoic" mass in the right medial superior breast with "irregular" shape.

Answers

1. Mass in the superior medial right breast that is new since prior mammogram. The mass in the upper outer quadrant is stable since 2 years and therefore benign.

2. Two years prior mammogram is the key image to compare a screening mammogram with. Any well-circumscribed mass stable since 2 years or any asymmetry without distortion, stable since 2 years, can be considered to be benign. Remember, we use 2-year time period to follow "probably benign" lesions before converting the assessment into "benign."

3. Some breast cancers grow relatively slow. Average double time of breast cancer cells is about 90 days. Therefore, it is recommended to look back 2 years—this will improves sensitivity.

4. Lesion is located in the medial breast and in the central breast at the level of the nipple as seen on the MLO view. Therefore, it will be higher on the ML view in comparison with the MLO view because it is located in the medial breast. Thus, 2:00 is correct.

5. Cyst aspiration would be an appropriate first step. If the cyst pops and disappears and typical cyst-like fluid is aspirated, the fluid can be discarded repeat mammogram should be obtained to prove resolution of the new mass. If the fluid does show bloody fluid, a clip marker should be placed, the aspirate should be sent for cytological analysis, and depending on the outcome, the patient might be sent for surgical excision.

Pearls

- Any developing mass remains concerning, unless it can be explained by simple cyst or other benign finding.
- Even if the ultrasound finding shows corresponding circumscribed solid mass with smooth margins, the finding has to be biopsied if it correlates to a new mass seen on mammogram, since it can be assumed that it has grown in the past.

Suggested Reading

D'Orsi CJ, Bassett LW, Berg WA, et al. *Breast Imaging Reporting and Data System: ACR BI-RADS–Mammography.* 4th ed. Reston, VA: American College of Radiology; 2003.

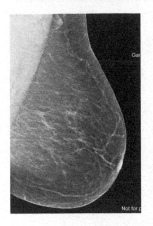 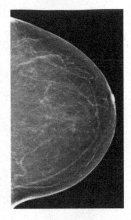 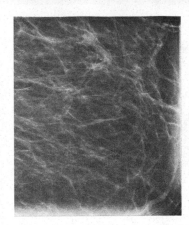 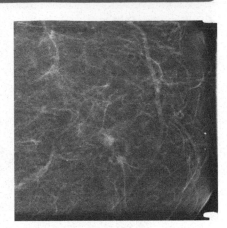

1. What is the finding on the mammogram?

2. Why is "focal asymmetry" better descriptor than nodular density?

3. Where are most breast cancers found in the breast?

4. What would be the appropriate assessment if ultrasound is normal and finding is new?

5. What is the significance of the ultrasound finding?

Case ranking/difficulty: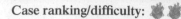

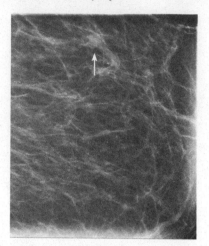

Diagnostic mammogram, left MLO spot compression view demonstrates subtle focal asymmetry.

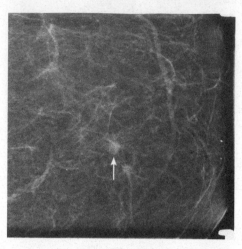

Diagnostic mammogram, left CC spot compression view demonstrates subtle focal asymmetry.

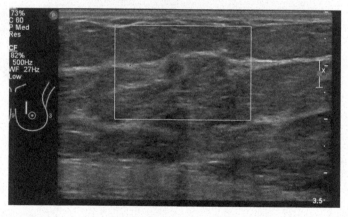

Gray-scale ultrasound demonstrates small mass.

Pearls

- This case illustrates that any "focal asymmetry"— especially in the medial breast—should raise concern, since that area in general does not contain much fibroglandular tissue.
- Other problem zone in the breast is the so-called milky way, the area behind the fibroglandular tissue on MLO or CC view.

Suggested Reading

Brown M, Eccles C, Wallis MG. Geographical distribution of breast cancers on the mammogram: an interval cancer database. *Br J Radiol*. 2001;74(880):317-322.

Answers

1. Given its concave margin, the BI-RADS term "focal asymmetry" could be used in place of "mass" which would have a convex margin.

2. Nodular density is not part of the BI-RADS lexicon.

3. Most breast cancers are located in the upper outer quadrant. This is simply due to the fact that there is the most tissue, in general.

4. BI-RADS 4, if this is a new finding, would be appropriate assessment—if it is an asymmetry on first screening mammogram, BI-RADS 3 would be appropriate.

5. Ultrasound finding does correlate to the mammogram and ultrasound-guided biopsy is recommended.

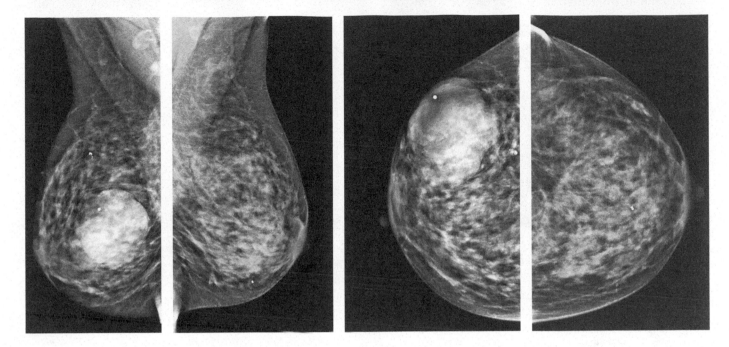

1. What is the BI-RADS category for this diagnostic exam?

2. What is the likely underlying pathology?

3. What is the risk of lymph node spread in malignant phyllodes tumors?

4. What type of biopsy should be performed?

5. The biopsy comes back as dense fibrous tissue with no epithelium. What is your recommendation?

Case ranking/difficulty:

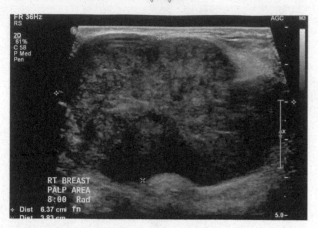

Ultrasound—the mass appears "bi-phasic" on ultrasound, with an echogenic upper portion, and a more hypoechoic portion below.

Doppler ultrasound shows prominent vascular channels, but without a specific characteristic distribution.

Answers

1. This is not a screening exam, and therefore not BI-RADS 0. Phyllodes tumors, if small, can simulate classic fibroadenomas, and can look benign. This lesion is large and atypical on ultrasound; therefore, a BI-RADS 4: suspicious assessment is appropriate.

2. While occasionally cysts and sarcoid appear this way, the size and lobulated features narrow down the differential to fibroadenoma or phyllodes tumor. Occasionally a special type of IDC variant can give these appearances, including mucinous, colloid/medullary carcinoma.

3. Although extremely rare and said to be "locally" malignant, metastases from malignant phyllodes still can occur—but very rare indeed.

4. A combination of palpation and ultrasound is probably the best way to direct the sampling of a tumor of this size. Multiple samples from different areas of the mass should be taken to give the pathologist a good chance at making the diagnosis. Stabilizing a mobile tumor using finger pressure is a useful technique to learn, as when you are already holding the probe in one hand and the biopsy device in the other, the mass may move under the probe, and satisfactory sampling may sometimes be challenging. FNAC may have a role in centers with expert breast cytopathologist.

5. There are two main options. You need more tissue, so move to a larger lesion, for example, to an 8-gauge vacuum-assisted needle from a 14-gauge core biopsy. If you have had no success with vacuum-assisted biopsy, then surgical excision is the next logical step. You need

to inform the surgeon who is performing the procedure that you suspect a phyllodes tumor, and then they will take a healthy formal margin, rather than "shelling it out" of the breast tissue.

Pearls

- Mainly affects premenopausal females.
- Has benign and malignant spectrum.
- May have precursor lesion of fibroepithelial lesion.
- Treatment by wide excision.
- High risk of local recurrence of 20 to 30%.

Suggested Readings

Abe M, Miyata S, Nishimura S, et al. Malignant transformation of breast fibroadenoma to malignant phyllodes tumor: long-term outcome of 36 malignant phyllodes tumors. *Breast Cancer.* 2011;18(4):268-272.

Gould DJ, Salmans JA, Lassinger BK, et al. Factors associated with phyllodes tumor of the breast after core needle biopsy identifies fibroepithelial neoplasm. *J Surg Res.* 2012;178(1):299–303.

Jang JH, Choi MY, Lee SK, et al. Clinicopathologic risk factors for the local recurrence of phyllodes tumors of the breast. *Ann Surg Oncol.* 2012;19:2612-2617.

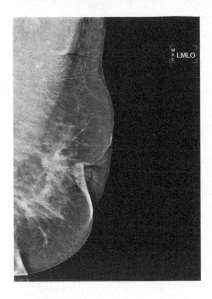
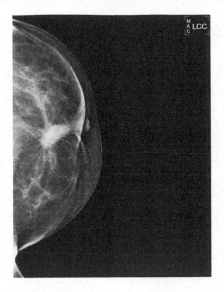
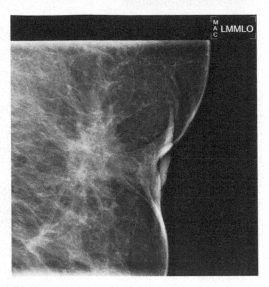

1. What is the appropriate workup of a patient after lumpectomy?

2. What is the role of ultrasound after lumpectomy?

3. If there is questionable recurrent new density in the lumpectomy bed, what is the best exam?

4. What could decrease sensitivity of the MRI in assessing recurrent malignancy?

5. What are the expected morphological findings after lumpectomy?

Case ranking/difficulty:

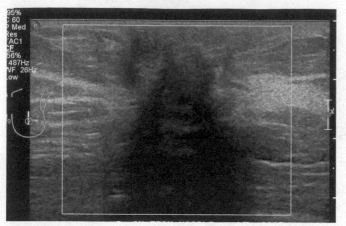

Ultrasound of left breast demonstrating the scar from prior surgery done in 2010.

Answers

1. Oftentimes, mammography after lumpectomy is performed as a diagnostic mammogram and spot compression view of the scar is included.

2. Ultrasound, in general, does not add any information about the lumpectomy site but could be helpful in detecting recurrent malignancy in dense breast tissue. It might also be helpful to detect recurrent lymphadenopathy.

3. The best exam to assess possible recurrent malignancy would be MRI with contrast.

4. In a premenopausal female, the strongest enhancement of the breast parenchyma will be in the first and last week of the cycle. Also up to 6 months after surgery, there will be postsurgical enhancement due to granulation tissue.

5. Postlumpectomy we expect to see distortion, densities that could represent irregular margin due to the scar—but no new linear calcifications or segmental distribution of suspicious calcifications.

Pearls

- After history of lumpectomy, mammograms are oftentimes performed as diagnostic mammograms and include spot compression magnification view of the lumpectomy site.
- In this case, the lumpectomy site demonstrates architectural distortion and was stable since prior studies—BI-RADS 2: there is no need for additional ultrasound.
- However, if ultrasound is requested, the scar tissue from prior lumpectomy on ultrasound appears to be indeterminate and, if mammogram is stable, would trigger BI-RADS 3 and subsequent follow-up.
- If there is concern for recurrent malignancy, MRI would be the best test to investigate the lumpectomy site if there is a focal abnormality showing suspicious enhancement.

Suggested Reading

Dershaw DD, McCormick B, Cox L, Osborne MP. Differentiation of benign and malignant local tumor recurrence after lumpectomy. *AJR Am J Roentgenol.* 1990;155(1):35-38.

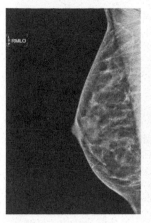 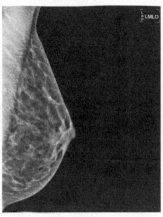 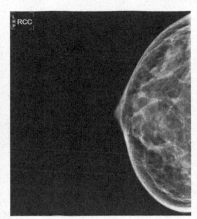 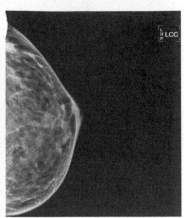

1. What is the BI-RADS category for this screening exam?

2. Which view is the best mammogram to include the most breast tissue?

3. What are the danger areas to review if you cannot spot the abnormality?

4. If you perceive an abnormality on one view only (asymmetry), what views do you recommend to localize the lesion prior to ultrasound?

5. Now the asymmetry has been found on mammography, what imaging test do you recommend?

Category: Screening

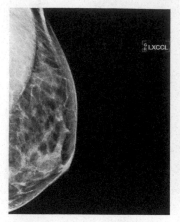

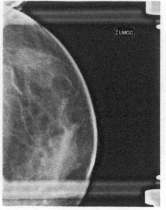

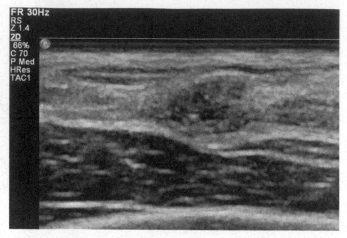

Left XCCL—an asymmetry is just about visible at the edge of the breast disc. A right XCCL was also taken for comparison, as it was thought that this may just be some asymmetrical tissue.

Left spot magnification in XCCL position confirms an ill-defined mass at this site.

Careful ultrasound revealed a subtle mass with calcifications that was biopsied. Final pathology: Grade 3 invasive ductal carcinoma.

Answers

1. There is a possible asymmetry on the lateral margin of the left CC film. Needs further workup. Therefore, this is a BI-RADS 0 exam.

2. The mediolateral mammogram was identified as the best view to get the majority of the breast tissue on one film. Up to then, standard orthogonal radiological views were performed CC and lateral exams. Some European organizations, such as the UK NHS Breast Screening Programme, started to reduce costs and radiation dose based on a single MLO mammogram. This was reversed later.

3. There are four danger areas, but the finding does not lie in any of them.

   i. Inframammary fold on MLO
   ii. Medial aspect of CC film, adjacent to sternum
   iii. Subareolar region
   iv. 1 cm below the pectoral muscle on the MLO

4. If you have tomosynthesis, then only that may be required, unless the lesion happens to be off the image plane. Effectively you have to think first where the asymmetry may possibly lie, then target the appropriate areas. On the MLO, it is seen in the upper half, but this could be either lateral breast or medial breast. The extended views, lateral and medial (XCCL and XCCM), may reveal the location. Otherwise trying additional views may help. Two particular techniques may help as well: (a) stepped obliques and (b) rolled views.

5. Targeted ultrasound should be the first step following mammography to fully characterize the asymmetry, and determine if this is a mass that can be targeted for biopsy. Either FNAC or core biopsy may be appropriate once that has been done. For a small lesion such as this, MRI may not be required for staging purposes, as it is unlikely to influence surgical management.

Pearls

- Evaluate a film for danger areas, if you think that the mammogram is otherwise normal, and a finding is expected (oral exam situations).
- The edges of a film sometimes provide high pick-up rates for incidental cancers, as the dynamic range can be affected at the edge of the receptor. This was much more prevalent in the age of analog mammography.

Suggested Readings

Leung JW, Sickles EA. Developing asymmetry identified on mammography: correlation with imaging outcome and pathologic findings. *AJR Am J Roentgenol.* 2007;188(3):667-675.

Sickles EA. The spectrum of breast asymmetries: imaging features, work-up, management. *Radiol Clin North Am.* 2007;45(5):765-771, v.

Venkatesan A, Chu P, Kerlikowske K, Sickles EA, Smith-Bindman R. Positive predictive value of specific mammographic findings according to reader and patient variables. *Radiology.* 2009;250(3):648-657.

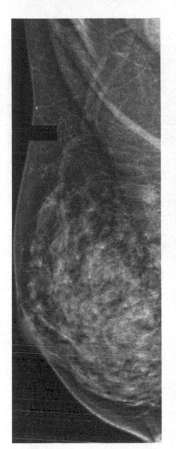
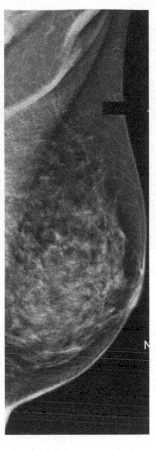
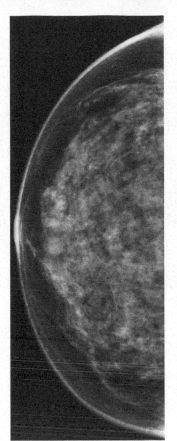
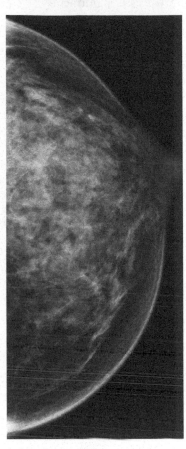

1. What is the finding on the screening mammogram?

2. What is the next step on the screening mammogram?

3. What is the next step in workup?

4. What does the spot compression view (next page) confirm?

5. What do you expect the outcome of an ultrasound scan to be?

Case ranking/difficulty:

Category: Screening

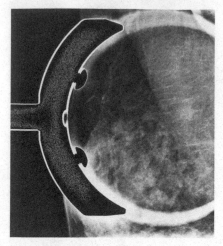

Diagnostic mammogram, right spot compression MLO view demonstrating "focal asymmetry" projecting over the pectoralis muscle.

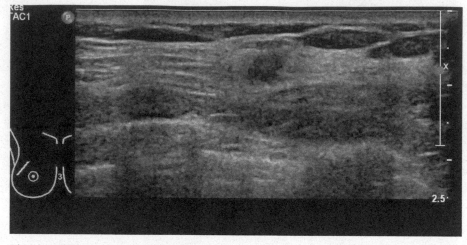

Ultrasound of right breast demonstrates the corresponding, small (5 mm), "irregular"-shaped mass with mixed echogenicity.

Answers

1. Finding is consistent with "focal asymmetry" given its concave shape of the margin—it should not be called mass because it was seen only on one projection.

2. Patient has to be worked up. BI-RADS 3 should never be used on screening mammogram. The only BI-RADS assessment on screening mammogram is BI-RADS 1 (negative).

3. Since it is not clearly seen on CC view and it could be outside the scan field, XCCL view is a good choice—also patient needs spot compression view MLO. ML view could also be added to further assess the localization of the lesion. However, ML view might not be able to get as far back to include the lesion.

4. The spot compression view confirms that the finding is real and needs to be further worked up with ultrasound.

5. Ultrasound confirms the finding of a small "focal asymmetry" and therefore is BI-RADS 4 and biopsy is recommended—and did confirm the presence of invasive ductal carcinoma.

Pearls

- Further evaluation with spot compression MLO view and right XCCL view is the next step. Since the lesion is not definitely seen on the CC view, it could be outside the scan field and additional XCCL view was recommended.
- The "focal asymmetry" was not well seen on the additional XCCL view (not submitted) but persists on the spot compression MLO view and subsequently an ultrasound was performed.
- Ultrasound demonstrates small 7-mm mass with "angular" margin and subsequently ultrasound-guided biopsy was performed for the BI-RADS 4 lesion and showed the presence of invasive ductal carcinoma.

Suggested Reading

Leung JW, Sickles EA. Developing asymmetry identified on mammography: correlation with imaging outcome and pathologic findings. *AJR Am J Roentgenol.* 2007;188(3):667-675.

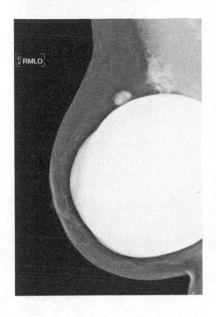
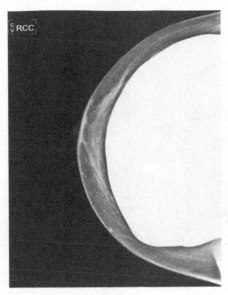
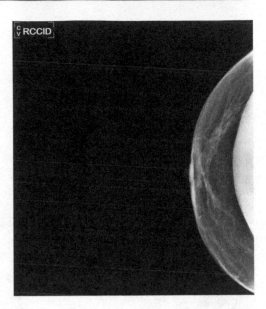

1. What is the abnormality on the mammogram?

2. What is the gold standard modality to assess
   if implant is intact?

3. What is the typical appearance of intracapsular
   rupture on imaging?

4. What are typical signs for extracapsular
   implant rupture?

5. What defines the capsule of the implant?

Case ranking/difficulty:

Category: Screening

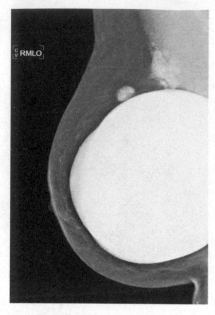

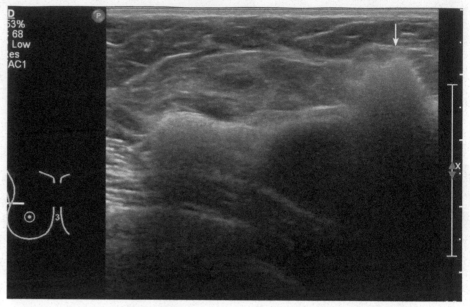

Right screening mammogram MLO view demonstrating extracapsular free silicone in superior right breast.

Ultrasound demonstrates area of abnormal echo with strong posterior shadowing ("snowstorm sign"), correlating to the area of concern seen on the mammogram (*arrow*) consistent with extracapsular rupture.

Answers

1. This is a patient with subglandular, prepectoral silicone implant and two area of high density superior to the implant highly suspicious for extracapsular rupture.

2. The gold standard is breast MRI to prove the presence of silicone implant rupture. It can show intracapsular rupture better than ultrasound. However, it can be tricky to prove subtle intracapsular rupture, since complex folds can have very similar appearance. Extracapsular rupture can be detected on mammogram and ultrasound, but MRI again is the most sensitive and specific exam. For saline implants, there is, in general, no need for imaging to show rupture. A mammogram is sufficient to show deflation of the implants.

3. Intracapsular rupture can be very subtle and is oftentimes more questionable clinical significance. It cannot be detected on mammogram, might show up as "step ladder" sign on ultrasound, and can be diagnosed with confidence if there is a "linguini sign" on MRI. "Step ladder" sign can be called when there are several linear structures that are interrupted, forming steps. "Linguini" sign indicates the presence of multiple linear structures in the implant.

4. Extracapsular implant rupture is the most significant injury to the implant. It might result in symptoms and possible implant replacement. On mammogram, area of high, silicone-like density is seen apart from the implant.

This can be seen on ultrasound as an area of hyperechoic signal with posterior shadowing (snow storm sign). MRI is performed to assess implants without contrast.

5. The capsule is formed as a physiological response in the form of fibrous tissue surrounding the implant. Intracapsular rupture refers to rupture of the shell of the implant, but silicone is defined by the fibrous capsule. Extracapsular rupture is defined by penetration of silicone through the fibrous capsule.

Pearls

- Screening mammograms for patients with breast implant require to add additional so-called implant displacement views bilateral in MLO and CC projections to better assess the breast parenchyma.
- This case demonstrates extracapsular rupture, stable for many years in an asymptomatic patient. In this particular situation, this had no consequence and the implant was not removed.

Suggested Reading

Everson LI, Parantainen H, Detlie T, et al. Diagnosis of breast implant rupture: imaging findings and relative efficiencies of imaging techniques. *AJR Am J Roentgenol.* 1994;163(1):57-60.

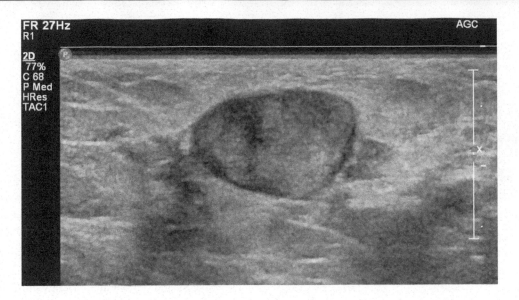

1. What BI-RADS classification should be used here?

2. What mammographic views would you perform?

3. What is the likely pathology of the mass?

4. What is the appropriate diagnostic interventional tool you would recommend?

5. The ultrasound is now shown to contain reflective echoes suggesting microcalcification. What additional test would you perform?

Case ranking/difficulty:

Category: Diagnostic

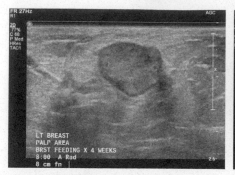

Ultrasound shows gentle lobulations to the mass.

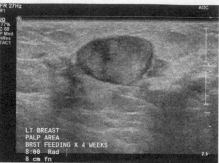

Ultrasound shows the echo pattern to have both hyperechoic debris within the "cyst" and some lower echo areas.

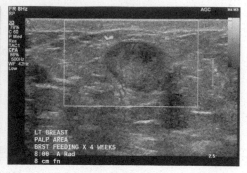

Power Doppler. The lesion is shown to be avascular.

Answers

1. This is not a screening examination, so BI-RADS 0 is not appropriate. The findings within context are benign, but if you are uncertain, or if you are swayed by the lesion being palpable, then give it a BI-RADS 4 and make the diagnosis by aspirating the milky fluid.

2. Unless the ultrasound was suspicious of malignancy, or showed the presence of microcalcification, mammography is usually of extremely low yield. A high kV technique will not improve the chances of seeing through extremely dense breast tissue in a lactating woman.

3. These appearances, in a lactating breast, are of a galactocele. Simple cysts can occur, but are anechoic. Fibroadenomas usually appear as a hypoechoic mass against the bright background glandular tissue. Mucinous carcinoma usually has indistinct margins and occurs in an older age group. Lactational adenoma tends to present during pregnancy itself.

4. Galactoceles are not malignant. Surgical excision is disfiguring, but may be required for lesions that cannot be treated by multiple aspirations. There is inflammatory change associated with galactoceles, and if they leak then they can be a cause of an abscess, which may then need a drain placed. Surgical treatment with healing by granulation would give a horrendous cosmetic effect, and is therefore not performed.

5. You are concerned about the possibility of DCIS; therefore, regardless of age in the presence of a particular suspicious finding on ultrasound, unilateral mammograms should be performed. MRI is unlikely to help, as lactating breasts may enhance so strongly that clumped ductal or linear enhancement would be masked. Elastography has not been shown to be of help in this situation yet. PEM and BSGI are isotope-based tests that should be avoided in a nursing mother wherever possible.

Pearls

- Galactoceles are common findings toward the end of breast feeding in lactating women.
- Diagnosis is usually by ultrasound and possibly aspiration that shows milk.
- Surgical treatment is usually avoided.
- Multiple aspirations are a better alternative.

Suggested Readings

Engohan-Aloghe C, Bucella D, Boutemy R, Noël JC. Giant galactocele in a lactating woman [in French]. *Ann Pathol.* 2008;28(6):526-528.

Perez-Bóscollo AC, Dutra RA, Borges LG, et al. Galactocele: an unusual cause of breast enlargement in children. *J Pediatr Surg.* 2009;44(7):e1-e3.

Sabate JM, Clotet M, Torrubia S, et al. Radiologic evaluation of breast disorders related to pregnancy and lactation. *Radiographics.* 2007;27(Suppl 1):S101-S124.

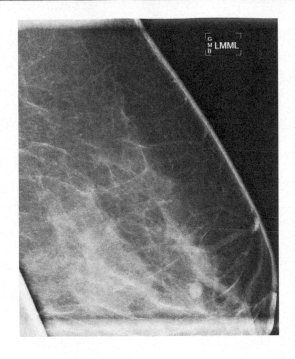 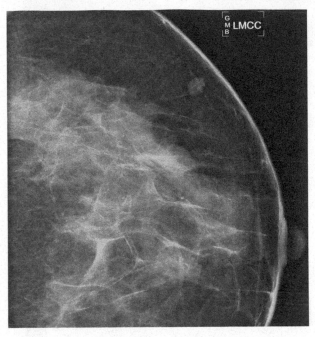

1. How would you describe the calcifications in the left breast?

2. What is the assessment if the calcifications are new?

3. What would be the assessment if the calcifications are seen on first mammogram?

4. What are other findings on a first mammogram typically called benign?

5. What are other findings on first mammogram that after diagnostic workup can be called probably benign?

Case ranking/difficulty:

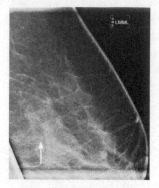

Diagnostic mammogram, left ML magnification view.

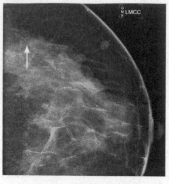

Diagnostic mammogram, left CC magnification view.

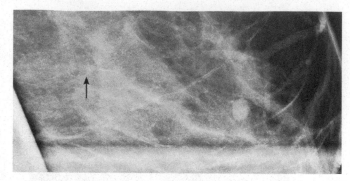

Diagnostic mammogram, left magnification ML view (additional electronic magnification) demonstrating group of "round and oval" calcifications.

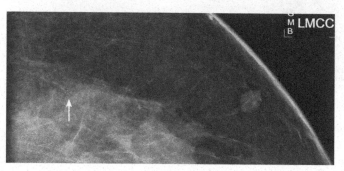

Diagnostic mammogram, left CC view (additional electronic magnification).

Answers

1. This is a group of "oval and round" calcifications.

2. A new group of "round and oval" calcifications is suspicious and can be called BI-RADS 4 and biopsy should be performed.

3. This finding of a group of calcification, oval and round on first screening mammogram, after diagnostic workup, is a typical BI-RADS 3 finding and 6-month follow-up can be recommended. After 2 years of stability, they can be called benign.

4. Only the mole and the popcorn-type calcifications can be called benign on a screening mammogram; Popcorn-type calcifications, typical eggshell type calcifications or secretory calcifications can be called benign on a screening mammogram.

5. There are three classical BI-RADS 3 findings on first mammogram after diagnostic workup: a "focal asymmetry," "round well-circumscribed mass," and "oval and round" calcifications. The diagnostic workup of the mass and the asymmetry does include ultrasound.

Pearls

- Treatment of patients with diagnosis of lobular carcinoma in situ (LCIS) or atypical lobular hyperplasia (ALH) is controversial.
- Since upgrade to invasive carcinoma or DCIS after diagnosis of LCIS or ALH was reported to be between 17% and 30%, there is increasing consensus to perform surgical excision of the area after diagnosis on core needle biopsy.

Suggested Readings

Choi BB, Kim SH, Park CS, Cha ES, Lee AW. Radiologic findings of lobular carcinoma in situ: mammography and ultrasonography. *J Clin Ultrasound*. 2011;39(2):59-63.

Foster MC, Helvie MA, Gregory NE, Rebner M, Nees AV, Paramagul C. Lobular carcinoma in situ or atypical lobular hyperplasia at core-needle biopsy: is excisional biopsy necessary? *Radiology*. 2004;231(3):813-819.

Hussain M, Cunnick GH. Management of lobular carcinoma in-situ and atypical lobular hyperplasia of the breast—a review. *Eur J Surg Oncol*. 2011;37(4):279-289.

Lump found in armpit while washing

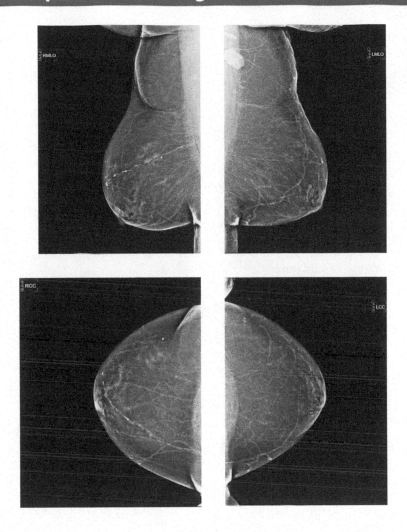

1. What BI-RADS classification should be used here?

2. What is the most likely pathology based on the imaging?

3. What is the next best imaging test?

4. What are the physical findings of a hamartoma?

5. What would be the best way to biopsy this lesion.

Case ranking/difficulty:

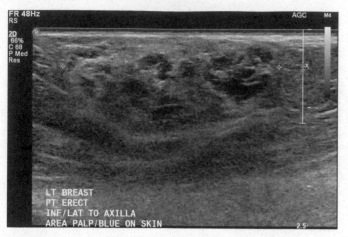

Mixed echo mass with a capsule. Mixture of solid and cystic elements. Ultrasonographically would fit with a hamartoma, with a predominantly solid component, but the mammographic appearances do not fit and it was hard on physical examination, and therefore a biopsy was performed, which revealed the diagnosis.

Answers

1. This was a hard lump to palpate the lower axilla, which does not look like a standard lymph node, as it neither is smooth in contour nor has a hilum. Ultrasound is needed for further evaluation.

2. The mass does not look like a lymph node or accessory breast tissue. Invasive lobular carcinoma usually presents with minimal change of distortion. DCIS usually presents with microcalcifications, although it can present with a mass, which usually is hypoechoic and circumscribed (simulates fibroadenoma).

3. The cheapest and nonionizing examination is ultrasound, which can be targeted to the palpable or mammographic abnormality. If tomosynthesis has already been performed, the margins of the mass may have been identified.

4. A hamartoma is composed of normal breast tissue (think of breast within a breast). As a result, physical examination either is normal or shows a soft mass.

5. FNAC may not give a definitive answer, and relies on your site having trained cytopathology staff. Core biopsy of either type may work here. Surgical excision should be avoided if possible, until a preop diagnosis has been obtained. Punch biopsy is good only for dermal lesions.

Pearls

- Rare, special type of variant IDC.
- Poorer prognosis.
- May appear with relatively benign imaging appearances.

Suggested Readings

Choi BB, Shu KS. Metaplastic carcinoma of the breast: multimodality imaging and histopathologic assessment. *Acta Radiol.* 2012;53(1):5-11.

Joshi D, Singh P, Zonunfawni Y, Gangane N. Metaplastic carcinoma of the breast: cytological diagnosis and diagnostic pitfalls. *Acta Cytol.* 2011;55(4):313-318.

Nonnis R, Paliogiannis P, Giangrande D, Marras V, Trignano M. Low-grade fibromatosis-like spindle cell metaplastic carcinoma of the breast: a case report and literature review. *Clin Breast Cancer.* 2012;12(2):147-150.

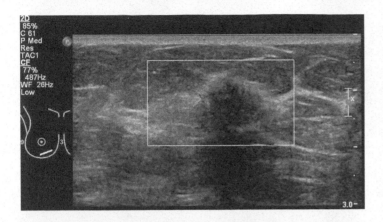
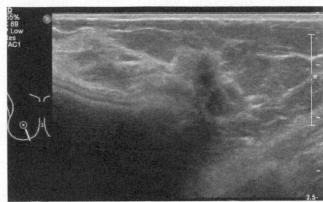
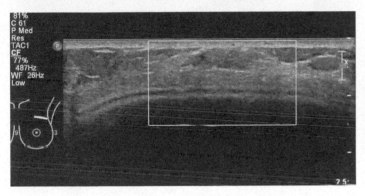
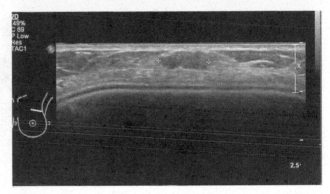

1. What could be the next step to evaluate multiple indeterminate masses?

2. What is the description of the finding in the two figures (left and right) on the top?

3. What is the best way to biopsy a lesion when patient has implants?

4. What is a tubular adenoma?

5. What is the consequence of biopsy demonstrating tubular adenoma?

Case ranking/difficulty:

Category: Diagnostic

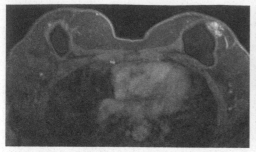

MRI T1-weighted sequence after IV contrast demonstrating heterogeneously enhancing mass in the left superior breast near implant.

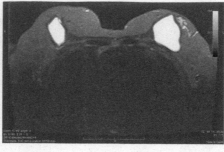

MRI T2-weighted sequence demonstrating mass high in signal near implant left breast.

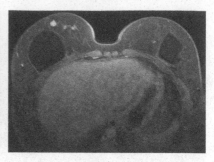

MRI T1-weighted sequence after IV contrast demonstrating mass in the right inferior breast.

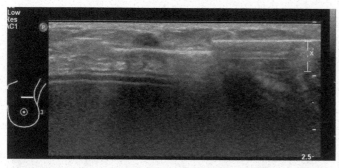

Ultrasound-guided biopsy of the abnormality in the left superior breast as seen on ultrasound, which correlates to MRI.

Answers

1. Any finding—if masses, calcifications, and so on—scattered bilaterally decreases the suspicion for malignancy. MRI is a helpful problem-solving modality to determine which of the abnormalities is more concerning.

2. "Hypoechoic" mass, hypoechoic in comparison with the anterior fat, demonstrates posterior shadowing.

3. Ultrasound-guided biopsy is the best way to biopsy lesion when patient has breast implant, since it is done in real time and needle can be inserted more flexibly than it is by MRI or stereotactic biopsy.

4. Tubular adenoma is a proliferative change similar to fibroadenoma but with more tubular and less stromal elements. It is a benign lesion.

5. This is benign proliferative change—no need for further treatment.

Pearls

- Tubular adenoma, phyllodes tumor, and lactating adenoma are all entities related to fibroadenoma.
- This is an example that ultrasound-guided biopsy can be performed safely in patients with implants; in this case, patient had bilateral saline implants.

Suggested Reading

Barsky, Gradishar, Recht, et al. *The Breast.* 4th ed. Philadelphia, PA: Saunders Elsevier; 2009.

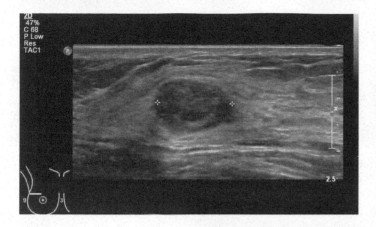

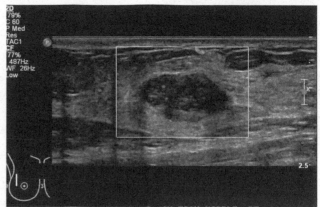

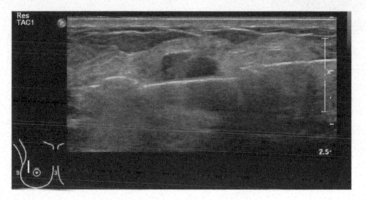

1. What is the first exam when a 23-year-old patient reports palpable lump?

2. What is the next step if ultrasound does not demonstrate any abnormality?

3. What is the management of a palpable mass that has benign features on ultrasound?

4. What would be the management, if multiple masses are seen?

5. What other histology could have findings similar to fibroadenoma?

Case ranking/difficulty:

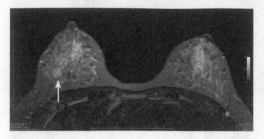

MRI, T2-weighted images demonstrate mass in the right lateral breast with mild increased signal on T2-weighted images.

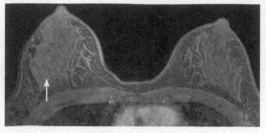

MRI, T1-weighted sequence after IV contrast demonstrates no enhancement within the mass. The mass demonstrates low signal.

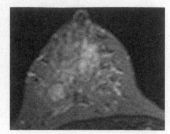

MRI, T2-weighted sequence demonstrates mass with septations of low signal, as described as "dark septations."

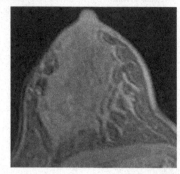

MRI, T1-weighted sequence demonstrates mass without enhancement.

Answers

1. The first step is ultrasound. Mammography is avoided—because of the fact that young patients are more sensitive to radiation—and that in this age there is, very dense fibroglandular tissue that limits the value of mammography. Mammography would be the second step if ultrasound does not explain the palpable abnormality. Five percent of all breast cancers occur in the age group younger than 40 years. These are usually the more aggressive tumors.

2. Next step is to perform a mammogram. While some breast imagers would argue that one single image—for example, a MLO view—would be good enough, while some would favor even to perform a bilateral baseline exam. The former would argue that the lack of a mass on ultrasound makes the presence of mass on mammogram very unlikely and the purpose of the mammogram would be to find calcifications. This can be achieved by one view only. The latter point of view is that focal asymmetries might be missed on an ultrasound and on a single view mammogram. A reasonable approach is to start with a unilateral standard mammogram first and if there is any remaining concern then to include the contralateral side.

3. If mass is palpable—despite benign features on imaging—conservative approach is to call it suspicious

and to perform biopsy (BI-RADS 4) or send patient to surgical excision. However, Harvey et al. published in 2009 a paper arguing that follow-up of palpable masses is more cost-effective and safe.

4. If there are additional incidental masses found at the time of ultrasound, ultrasound-guided biopsy can be performed for the palpable mass and the remainder of the masses can be followed in 6 months. This would also apply if a patient on a "screening ultrasound" presents with incidental finding of benign-appearing mass. We would call it BI-RADS 3 and follow it in 6 months. If there are multiple benign appearing palpable masses it is not practical to biopsy several masses and can be followed.

5. Papillomas or even malignancies such as mucinous carcinomas, tubular and medullary carcinomas and can be well circumscribed.

Pearls

- Palpable masses in young patients are not uncommon, and if it correlates to a benign-appearing mass, most likely fibroadenoma, management is controversial.
- A more conservative approach is to recommend biopsy or surgical excision.
- If the mass does show all typical findings of fibroadenoma, the other, not infrequently used, approach is to follow the mass over 2 or 3 years.

Suggested Reading

Harvey JA, Nicholson BT, Lorusso AP, Cohen MA, Bovbjerg VE. Short-term follow-up of palpable breast lesions with benign imaging features: evaluation of 375 lesions in 320 women. *AJR Am J Roentgenol.* 2009;193(6):1723-1730.

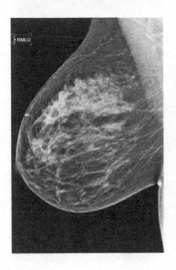 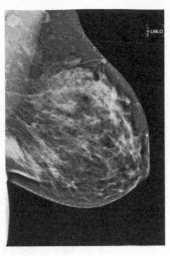 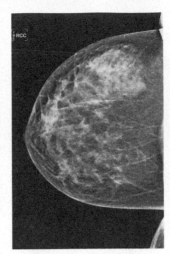 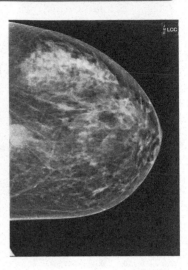

1. What is the BI-RADS category for this screening exam?

2. What are the "danger areas" in mammography?

3. What is the positive predictive value of a developing focal asymmetry?

4. What is the definition of a focal asymmetry?

5. What is the best imaging examination in the workup of this patient?

Case ranking/difficulty:

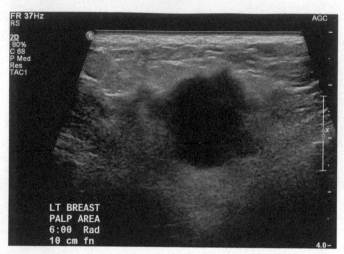

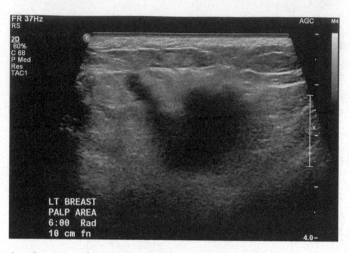

Although this mass appears round on mammography (a benign descriptor), it has "angular margins" on ultrasound (a suspicious descriptor).

Another view of the same mass shows that there is "duct extension," which is extending anteriorly to the surface of the glandular tissue.

Answers

1. This patient has an asymmetry in the lower half of the left breast in the inferior mammary fold, which is a well-known "danger area." As the patient needs workup with further films and ultrasound, this patient should be given a BI-RADS 0.

2. There are four main danger areas: (a) The immediate prepectoral area, where we frequently see intramammary lymph nodes. If a mass develops or there is a mass without a hilum, you should be suspicious and work the thing up. (b) The inferior mammary fold: although it is not uncommon for a developing sebaceous cyst to mimic the development of a carcinoma at this site. (c) Medial aspect of the breast on a CC film. (d) Subareolar—often difficult to pick up a mass in this area, which typically has a lot going on.

3. UCSF data showed that the PPV for a developing asymmetry was 12%, and that if not a skin lesion such as a sebaceous cyst, then it deserves a full workup and biopsy.

4. The definition of a focal asymmetry is a density present on two views (ie, localized to a part of the breast). An asymmetry is a density that is not a space-occupying lesion, on one projection only (either CC or MLO). A space-occupying lesion is a mass rather than an asymmetry or focal asymmetry.

5. If you are unlikely to get better images of the area, and you have a mass lesion, going direct to ultrasound to characterize the lesion works well. Tomosynthesis or spot views (+/− magnification) can be performed for more complete mammographic workup. This lesion may be adherent to the chest wall, and if there is any doubt, an MRI could be performed, but this is not the best first-line exam in this case.

Pearls

- Inferior mammary fold is a danger area for developing malignancy.
- A developing asymmetry in this area should be taken seriously.

Suggested Readings

Leung JW, Sickles EA. Developing asymmetry identified on mammography: correlation with imaging outcome and pathologic findings. *AJR Am J Roentgenol.* 2007;188(3):667-675.

Sickles EA. The spectrum of breast asymmetries: imaging features, work-up, management. *Radiol Clin North Am.* 2007;45(5):765-771, v.

Venkatesan A, Chu P, Kerlikowske K, Sickles EA, Smith-Bindman R. Positive predictive value of specific mammographic findings according to reader and patient variables. *Radiology.* 2009;250(3):648-657.

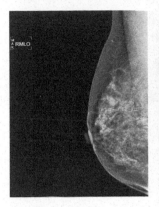 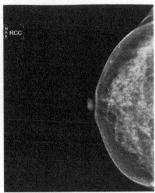 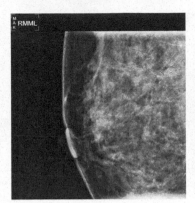 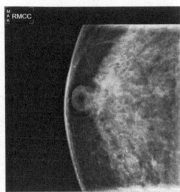

1. What is the best description of the calcifications?

2. What is the best management?

3. What is the consequence if the pathology shows adenosis?

4. How good is mammography to detect recurrent DCIS and how likely is the recurrence of DCIS?

5. What is the prognosis of recurrent DCIS after lumpectomy?

Case ranking/difficulty:

Category: Diagnostic

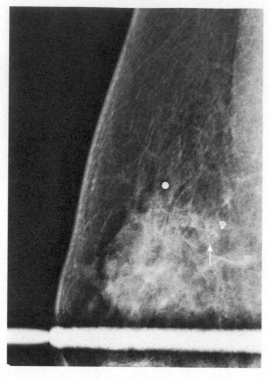

Postlumpectomy mammogram, right ML magnification view.

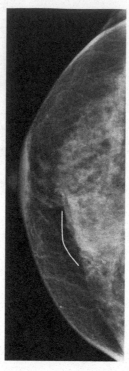

Postlumpectomy mammogram, right CC view with scar marker. Calcifications not covered.

Answers

1. This is an example of a group of "pleomorphic" calcifications in segmental distribution.

2. The best workup would include, at this point, ultrasound to assess possible invasive solid component—if ultrasound does not show solid component, stereotactic biopsy is the next step, since the finding is highly suspicious (BI-RADS 5). MRI would be helpful preoperative to assess for additional disease; lumpectomy is the most likely surgical treatment.

3. Since a new group of pleomorphic calcifications can be classified as BI-RADS 5 (highly suspicious), it has to be excised—even if pathology after stereotactic biopsy demonstrates a "benign" findings.

4. Mammography is very effective (97% sensitivity) to detect recurrent DCIS at lumpectomy site. This is in particular true, since recurrent calcifications due to recurrent DCIS in general present with same morphology of the initial calcifications. Recurrence rate is about 7% at 5 years after lumpectomy and not significantly different from mastectomy.

5. Prognosis of recurrent DCIS in lumpectomy bed is usually excellent and most likely stage 0 or 1.

Pearls

- Most patients who presented with calcifications consistent with DCIS at the time of initial diagnosis and who develop recurrence will present with suspicious calcifications as well at the time of recurrence.
- Mammography is very effective in detecting recurrence (sensitivity of 97%).
- Recurrent malignancy of DCIS is in general stage 0 or 1 and therefore the prognosis is excellent.
- In 90% of the cases, the morphology of the recurrent calcifications is similar to the morphology of the initial calcifications.
- Mean time between the initial diagnosis and recurrence is about 4.5 years with range from 1 to 12 years and clustering between 1 and 7 years.

Suggested Reading

Pinsky RW, Rebner M, Pierce LJ, et al. Recurrent cancer after breast-conserving surgery with radiation therapy for ductal carcinoma in situ: mammographic features, method of detection, and stage of recurrence. *AJR Am J Roentgenol.* 2007;189(1):140-144.

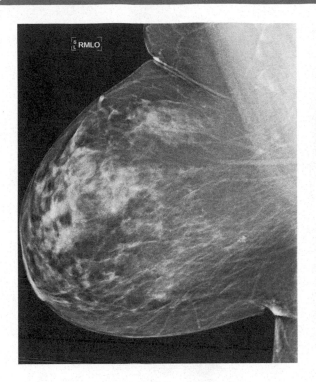
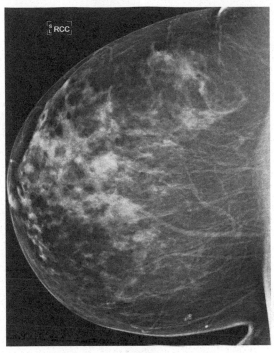

1. What is the finding on the mammogram?

2. If the histology is tubular adenoma, in this case, what is your next step?

3. Why do some authors suggest that there is no need for 6-month follow-up after benign concordant biopsy?

4. What is the difference between tubular adenoma and fibroadenoma?

5. What is the difference between tubular adenoma and lactating adenoma?

Case ranking/difficulty:

Category: Diagnostic

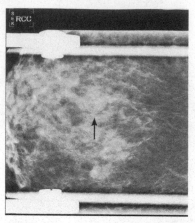

Diagnostic mammogram, spot compression right CC view confirming mass in the right breast subareolar in location.

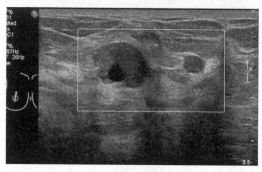

Ultrasound with duplex demonstrating mass with increased flow.

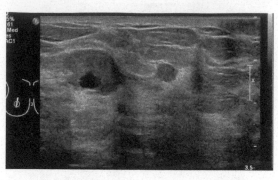

Gray-scale ultrasound images demonstrating corresponding mass.

Answers

1. Noted is a "partially obscured" mass in the right upper outer quadrant of the right breast. It is best appreciated on the CC view. Additional spot compression view confirms "well-circumscribed" margin of the mass.

2. This is a concordant benign finding and 6-month follow-up is, in general, the standard in most practices.

3. The likelihood of malignancy in a screening population is about 3 to 4 per 1000, which is 0.3% to 0.4%. The likelihood of malignancy less than 2% is considered as probably benign (BI-RADS 3). Salkowski et al. (2011) found that PPV of rebiopsy did not differ between 6 and 12 months after benign and concordant biopsy and that the incidence of malignancy was close to normal incidence in screening population.

4. Tubular adenoma has less stromal and more epithelial elements.

5. It is believed that both are similar lesions in different physiologic states of the patient. Lactating adenoma is found in pregnant or breast-feeding women, whereas tubular adenoma is found in premenopausal females. Some theories believe that tubular adenomas are present before pregnancy and then appear as lactating adenomas during pregnancy.

Pearls

- Tubular adenoma and lactating adenoma are histologically similar lesions, related to fibroadenoma, seen in different phases of life. Tubular adenomas occur during reproductive years and lactating adenomas occur during lactation and during pregnancy.
- Tubular adenomas are indistinguishable from fibroadenomas on imaging.
- Tubular adenomas have, in comparison with fibroadenomas, almost no stromal components but only epithelial components and can undergo infarction and may produce acoustic shadowing.
- Necessity of 6-month follow-up after benign and concordant biopsy is debatable—according to Salkowski et al. (2011), rebiopsy rate was 0.8% at 6-month interval and 0.5% at 12-month interval.

Suggested Readings

Salkowski LR, Fowler AM, Burnside ES, Sisney GA. Utility of 6-month follow-up imaging after a concordant benign breast biopsy result. *Radiology*. 2011;258(2):380-387.

Stavros AT. Breast Ultrasound. 1st ed. Philadelphia; PA: Lippincott Williams & Wilkins; 2004.

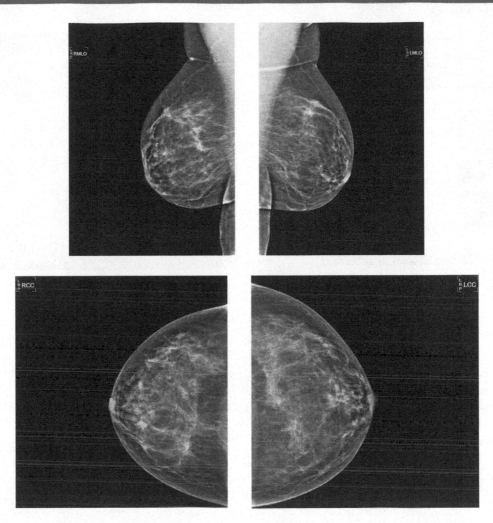

1. What is the BI-RADS category for this screening exam?

2. What additional mammographic views do you recommend?

3. Is there another test that should also be performed?

4. Is this a mass or a type of asymmetry?

5. If this patient has a history of prior right-sided breast surgery, what is the differential diagnosis?

Case ranking/difficulty:

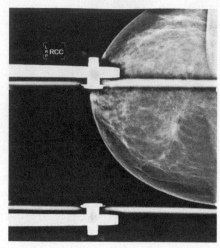

RCC spot magnification pushes away normal tissue and allows the mass to be seen more clearly.

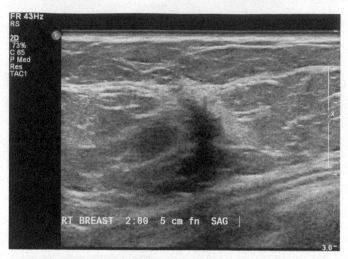

Ultrasound shows "irregular mass" with "ill-defined margins," taller than wide ("not parallel").

Answers

1. There is a focal asymmetry in the right breast, which needs further workup. BI-RADS 4 or 5 should not be used for a screening exam, as the patient may have fat necrosis, or a benign finding including superimposition to account for the findings. If given a BI-RADS 4 or 5, and referred to a surgeon, these often end up in surgery for biopsy or treatment, without tissue biopsy.

2. Although there is an argument for performing the above views, simply performing a lateral exam (in the projection with the abnormality nearest to the bucky) and spot views may be all that is required. Many breast imagers recommend that if you perform spot films, you should also do it with magnification to get the best possible resolution, and to further characterize the calcific particles or margins of a mass.

3. Use of a cheap nonionizing exam such as ultrasound is the most useful first-line additional modality in this situation.

4. Unless there is definite space-occupying lesion, then it should be called a focal asymmetry rather than a mass at this point. Spot films and ultrasound may assist to further identify if this is truly a mass. If visible in one plane, it should be called an asymmetry rather than a focal asymmetry.

5. Regardless of the history, the findings of a focal asymmetry in the absence of evidence on prior films mean that the patient should be worked up. If the patient

has had surgery, repeat mammograms with a scar marker may be helpful to differentiate. Fat necrosis is more likely if fat lucency is present, associated with the scar, or with characteristic dystrophic calcifications. Cancer recurrence should be suspected if the scar is getting denser over time.

Pearls

- Treat medial densities, especially if developing, with caution.
- Do full workup.
- Have a low threshold for biopsy.

Suggested Readings

Leung JW, Sickles EA. Developing asymmetry identified on mammography: correlation with imaging outcome and pathologic findings. *AJR Am J Roentgenol.* 2007;188(3):667-675.

Sickles EA. The spectrum of breast asymmetries: imaging features, work-up, management. *Radiol Clin North Am.* 2007;45(5):765-671, v.

Venkatesan A, Chu P, Kerlikowske K, Sickles EA, Smith-Bindman R. Positive predictive value of specific mammographic findings according to reader and patient variables. *Radiology.* 2009;250(3):648-657.

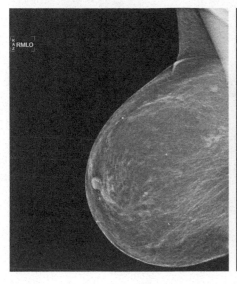 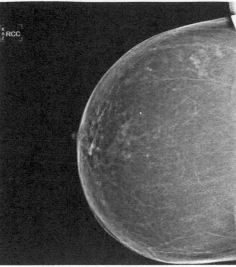 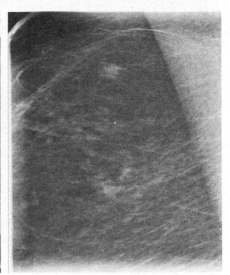

1. What is the appropriate workup of a new asymmetry?

2. What is the next step after finding of a hyperechoic mass?

3. What would be the next step if ultrasound was normal?

4. What is the most likely histology for a hyperechoic mass?

5. What is the most likely histology if there is a suspicious corresponding finding on mammogram?

Case ranking/difficulty: **Category:** Diagnostic

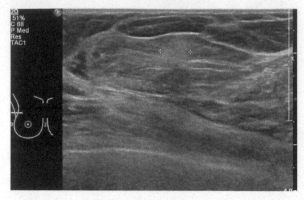

Ultrasound directed to the area with corresponding finding. Hyperechoic mass, slightly "irregular" in shape.

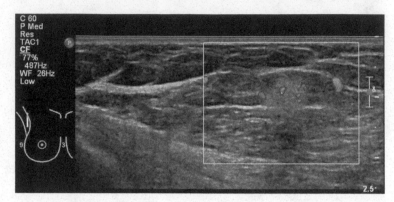

Ultrasound with duplex with corresponding mass with increased flow on duplex.

Answers

1. Next steps are spot compression views, MLO, and CC followed by ultrasound.

2. Despite the fact that hyperechoic masses seen on ultrasound are overwhelmingly benign—if "hyperechoic" mass correlates to a new "focal density" on mammogram—it needs to be biopsied, especially if it presents with "irregular margins."

3. Given that the density was not seen on prior study, this is suspicious and biopsy is recommended.

4. The majority of findings will be benign. If there is no corresponding denisty on mammogram it could be a lipoma, differential diagnosis could include fat necrosis or hematoma.

5. Metastasis, liposarcoma, angiosarcoma, and lymphoma are very rare entities—given the suspicious morphology (new density), the most likely malignancy will be invasive ductal carcinoma.

Pearls

- Findings on ultrasound, which are hyperechoic, are in general not very likely to represent malignancy—according to Linda et al. (2011), of 1849 biopsied lesions showing malignancy, only 9 were hyperechoic.
- However, if hyperechoic lesion corresponds to new mammogram finding or is palpable, biopsy is strongly recommended.
- Malignant hyperechoic lesions include lymphoma, angiosarcoma, metastasis, however, the most likely pathology would be an invasive ductal carcinoma.
- None of the nine hyperechoic malignancies described by Linda et al. (2011) was a purely sonographic lesion.

Suggested Reading

Linda A, Zuiani C, Lorenzon M, et al. Hyperechoic lesions of the breast: not always benign. *AJR Am J Roentgenol*. 2011;196(5):1219-1224.

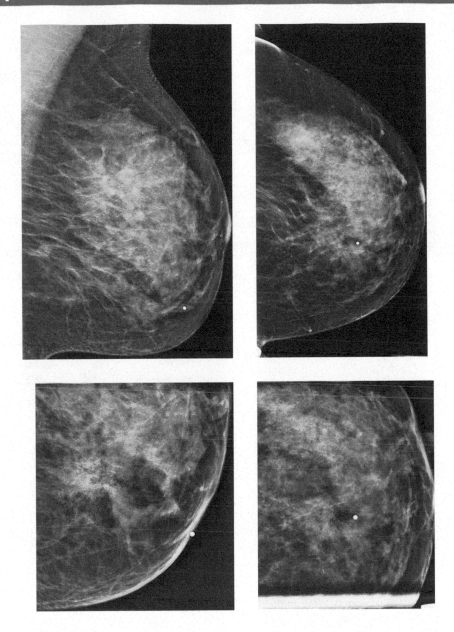

1. What is the pertinent mammogram finding?

2. What is the next step?

3. What is a radial scar?

4. What is the consequence if pathology demonstrates radial scar?

5. Is MRI of any help in the assessment of radial scar?

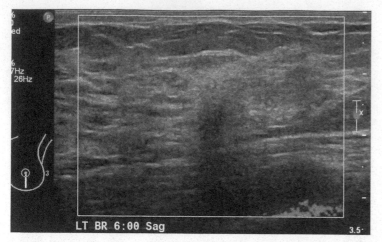

Ultrasound duplex demonstrating "irregular" mass with "spiculation."

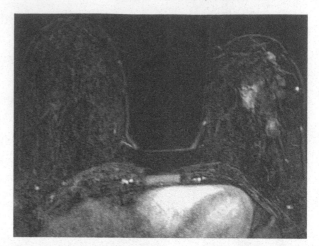

MRI, postcontrast, subtracted images demonstrating area of increased enhancement in the left central inferior breast correlating to the mammogram and ultrasound.

Answers

1. Noted is a subtle area of architectural distortion in the left inferior breast as best seen on the spot compression views.

2. Next step is ultrasound. It is also important to correlate the findings with possible history of prior surgery or biopsy.

3. Radial scar has been described in the literature under several different names, such as "radial sclerosing lesion" and "complex sclerosing lesion." It is a form of benign proliferative breast tissue, which mainly consists of ductal elements. This results in tubular structures/focal asymmetry on mammography.

4. Despite the fact that radial scars are a form of benign proliferative disease, excisional biopsy is recommended since it is associated with a malignancy rate of up to 40% on surgical excision. The recommended reason for excision is also due to the fact that radial scar is usually extending outside the sample obtained by the core biopsy.

5. MRI is not very specific. If there is enhancement, it does not indicate that there is malignancy. However, it can screen for additional malignancy in the breast. It is not established at this point if biopsy-proven radial scar could be left alone and MRI does not show enhance. After biopsy, there is, in general, always some iatrogenic enhancement that impairs assessment.

Pearls

- Radial scar is a benign proliferative lesion characterized by a central fibroelastotic core with ducts and lobules radiating outward, giving lesion typical stellate appearance.
- Literature suggests that radial scars are associated with surrounding malignancy in up to 40% at the time of surgical excision.
- MRI cannot predict the likelihood of associated malignancy.
- Surgical excision is recommended after the diagnosis of radial scar on all core biopsies, including MRI-guided biopsy.

Suggested Readings

Linda A, Zuiani C, Furlan A, et al. Radial scars without atypia diagnosed at imaging-guided needle biopsy: how often is associated malignancy found at subsequent surgical excision, and do mammography and sonography predict which lesions are malignant? *AJR Am J Roentgenol.* 2010;194(4):1146-1151.

Sringel RM, Eby PR, Demartini WB, et al. Frequency, upgrade rates, and characteristics of high-risk lesions initially identified with breast MRI. *AJR Am J Roentgenol.* 2010;195(3):792-798.

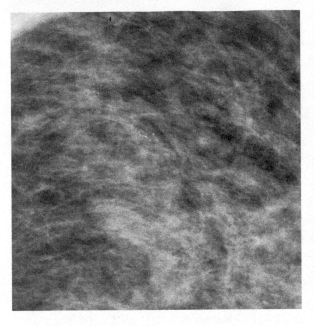 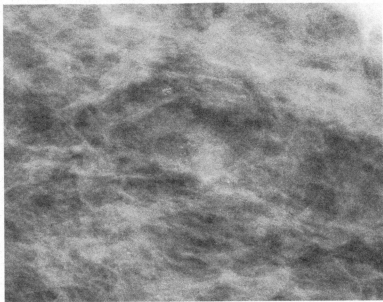

1. Which of the BI-RADS descriptors most accurately represents the findings?

2. What is the most likely pathology based on the imaging?

3. What is the next best imaging test?

4. What are the biochemical types of calcifications found in the breast?

5. Which compartment of the breast are these calcifications likely to originate?

Answers

1. Although some of the individual calcific particles have a round or curvilinear margin, the best description here would be amorphous. BI-RADS is still the best lexicon we have for the description of calcium in the United States.

2. These types of calcifications are commonly found in benign breast conditions, but can also be associated with lobular neoplasia because the biopsy was prompted. Low-grade DCIS calcifications are very similar to benign causes of calcifications, and if your threshold for biopsy is set too high, you may miss diagnoses of low-grade DCIS.

3. If the calcification looks like DCIS, and the patients have dense breast tissue, then an ultrasound may be a good test to determine if it is an associated mass. Targeting the mass will also increase the yield for invasive cancer, if present. If you suspect DCIS, some say that you should perform MRI to determine extent and any associated mass to assist targeting biopsy. Best test would be to perform a stereotactic core biopsy.

4. Calcium particles can be made up of virtually any calcium salt found in the body. Calcium pyrophosphate and calcium oxalate may be difficult to see on pathology without polarizing light because of their birefringence.

5. These types of amorphous calcifications are indeterminate and are found in a variety of compartments within the breast. The terminal ductal lobular unit is a common site, as is the stroma in simple calcifications associated with diseases such as sclerosing adenosis. Calcifications within ducts frequently represent DCIS. Differential is secretory calcifications that have a characteristic appearance.

Pearls

- Specimen x-ray can see calcifications but may not be appreciated on conventional pathology stains.
- They are not pink-staining crystals as H&E stain.
- Need polarized light to identify birefringent calcifications.

Suggested Readings

Corben AD, Edelweiss M, Brogi E. Challenges in the interpretation of breast core biopsies. *Breast J.* 2010;16 (Suppl 1):S5-S9.

Grimes MM, Karageorge LS, Hogge JP. Does exhaustive search for microcalcifications improve diagnostic yield in stereotactic core needle breast biopsies? *Mod Pathol.* 2001;14(4):350-353.

Tornos C, Silva E, el-Naggar A, Pritzker KP. Calcium oxalate crystals in breast biopsies. The missing microcalcifications. *Am J Surg Pathol.* 1990;14(10):961-968.

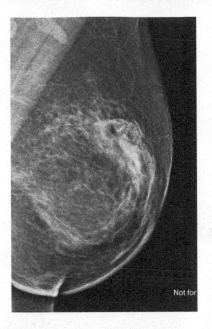
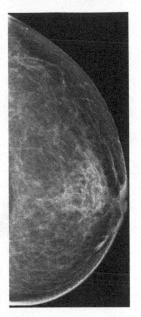

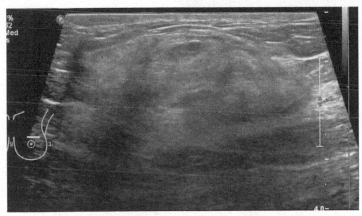
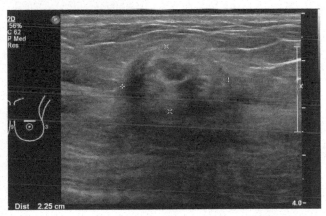

1. What is the most likely reason for palpable lump?

2. What are the features of fat necrosis on ultrasound?

3. What are the features of fat necrosis on MRI?

4. What is the time frame when fat necrosis occurs after lumpectomy?

5. What are the features of fat necrosis on mammogram?

Case ranking/difficulty:

Category: Diagnostic

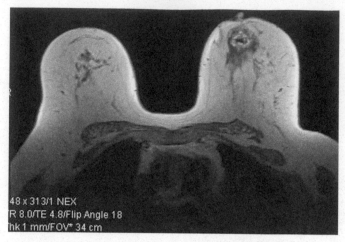

MRI of the breast, non–fat-suppressed T1-weighted images showing mass in the left breast containing fat.

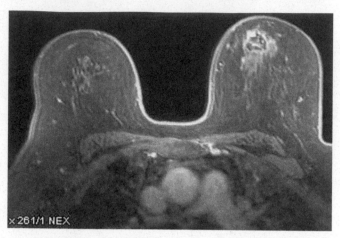

Fat-suppressed postgadolinium image showing enhancement in the periphery of the mass with mixed kinetics.

Answers

1. Mammogram fails to show any suspicious abnormality. Ultrasound demonstrates heterogeneous mass with posterior shadowing. Given the history of recent benign biopsy with vacuum-assisted 9-gauge device, this is most consistent with fat necrosis.

2. Fat necrosis again can show up in many different forms. Well-circumscribed mass may be classified as BI-RADS 3, while heterogeneous mass or ill-defined masses are unspecific and malignancy is difficult to exclude.

3. MRI can be relatively specific if there is fat identified within the abnormality. The enhancement kinetics can be very different and are not specific.

4. Fat necrosis can occur almost any time after surgery. More than 3 years after surgery, however, is unusual.

5. Fat necrosis can present in many different forms. Some findings are specific and can be classified as BI-RADS 2 (benign), for example, fat-containing oil cysts and curvilinear calcifications associated with "radiolucent mass." Some findings are more indeterminate such as "coarse and heterogeneous" calcifications. Some findings cannot be differentiated from malignancy and biopsy cannot be avoided, for example, in case of spiculated mass. MRI can be helpful in this particular case, if there is at least a time period of 6 months since biopsy.

Pearls

- Fat necrosis may be due to trauma, prior biopsy, or surgery.
- It can appear as long as 3 years after surgery.
- Appearance on imaging depends on the amount of fibrotic reaction. No fibrosis results in oil cyst—more fibrotic reaction results in fat necrosis and is difficult to differentiate from malignancy.
- MRI can be specific if fat signal is identified.

Suggested Readings

Solomon B, Orel S, Reynolds C, Schnall M. Delayed development of enhancement in fat necrosis after breast conservation therapy: a potential pitfall of MR imaging of the breast. *AJR Am J Roentgenol.* 1998;170(4):966-968.

Taboada JL, Stephens TW, Krishnamurthy S, Brandt KR, Whitman GJ. The many faces of fat necrosis in the breast. *AJR Am J Roentgenol.* 2009;192(3):815-825.

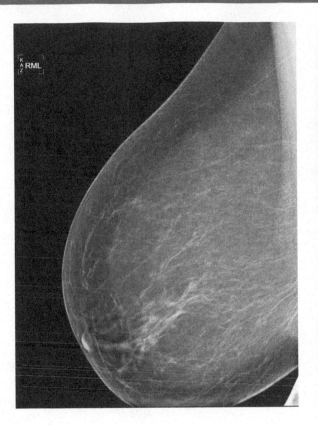
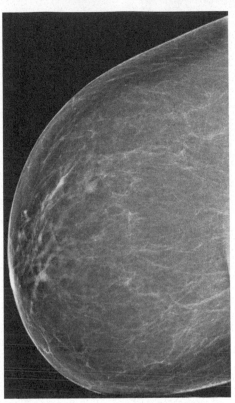

1. What is the pertinent finding?

2. What is juvenile papillomatosis?

3. What is the recommendation after biopsy showing papilloma?

4. What is the management of the incidental finding of "juvenile papillomatosis"?

5. What are the typical imaging features of a papilloma?

Case ranking/difficulty:

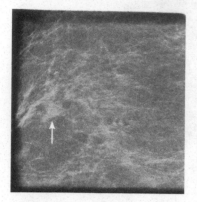

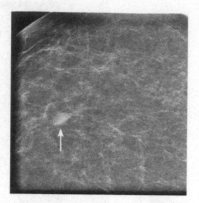

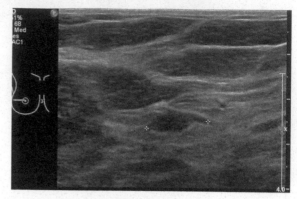

Diagnostic mammogram, right spot compression MLO view confirming the presence of small mass.

Diagnostic mammogram, right spot compression CC view confirming small "well-circumscribed" mass.

Ultrasound, right lateral breast demonstrating small mass with "ductal extension" (Stavros).

Answers

1. Noted is the focal asymmetry in the right lateral breast.

2. Proliferative breast change with the presence of ductal hyperplasia and multiple associated cysts in young patients. Patients oftentimes have family history of breast cancer and increased risk of developing breast cancer in older age.

3. Since there is evidence that by surgical excision a "benign" papilloma gets upgraded to malignancy in more than 2% (definition of BI-RADS 3), surgical excision is recommended. However, the issue remains controversial, and in some institutions not all "benign papillomas" (without atypia, etc.) get surgically resected.

4. Patients with juvenile papillomatosis have likely an increased risk of breast cancer affecting their family as well as an approximately threefold increased personal risk of breast cancer. It is debatable if additional screening with breast MRI should be recommended.

5. It is a benign lesion related to the ductal system, which oftentimes causes nipple discharge. It is being debated if centrally located papillomas have a higher risk of malignancy than papilloma in the periphery.

- This is based on recent publications suggesting upgrading of papillomas in up to 16% after surgical excision, in particular of centrally located papillomas.
- Papillomas in the periphery, located in the terminal ductal lobular units (TDLU), are less likely to cause nipple discharge and are supposed to have less risk of associated malignancy.
- "Juvenile papillomatosis" occurs in young women and is characterized by duct hyperplasia and the presence of multiple cysts. It oftentimes presents as palpable mass. Patients oftentimes have family history of breast cancer and increased lifetime risk, especially in older age. Close imaging surveillance is recommended including of the family of the patient.

Suggested Readings

Jaffer S, Nagi C, Bleiweiss IJ. Excision is indicated for intraductal papilloma of the breast diagnosed on core needle biopsy. *Cancer.* 2009;115(13):2837-2843.

Mercado CL, Hamele-Bena D, Oken SM, Singer CI, Cangiarella J. Papillary lesions of the breast at percutaneous core-needle biopsy. *Radiology.* 2006;238(3):801-808.

Muttarak M, Lerttumnongtum P, Chaiwun B, Peh WC. Spectrum of papillary lesions of the breast: clinical, imaging, and pathologic correlation. *AJR Am J Roentgenol.* 2008;191(3):700-707.

Pearls

- In recent years, there is growing tendency to support surgical excision of "benign" papillomas, diagnosed on core biopsy. However, the issue remains controversial and management differs depending between centers.

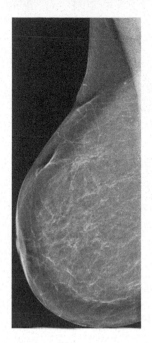
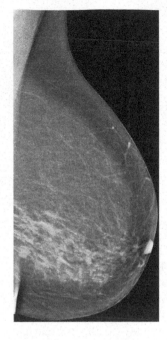
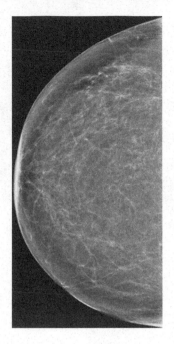
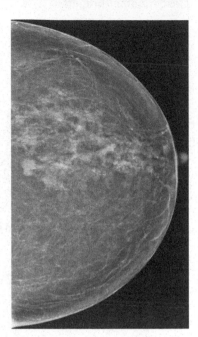

1. What BI-RADS classification should be used here?

2. How would you describe the asymmetry in the left breast?

3. What is the risk of malignancy associated with an asymmetry?

4. This area is diffuse, so what imaging should be considered to work this up?

5. What type of biopsy would you recommend?

Case ranking/difficulty: **Category:** Screening

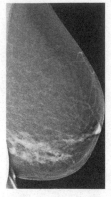
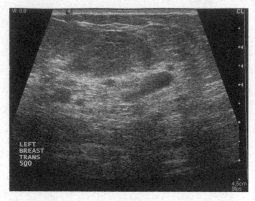
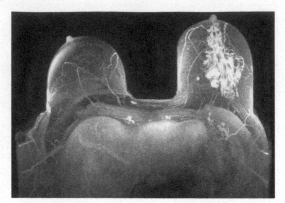

Left lateral showing segmental nodular asymmetry.

Ultrasound showing multiple solid "intraductal masses."

MRI—MIP axial reconstruction (subtracted).

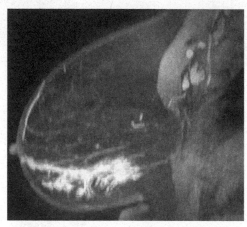

Left breast—Sagittal thin MIP reconstruction to show extent of disease to nipple.

Answers

1. The patient is having a screening exam, despite the fact she has had prior surgery, so an abnormal exam like this should be given a BI-RADS 0.

2. The asymmetry is rather large in the CC plane to describe it as a simple focal asymmetry. However, it could be used if stated as "large segmental focal asymmetry." Some may prefer to describe it as a regional asymmetry, which has segmental features. Either way, you need to emphasize in the report that this is abnormal and needs workup. A BI-RADS 0 would be fine in a screening patient. If this were a diagnostic mammogram, then I would continue ultrasound, and give a suspicious BI-RADS impression after ultrasound was performed.

3. For a simple asymmetry, the risk of malignancy is less than 2%. The risk is higher for a focal asymmetry (10–15%), but much higher for a developing focal asymmetry, such that further workup is indicated in patients with this entity.

4. Initial workup with diagnostic mammograms or tomosynthesis (depending on availability), followed by ultrasound and biopsy. Consider performing at least two biopsies of either one anterior and one posterior lesion or one medially and one laterally. If breast conservation is being considered, an MRI will give a better idea of the extent of the disease. In this case, compare the MRI findings with the mammograms, and see how the MRI delineates the extent of the disease much more clearly, in a very visual way.

5. If the lesions can be seen clearly on ultrasound, then this is the best method for biopsy. In diffuse disease, when you are trying to mark the boundaries of the disease, stereotactic core biopsy may be preferred.

Pearls

- "Developing focal asymmetry" is suspicious, until proven otherwise.
- An "asymmetry" that does not look like normal glandular tissue should be worked up fully.

Suggested Readings

Leung JW, Sickles EA. Developing asymmetry identified on mammography: correlation with imaging outcome and pathologic findings. *AJR Am J Roentgenol.* 2007;188(3):667-675.

Sickles EA. Mammographic features of "early" breast cancer. *AJR Am J Roentgenol.* 1984;143(3):461-464.

Venkatesan A, Chu P, Kerlikowske K, Sickles EA, Smith-Bindman R. Positive predictive value of specific mammographic findings according to reader and patient variables. *Radiology.* 2009;250(3):648-657.

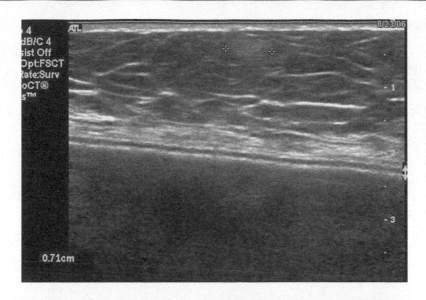

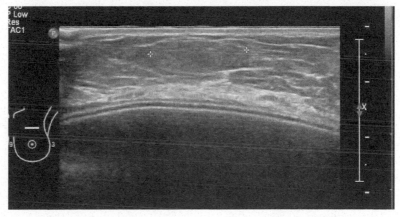

1. What is the next step in a patient with bilateral mastectomy and palpable mass?

2. What is the differential diagnosis of a well-circumscribed hyperechoic mass?

3. What is the typical ultrasound-guided biopsy procedure?

4. What are the techniques to differentiate mass from fat lobules?

5. What scenario decreases sensitivity in ultrasound?

Case ranking/difficulty: 🌸🌸

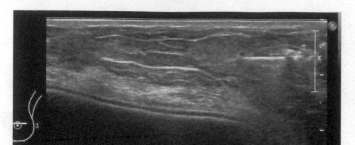

Ultrasound-guided biopsy of the mass with 11-gauge core biopsy needle.

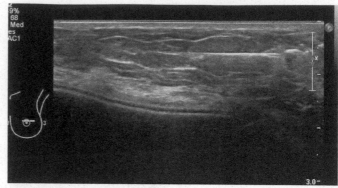

Ultrasound-guided biopsy.

Answers

1. Ultrasound is the first choice.

2. In general, a well-circumscribed homogeneously hyperechoic mass in the breast is a benign finding. In a fatty replaced breast, it can be classified as BI-RADS 2—if there is any doubt or if it correlates to dense fibroglandular tissue, it could be followed over 2 years and called BI-RADS 3 ("probably benign"). As soon as it is palpable, it is more of a concern but again is most likely benign. In this particular case, biopsy was performed because it has grown since prior ultrasound. In rare cases, malignancy, for example, lobular carcinoma, can present in the form of a hyperechoic mass.

3. FNA can be performed in selected cases—for example, fibroadenomas can be diagnosed in the experienced hand. However, in most practices in the ultrasound, core biopsies are the standard for ultrasound-guided biopsies. Spring-loaded 14-gauge needle systems have been the standard for many years. These days, there is a tendency to use vacuum-assisted core biopsy needles that are in general slightly larger and are 12 or 11 gauges in diameter. The smaller the lesion, the more samples will be necessary to be certain that an adequate sample has been obtained.

4. Harmonic imaging can improve contrast between mass and surrounding tissue. Power Doppler with patient humming a deep sound (vocal fremitus) can help to distinguish mass from surrounding tissue. Since fat is well perfused in general, duplex and power Doppler are of limited help. Increased pressure can help to see if the suspected mass is real. Fat demonstrates deformity under pressure. A solid nodule does not show similar deformity.

5. Large breast with fatty replaced tissue does decrease sensitivity of ultrasound to find small mass. Fat is hypoechoic on ultrasound and most masses are hypoechoic as well. Therefore, the contrast is diminished and masses can be disguised much easier. Fibrocystic changes also impair the ability to find malignancy.

Pearls

- Angiolipomas account for 5% to 8% of benign fatty tumors and are a variant of lipomas.
- Since the hallmark of an angiolipoma is the presence of scattered microthrombi in small blood vessels, they can cause some pain.
- The etiology of angiolipomas is unknown, but some investigators see an association with repetitive trauma.

Suggested Reading

Weinstein SP, Conant EF, Acs G. Case 59: Angiolipoma of the breast. *Radiology.* 2003;227(3):773-775.

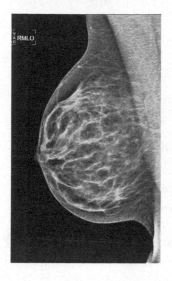
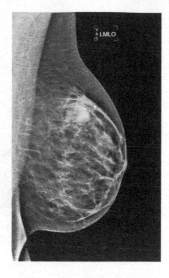
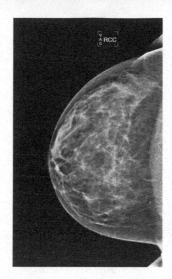
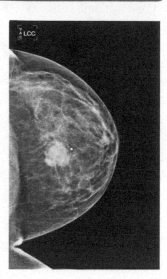

1. What BI-RADS classification should be used here?

2. What is the most likely pathology based on the imaging?

3. What is the next best examination in a young woman?

4. If a biopsy is performed for this lesion and core biopsy shows fibroepithelial lesion, what do you recommend?

5. If ultrasound shows a solid mass and core biopsy shows fibroadenoma, what is the management?

Case ranking/difficulty:

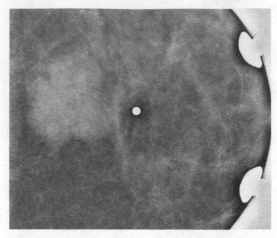

Spot magnification views for better characterization of margins and to look for associated calcifications. Note how the margins have "microlobulations" and angulations.

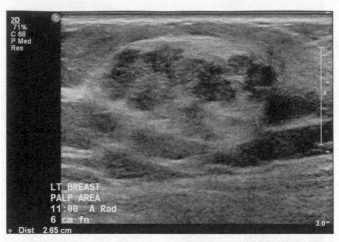

Ultrasound of the palpable mass. This confirms the circumscribed nature felt on palpation. The appearances are similar to a hamartoma, with both hyperechoic and hypoechoic areas, and no shadowing. They are sometimes difficult to perceive against the prominent glandular tissue in young women.

Answers

1. The finding of a mass in a young woman with what appears to be a circumscribed mass at first viewing, but on further evaluation of the margins shows irregularity or any other suspicious feature, should prompt a BI-RADS 4 and biopsy.

2. There are enough findings on imaging to indicate that this is not a fibroadenoma, which is usually round or more frequently oval, with circumscribed margins. There is no calcification to indicate DCIS, although in younger women DCIS can present as a noncalcified mass. Mucinous carcinoma usually has indistinct margins, and is easier to confuse with a benign lesion on ultrasound. It is more common in the elderly. There is no history of trauma or bruising on the skin to indicate hematoma formation.

3. A single tomosynthesis view may outline the margins more clearly. Ultrasound is the best examination in young women, especially as it is a nonionizing radiation exam. MRI may help if proven cancer, and extent difficult to judge, but as the next step, it is expensive and not really indicated. PEM and BSGI may have a role in really dense breasts in young women, but the downside is the radiation dose.

4. A fibroepithelial lesion is a relatively new pathological entity, which can be under-sampled using core biopsy or vacuum biopsy, and surgical excision is recommended.

5. If the imaging appearances are concordant with a fibroadenoma, many groups will discharge the patient to routine screening. Some groups would perform short-term clinical follow-up with appropriate imaging for

stability. Others advocate excision of the fibroadenoma with vacuum-assisted biopsy (especially if less that 2 cm in max diameter). This is usually done as part of the initial biopsy. Surgical excision is not medically required, but many young patients request excision, even when proven benign.

Pearls

- Cancers may present with circumscribed margins in young women.
- Noncalcified DCIS masses can present in this manner.
- Evaluate margins of mass to determine if any suspicious features to prompt biopsy or suggest a diagnosis other than fibroadenoma.

Suggested Readings

Chung J, Son EJ, Kim JA, Kim EK, Kwak JY, Jeong J. Giant phyllodes tumors of the breast: imaging findings with clinicopathological correlation in 14 cases. *Clin Imaging.* 2011;35(2):102-107.

Gwak YJ, Kim HJ, Kwak JY, et al. Ultrasonographic detection and characterization of asymptomatic ductal carcinoma in situ with histopathologic correlation. *Acta Radiol.* 2011;52(4):364-371.

Yang WT, Hennessy B, Broglio K, et al. Imaging differences in metaplastic and invasive ductal carcinomas of the breast. *AJR Am J Roentgenol.* 2007;189(6):1288-1293.

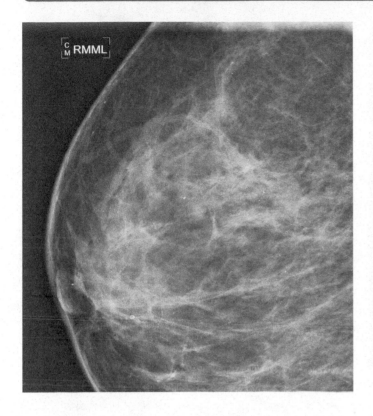
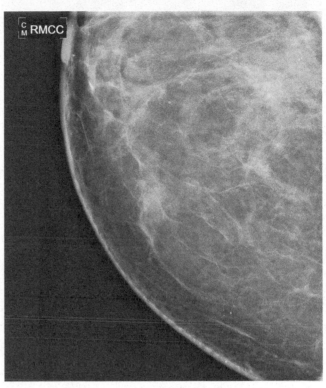

1. What is the significance of group of "round and oval" calcifications?

2. What are typical benign proliferative changes in the breast?

3. What is the difference between atypical ductal hyperplasia and DCIS?

4. What are important quality-assuring steps in stereotactic core biopsy?

5. Why does atypical ductal hyperplasia need to be surgically excised?

Case ranking/difficulty:

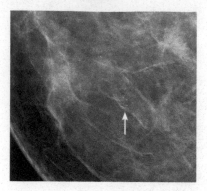

Right magnification view, with additional electronic magnification.

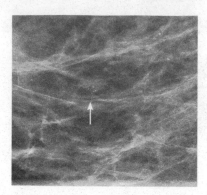

Right magnification view, with additional electronic magnification.

Answers

1. "Round and oval" calcifications as characterized on magnification views after workup of baseline screening mammogram are probably benign and can be followed over 2 years, given the likelihood of malignancy of less than 2%. Any developing group of "round and oval" calcifications is suspicious (BI-RADS 4) and ought to be biopsied. They can represent adenosis but also low-grade DCIS.

2. During the aging of the breast parenchyma, there is the process of involution with atrophy of fibroglandular tissue, and at the same time there is also a chance for proliferative processes that make the reading of mammograms difficult. The lobules can proliferate and form fibrocystic changes and adenosis, or if there is a dominant fibrotic component, even sclerosing adenosis. All these three processes can result in formation of calcium. Where "milk of calcium" is a typical benign finding, adenosis and sclerosing adenosis can form "oval and round" calcifications, and sclerosing adenosis can form even "pleomorphic" calcifications. This cannot be differentiated from DCIS, and biopsy is necessary.

3. It is only a quantitative difference between atypical ductal hyperplasia (ADH) and DCIS. If there are more than two lobules involved and a certain amount of cell layers that have proliferated, it is called DCIS.

4. The purpose of the stereotactic biopsy is not to remove all calcifications but to obtain a representative sample. It is important to obtain specimen radiograph to determine if the calcifications are sampled. To help the pathologist to reduce the amount of material, the core samples that contain the calcifications can be separated. Clip is left in the target zone to facilitate needle localization in case of subsequent lumpectomy. Postbiopsy mammogram is obtained to determine if the clip has not migrated and is in the correct location. One crucial step after obtaining the pathology report is to determine if the histology results are concordant with the imaging. If not the area has to be resampled or surgical excision is indicated.

5. If patients with ADH diagnosed on core biopsy subsequently obtain surgical excision, histology is being upgraded to DCIS in about 6% to 44%, dependent on the study—and also the size of the needle. But even if 9-gauge vacuum-assisted core biopsy needle was used, an upgrade will happen in more than 2%. Anything on mammography that has a likelihood of less than 2% can be followed according to the BI-RADS lexicon and can be classified as "probably benign"—BI-RADS 3. Since ADH does exceed the number in subsequent surgical excision, it cannot be followed and needs to be excised.

Pearls

- Suspicious (BI-RADS 4) calcifications can be due to benign proliferative changes such as adenosis or sclerosing adenosis or due to DCIS or even invasive ductal carcinoma. It is impossible to differentiate both etiologies based on mammographic criteria. Therefore, biopsy is required for differentiation.
- ADH is also a concordant finding. Differentiation to DCIS is based on the number of ducts and the amount of cell layers being involved.
- Since likelihood of upgrade of ADH to DCIS on excision biopsy exceeds the 2% rate required to qualify for BI-RADS 3, surgical excision is recommended.

Suggested Readings

Jackman RJ, Birdwell RL, Ikeda DM. Atypical ductal hyperplasia: can some lesions be defined as probably benign after stereotactic 11-gauge vacuum-assisted biopsy, eliminating the recommendation for surgical excision? *Radiology*. 2002;224(2):548-554.

Verkooijen HM, Peterse JL, Schipper ME, et al. Interobserver variability between general and expert pathologists during the histopathological assessment of large-core needle and open biopsies of non-palpable breast lesions. *Eur J Cancer*. 2003;39(15):2187-2191.

Stereotactic biopsy with 9-gauge vacuum-assisted needle for asymmetry 6 months ago; now patient complains of pain in that area

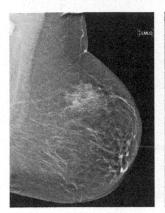 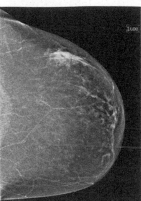 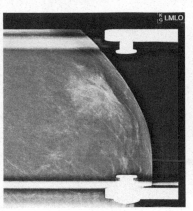 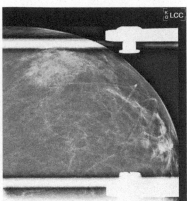

1. What is the finding on the spot compression views?

2. The patient had pain in the area of recent biopsy, what is the next step?

3. What do you expect to see on ultrasound after stereotactic biopsy?

4. If ultrasound shows a large scar, what would be an additional test to differentiate between scar and malignancy?

5. Why is ultrasound, in general, not performed as standard after surgery/biopsy?

Case ranking/difficulty: Category: Diagnostic

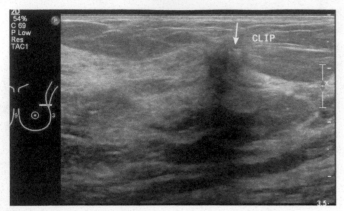

Gray-scale ultrasound of the area of concern, showing clip and "hypoechoic," "irregular-shaped" mass with "posterior acoustic shadowing."

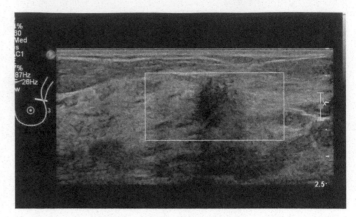

Duplex of the area does not show any flow.

Answers

1. The spot compression views demonstrate the asymmetric tissue with underlying "architectural distortion" but no other abnormality.

2. Next step is ultrasound directed to the area.

3. After 6-month biopsy with relatively large needle (9-gauge) we would expect a small scar. The scar, as seen on the ultrasound images, is relatively large. However, given the recent normal pathology and the fact that the reason for the biopsy was asymmetry, this was thought to be "probably benign"-BI-RADS 3 and 6-month follow-up mammogram and ultrasound was recommended. Given the symptoms of focal pain, MRI was suggested to better differentiate scar from questionable malignancy.

4. If the biopsy was performed at least 6 months ago, MRI with contrast would be helpful to differentiate between scar and possible malignancy. Scar or focal fibrosis would not enhance, whereas malignancy would enhance.

5. Ultrasound is not very good in differentiating scar from malignancy. It was performed because of the focal pain of the patient. Fat necrosis or scar (focal fibrosis) cannot be easily differentiated from malignancy on ultrasound.

Pearls

• On imaging, scar can be seen after benign, large-bore, vacuum-assisted biopsy.

• In case of concern about the appearance on imaging, it is helpful to review the recent prebiopsy images and the pathology results to reconfirm that the benign results were concordant with the imaging.

• If there is remaining concern, option can be to perform a repeat biopsy or short-term 6-month follow-up.

• MRI can also be helpful in case of concern to differentiate between scar and malignancy.

Suggested Readings

Aichinger U, Schulz-Wendtland R, Krämer S, Lell M, Bautz W. Scar or recurrence—comparison of MRI and color-coded ultrasound with echo signal amplifiers [in German]. *Rofo*. 2002;174(11):1395-1401.

Rosen EL, Soo MS, Bentley RC. Focal fibrosis: a common breast lesion diagnosed at imaging-guided core biopsy. *AJR Am J Roentgenol*. 1999;173(6):1657-1662.

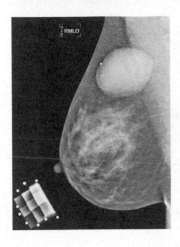
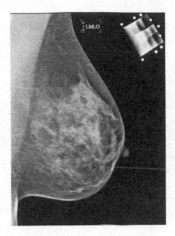
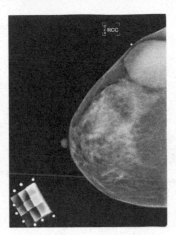
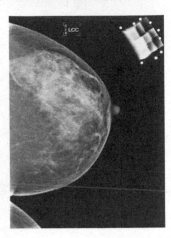

1. Which of the BI-RADS descriptors most accurately represents the findings?

2. What is the BI-RADS descriptor for the margin of this mass?

3. What is the most likely pathology?

4. This lesion turned out to be a spindle cell lipoma on core biopsy. What is the treatment?

5. Is any of the following advanced imaging tests indicated in this condition?

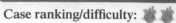
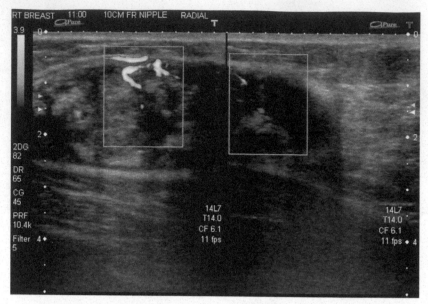

Vascular solid mass. Does not look like a fibroadenoma. BI-RADS 4—requires biopsy.

Answers

1. The shape of mass is the first BI-RADS descriptor. The description of the margins follows the shape.

2. Smooth margins with a "narrow zone of transition" from normal to abnormal.

3. Depends on age. In a postmenopausal woman, a developing circumscribed mass is more likely to be malignant than in a patient with active hormones.

4. The treatment of spindle cell tumors, even the lipoma variants, is similar to phyllodes tumor, with wide surgical excision. Full pathological analysis of the whole specimen will be able to distinguish between the benign and malignant variants of the disease.

5. The core biopsy and surgical excision is usually all that is required. There is no evidence that additional tests change the management of the patient.

Pearls

- Rare spindle cell variant lipoma.
- FNA not helpful.
- Core biopsy makes the diagnosis.
- Treatment by wide surgical excision.

Suggested Readings

Magro G, Bisceglia M, Michal M, Eusebi V. Spindle cell lipoma-like tumor, solitary fibrous tumor and myofibroblastoma of the breast: a clinico-pathological analysis of 13 cases in favor of a unifying histogenetic concept. *Virchows Arch.* 2002;440(3):249-260.

Magro G, Michal M, Bisceglia M. Benign spindle cell tumors of the mammary stroma: diagnostic criteria, classification, and histogenesis. *Pathol Res Pract.* 2001;197(7):453-466.

Mulvany NJ, Silvester AC, Collins JP. Spindle cell lipoma of the breast. *Pathology.* 1999;31(3):288-291.

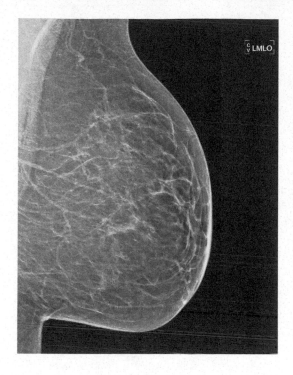 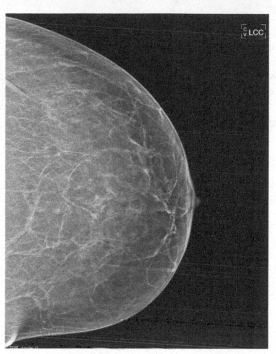

1. What is the finding on mammography?

2. Is there any situation where a finding can be called BI-RADS 3 on screening mammogram?

3. What calcification descriptors are high risk and imply the need for biopsy?

4. What would be the best way to address these calcifications as seen on magnification views?

5. What is the best technique to use in this case for the biopsy?

Case ranking/difficulty:

Category: Screening

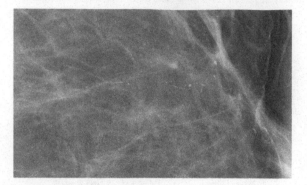

Diagnostic mammogram, right ML magnification view demonstrating "linear" calcifications.

Diagnostic mammogram, left CC magnification view demonstrating "linear" calcifications.

Answers

1. Noted is a subtle group of indeterminate calcifications in the left retroareolar breast. The consequence is to recall the patient for diagnostic mammogram with magnification views.

2. No. BI-RADS 3 is not an accepted conclusion for a screening mammogram. It is only acceptable after an appropriate workup in the form of a diagnostic mammogram.

3. "Lucent centered" calcifications are benign and usually in the skin. "Coarse and popcorn like" calcifications are benign and most likely due to a hyalinized fibroadenoma. "Dystrophic" calcifications are, in most cases, benign. "Pleomorphe and fine linear" are descriptors that imply "need for biopsy" because oftentimes these calcifications are related to DCIS.

4. In this case—fatty replaced breast parenchyma—ultrasound does not help, since it is almost impossible that there is any mass hiding. MRI can be performed after positive biopsy to search for additional disease—again it could be argued that in a breast with fatty replaced parenchyma, the need for an MRI is less. Surgical excision is not state of the art, without prior biopsy and histology. Ductogram does not help—based on the morphology, the calcifications are likely in a duct.

5. The preferred needle system is a 11- or 9-gauge vacuum-assisted core biopsy needle for calcifications. This is superior to a spring loaded 14-gauge needle system. The purpose is not to remove all calcifications but to sample a representative group. Based on the results, lumpectomy would take care of the abnormality. An FNA is not yielding a sufficient sample for diagnosis.

Pearls

- Certain BI-RADS descriptors for calcifications do imply malignancy and biopsy is required.
- In general, any description of calcifications as "pleomorphe" or "fine linear and branching" should never be followed by BI-RADS 2 (benign) or BI-RADS 3 (probably benign) assessment.
- If calcifications with suspicious form and shape are stable over 2 years, biopsy might still be required, since they could represent low-grade DCIS.
- Biopsy of calcifications should be performed with 9- or 11-gauge vacuum-assisted core biopsy needle.

Suggested Readings

Bird RE. Critical pathways in analyzing breast calcifications. *Radiographics.* 1995;15(4):928-934.

D'Orsi CJ, Bassett LW, Berg WA, et al. *Breast Imaging Reporting and Data System: ACR BI- RADS– Mammography.* 4th ed. Reston, VA: American College of Radiology; 2003.

Philpotts LE, Shaheen NA, Carter D, Lange RC, Lee CH. Comparison of rebiopsy rates after stereotactic core needle biopsy of the breast with 11-gauge vacuum suction probe versus 14-gauge needle and automatic gun. *AJR Am J Roentgenol.* 1999;172(3):683-687.

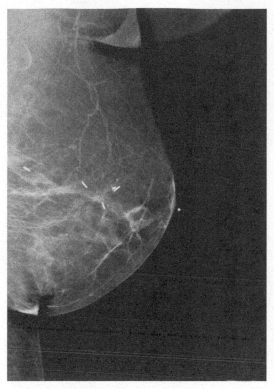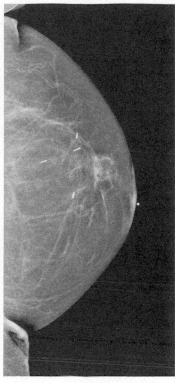

1. What BI-RADS is appropriate here?

2. What is the differential diagnosis for the scar changes in this patient?

3. In fat necrosis, what is the structure that calcifies?

4. What is the next best imaging test?

5. In patients who had breast conservation surgery, when is the time of maximum radiotherapy change in the treated breast?

Case ranking/difficulty:

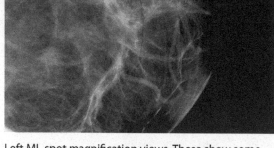

Left ML spot magnification views. These show some fatty lucency of the scar with fine calcifications seen around the periphery.

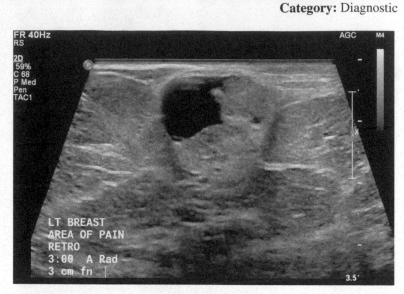

Cavitating fluid-filled lesion containing debris.

Answers

1. The findings are characteristic of fat necrosis following breast conservation therapy and intraoperative radiation therapy. There is no evidence of malignancy, and therefore a BI-RADS assessment of 2 (benign) is appropriate.

2. The findings of a circumscribed fatty lucency within a scar are typical of fat necrosis. In addition, calcifications develop in the periphery of the inflammatory change.

3. Classically, fat necrosis calcifies irregularly in the walled off liquefied center. There is chronic inflammation, and calcifications develop within the wall. Early microcalcifications can look very suspicious until they coarsen up and become classically dystrophic.

4. This finding is characteristic enough to leave alone. However, as it was also palpable on physical exam, an ultrasound was performed. MRI is not warranted, and a diagnostic mammogram has already been performed. Tomosynthesis may have a role in the initial diagnostic exam, as it should be able to differentiate between fat necrosis and a developing mass from local recurrence, but there are as yet no data on its use in this situation.

5. Following breast conservation, the risk of local recurrence has a peak approximately 2 to 3 years following completion of therapy. With patients on tamoxifen, there may be a second peak at around 6 to 7 years, but this has been mostly reduced by the use of aromatase inhibitors. The maximum radiation change occurs at 18 months and decreases over time.

Pearls

• Post–conservation surgery followed by radiation changes may be complicated by fat necrosis.

• There is increased risk of fat necrosis in patients undergoing intraoperative radiation with brachytherapy.

Suggested Readings

Budrukkar A, Jagtap V, Kembhavi S, et al. Fat necrosis in women with early-stage breast cancer treated with accelerated partial breast irradiation (APBI) using interstitial brachytherapy. *Radiother Oncol.* 2012;103(2):161-165.

Kuzmiak CM, Zeng D, Cole E, Pisano ED. Mammographic findings of partial breast irradiation. *Acad Radiol.* 2009;16(7):819-825.

Orecchia R, Leonardo MC. Intraoperative radiation therapy: is it a standard now? *Breast.* 2011;20(Suppl 3):S111-S115.

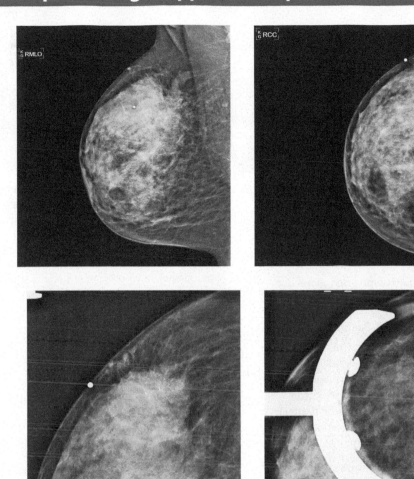

1. If there are suspicious calcifications in a palpable area, what is the next step?

2. What are the characteristics of a papillary cancer?

3. What is the next step after the imaging?

4. Why can highly differentiated tumors be a problem in MRI?

5. What is the role of duplex in ultrasound of the breast?

Case ranking/difficulty:

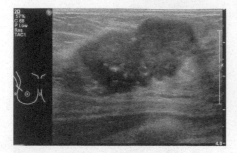

Ultrasound directed to the area demonstrates mass with associated calcifications and "microlobulated" margin.

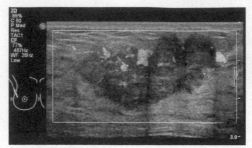

Ultrasound demonstrates increased flow in the mass.

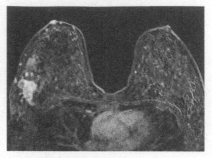

MRI of the breast with contrast demonstrating the index lesion in the right upper outer quadrant.

Answers

1. In our case, patient received spot compression views due to the distortion seen in the area of palpable abnormality. However, better would have been spot compression magnification views to assess the distribution of the calcifications and to better characterize the calcifications. In this particular case, it did not matter too much since calcifications were new and highly suspicious and ultrasound did confirm the presence of an associated mass. It is always helpful to perform ultrasound in the presence of dense tissue and highly suspicious calcifications to search for an invasive component of the malignancy.

2. Papillary cancers are a small fraction of invasive cancers of the breast (1–2%). They belong to the group of highly differentiated breast cancers and have a better prognosis then invasive ductal carcinoma. They usually are located in the retroareolar region and can occur in a cyst.

3. The best choice at this point is an ultrasound-guided biopsy. It is more convenient then stereotactic biopsy and will give the surgeon the information necessary to plan surgery to the maximum benefit of the patient.

4. Highly differentiated carcinomas are a subgroup of invasive ductal carcinoma including mucinous, tubular papillary, and medullary carcinomas. They can show more intermediate (tubular) or even high signal (mucinous) on T2-weighted images. These tumors can be round and well circumscribed (medullary, papillary, and mucinous carcinomas) and might have contrast enhancement patterns that are less specific; for example, they could increase enhancement over time.

5. Ultrasound with duplex can help to assess the degree of malignancy in an otherwise suspicious lesion. It should not sway the examiner into avoiding biopsy in case of lack of flow. There are low-grade malignancy not showing flow. Ultrasound with doppler can help to guide a biopsy needle to avoid bleeding and to help to differentiate between a cyst and a solid nodule if flow is seen.

Pearls

- Papillary and mucinous, tubular, and medullary carcinomas belong to the subgroup of well-differentiated invasive ductal carcinomas.
- They can present with increased signal on T2-weighted MRI images and can show increasing contrast enhancement kinetics.
- This case demonstrates importance of ultrasound in addition to mammography in situation of suspicious calcifications in dense breast tissue to search for solid invasive component of the malignancy.
- Increased flow on duplex images can reflect vascular neogenesis to supply fast-growing masses—however, finding is unspecific and can also be seen in benign masses, such as fibroadenomas.

Suggested Readings

Cosgrove DO, Kedar RP, Bamber JC, et al. Breast diseases: color Doppler US in differential diagnosis. *Radiology*. 1993;189(1):99-104.

Soo MS, Williford ME, Walsh R, Bentley RC, Kornguth PJ. Papillary carcinoma of the breast: imaging findings. *AJR Am J Roentgenol*. 1995;164(2):321-326.

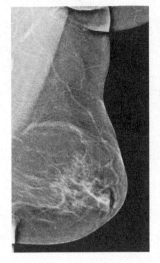
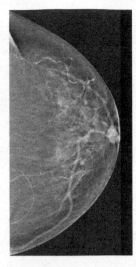
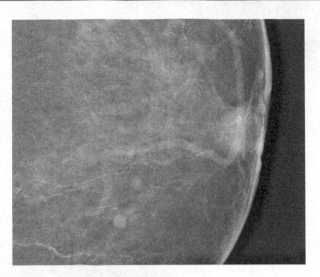

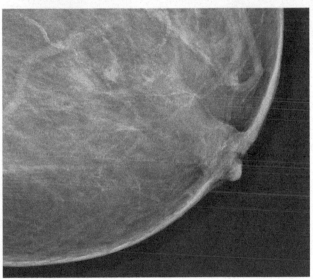

1. What BI-RADS classification should be used
   here?

2. Which of the following conditions can be
   a cause of nipple discharge?

3. What is the next best imaging test?

4. What are the clinical findings you anticipate
   finding in this patient?

5. What type of biopsy is best in Paget disease
   of the nipple?

Case ranking/difficulty:

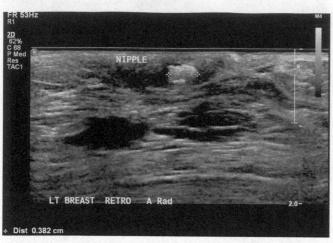

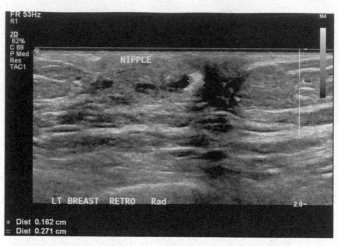

Targeted ultrasound. This is technically difficult in the subareolar area, especially when the patient has an inverted nipple.

Retroareolar ultrasound. Calcifications within the nipple are still remarkably well seen.

Answers

1. This patient has a bloody nipple discharge, and also calcifications in the nipple. Further investigation is warranted. The examination is a diagnostic exam, and so a BI-RADS 4 assessment is appropriate.

2. The answer is that virtually anything can be a cause of nipple discharge, which is very common condition, and has a low risk of associated malignancy. The only types of discharge you need to be concerned about are watery (from multiple papillomas, or DCIS) and bloody (papilloma, duct ectasia, periductal mastitis, etc.). Bloody nipple discharge associated with breast cancer is very rare.

3. Tomosynthesis may not help here, as the main findings are the calcifications in the nipple. Spot magnification views are therefore the best next test. If there is an associated mass, ultrasound may help. PEM does not have any utility when the patient has relatively fatty breasts. MRI is reported to increase the diagnostic accuracy for subareolar-associated cancer in Paget disease.

4. Slit-like nipple retraction is found in duct ectasia due to scaring and shortening of the central ducts. Flat nipple retraction is a presenting finding of retroareolar invasive cancer. She has presented with a bloody nipple discharge, so we may be able to see this spontaneously. Nipple discoloration along with purple patches on the nipple areolar complex (NAC) skin are found in Paget disease, and are the area for the punch biopsy or incisional biopsy to be performed to establish the diagnosis.

5. Nipple biopsy is the standard care for Paget disease. Ductal lavage, if available, can detect abnormal cells associated with DCIS, even if we cannot see it on imaging.

Pearls

- Calcifications within the nipple are unusual and should prompt investigation.
- Patient has associated nipple inversion that can be benign (most commonly) or malignant.
- Check nipple for discoloration, which might indicate the presence of Paget disease of the nipple, and prompt nipple biopsy for diagnosis.
- Paget disease is associated with DCIS.

Suggested Readings

Echevarria JJ, Lopez-Ruiz JA, Martin D, Imaz I, Martin M. Usefulness of MRI in detecting occult breast cancer associated with Paget's disease of the nipple-areolar complex. *Br J Radiol*. 2004;77(924):1036-1039.

Günhan-Bilgen I, Oktay A. Paget's disease of the breast: clinical, mammographic, sonographic and pathologic findings in 52 cases. *Eur J Radiol*. 2006;60(2):256-263.

Lim HS, Jeong SJ, Lee JS, et al. Paget disease of the breast: mammographic, US, and MR imaging findings with pathologic correlation. *Radiographics*. 2011;31(7): 1973-1987.

52-year-old patient with history of breast cancer and bilateral mastectomy—patient feels new lump in the right medial chest wall

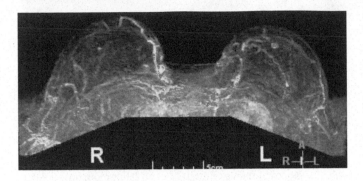 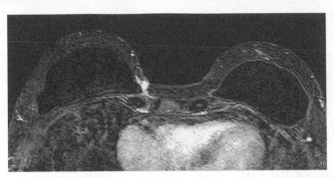

1. What is a an appropriate technique to follow patients after bilateral mastectomy?

2. Is clinical examination good enough to detect recurrent malignancy after mastectomy?

3. What it the finding seen on the submitted MRI images?

4. What is the next step?

5. What is the next step if ultrasound does not show the lesion?

Case ranking/difficulty: 🌸🌸

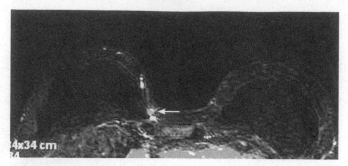

MRI after IV contrast and subtraction demonstrates an area of mixed contrast enhancement kinetics in the right medial breast.

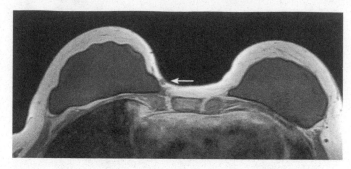

MRI T1-weighted images without IV contrast demonstrate small mass in the medial right breast.

Answers

1. A reasonable approach is to perform either ultrasound or MRI.

2. MRI and ultrasound are more successful in detecting local recurrence than clinical examination. Ultrasound is cheaper and more readily available and should be the first option. In case of suspicious findings on ultrasound, MRI could increase the specificity.

3. Noted is a 5-mm enhancing mass in the right chest wall near the medial contour of the silicone implant.

4. Second look ultrasound is the next step to see if we can see any correlate and if ultrasound-guided biopsy is feasible.

5. If the lesion is not seen on ultrasound, then we are in trouble—the only option left would be to send patient to breast surgeon. Breast surgeon will appreciate if we can mark the lesion by clip or even needle localize the lesion. The benefit to excise the lesion outweighs the danger to injure the implant.

Pearls

- Bilateral mastectomy does not 100% exclude the possibility of breast cancer in the future.
- Ultrasound or MRI can be used for screening of recurrent breast cancer in patients with bilateral mastectomy.

Suggested Readings

Vanderwalde LH, Dang CM, Tabrizi R, Saouaf R, Phillips EH. Breast MRI after bilateral mastectomy: is it indicated? *Am Surg.* 2011;77(2):180-184.

Yilmaz MH, Esen G, Ayarcan Y, et al. The role of US and MR imaging in detecting local chest wall tumor recurrence after mastectomy. *Diagn Interv Radiol.* 2007;13(1):13-18.

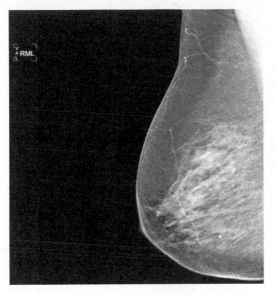
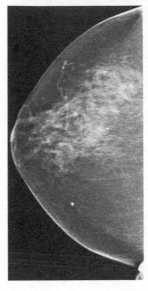
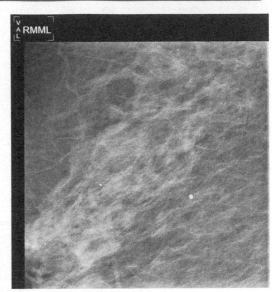

1. What is the consequence of the screening mammogram in this case?

2. Why are round and oval calcifications in this case not benign?

3. Why was in this case only one stereotactic biopsy performed?

4. Why was MRI performed?

5. What is the significance of multicentric and multifocal disease?

Case ranking/difficulty:

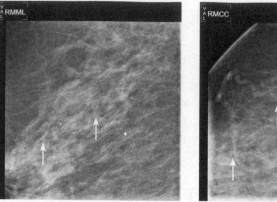

Diagnostic mammogram, right magnification ML view.

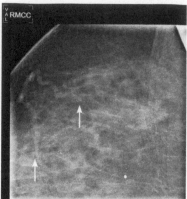

Diagnostic mammogram, right magnification CC view.

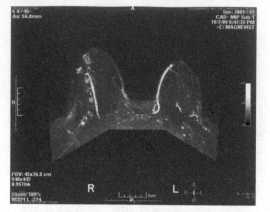

MRI MIP image after IV contrast demonstrates multifocal disease in the right breast.

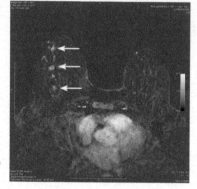

MRI, T1-weighted sequence after IV contrast with subtraction demonstrates multiple foci of increased enhancement correlating to the groups of calcifications.

Answers

1. For the assessment of screening mammogram, there are only three options available. Either the mammogram is normal (BI-RADS 1) or benign (BI-RADS 2), or there is an abnormality that needs further workup (BI-RADS 0) and the mammogram is labeled as "incomplete" and patient will be recalled for diagnostic mammogram. This is the appropriate assessment in this particular case.

2. Round and oval calcifications can be classified as BI-RADS 3 (probably benign) in a diagnostic workup with magnification views based on a first screening mammogram if there are no old exams available. Then they should be followed in 6 months and subsequently another 6 months and then a year later with magnification views to prove stability over 2 years. In this case, however, the calcifications were new and therefore suspicious BI-RADS 4. Remember, never classify a screening mammogram as probably benign (BI-RADS 3)—this can be done only after a diagnostic workup.

3. The goal of the biopsy is to prove the extent of the malignancy to guide the surgical procedure to avoid positive margins and to determine the appropriate surgical procedure. In this case, it would have been to biopsy two groups of the suspicious calcifications under stereotactic guidance. However, in this particular case, one biopsy was done with sterotaxis. The second was performed under MRI guidance based on the findings.

4. MRI is performed to assess the patient if there is additional disease, in particular, if there is additional disease in other quadrants (multicentric disease). Based on the mammogram, there is already evidence of multiple areas of disease in one quadrant (multifocal disease).

5. Multicentric disease (more than one quadrant is involved) requires, in general, mastectomy. Multifocal disease (more than one lesion in one quadrant) can oftentimes be addressed by lumpectomy. It is favorable to bracket the lesions at the time of needle localization to achieve best outcome.

Pearls

- In case of the presence of multiple suspicious groups of calcifications, stereotactic biopsy can be performed of two groups most apart from each other to prove the extent of the disease.
- If patient will get preoperative MRI, only one biopsy can be performed of the most suspicious group of calcifications and further biopsy can be determined based on the extent of disease as seen on MRI.

Suggested Reading

Esserman L, Hylton N, Yassa L, Barclay J, Frankel S, Sickles E. Utility of magnetic resonance imaging in the management of breast cancer: evidence for improved preoperative staging. *J Clin Oncol.* 1999;17(1):110-119.

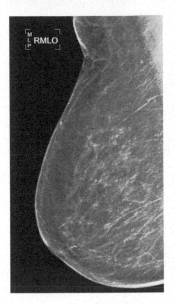
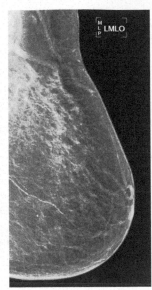
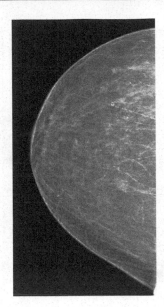
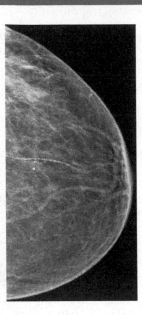

1. What is the risk of malignancy in an asymmetry?

2. What is the next best examination you recommend?

3. Which type of cancer can present with these findings?

4. What BI-RADS assessment would you give this finding?

5. What type of biopsy would you recommend?

Case ranking/difficulty:

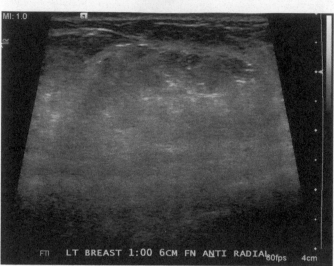

Targeted ultrasound—vague isoechoic mass at the site of mammographic abnormality.

Answers

1. Malignancy is very rare in an asymmetry, but this is modified by whether it is preexisting or new. A developing asymmetry is always suspicious and needs further evaluation. An asymmetry that has been stable on prior films for more than 3 years can be presumed to be benign.

2. The first thing that has to be addressed is the question of whether this is a real abnormality, and repeating the same views to see if still present (especially if young and at different stage of cycle). Second, does it press out. Once these questions have been addressed, then one can move on to ultrasound targeted to the mammographic finding. If this is still negative, but you still suspect an abnormality is present, then an MRI would help to include or exclude malignancy.

3. An asymmetry is usually a lobular cancer, although a developing focal asymmetry can be due to a high-grade invasive ductal cancer. Lobular cancer is hard to detect commonly presenting in atypical ways, such as vague distortion, a shrinking breast, or vague asymmetry.

4. The finding is suspicious, but this is a screening exam, so the correct answer is that this is a BI-RADS 0, recall for further workup. If this is a screening examination, then this finding should lead to a recall for further evaluation, and a hunt for prior mammograms.

5. FNA cytology is technically difficult with lobular carcinoma, and it is important to alert the pathologist to the potential for a lobular cancer at the time of the biopsy. Core biopsy is certainly the best way of both getting a diagnosis and performing routine tumor biomarkers. There are no significant calcifications associated with this tumor, and so stereotactic core biopsy is not indicated. The lesion is not palpable, so guidance will be required. Preoperative diagnosis should be performed rather than going direct to surgery.

Pearls

- Lobular cancer is well known for being subtle in presentation with atypical features at mammography.
- MRI is an important part of the diagnostic workup.
- Mammographic features of lobular cancer are as follows:
  - Asymmetry
  - Distortion
  - Reduction in breast volume of affected size.

Suggested Readings

Choi BB, Kim SH, Shu KS. Lobular lesions of the breast: imaging findings of lobular neoplasia and invasive lobular carcinoma. *J Reprod Med.* 2012;57(1-2):26-34.

Heller SL, Moy L. Imaging features and management of high-risk lesions on contrast-enhanced dynamic breast MRI. *AJR Am J Roentgenol.* 2012;198(2):249-255.

Kim SH, Cha ES, Park CS, et al. Imaging features of invasive lobular carcinoma: comparison with invasive ductal carcinoma. *Jpn J Radiol.* 2011;29(7):475-482.

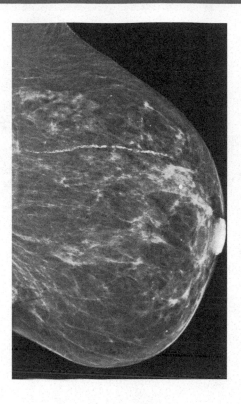 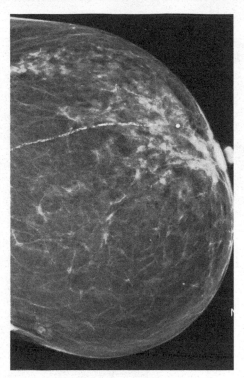

1. What is Paget disease of the breast?

2. What is the percentage of Paget disease among all breast malignancies?

3. Is there is risk of additional disease?

4. What could be the next step in this particular case?

5. Is there any abnormality seen around the nipple on the current exam?

Category: Diagnostic

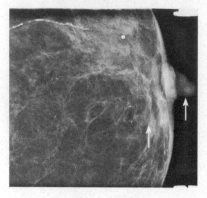

Spot compression view of left CC showing protruding mass in the left nipple and suspicious calcifications.

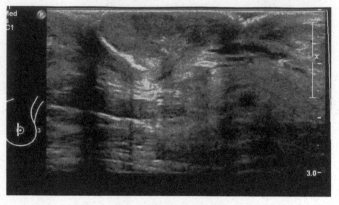

Ultrasound of left retroareolar breast demonstrates the mass within the nipple.

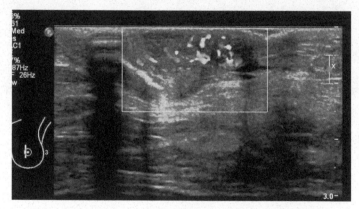

Ultrasound of left retroareolar breast with duplex demonstrates mass within the nipple with strong increased flow on duplex.

Answers

1. Paget disease is an uncommon form of breast cancer with typical appearance.

2. One to five percent of all breast carcinomas are Paget disease.

3. Paget disease is oftentimes associated with DCIS or invasive ductal carcinoma. DCIS is oftentimes high grade (comedo type). Fifty percent of patients have additional abnormalities on the mammogram in the same breast.

4. When mammogram confirms lack of additional abnormality, patient can be send to breast surgeon for biopsy. The lesion is accessible to inspection and does not require imaging guidance.

5. Noted best on the CC view is a mass extending out of the nipple as well as suspicious calcifications. They are in "linear distribution" and "fine and linear" in shape.

Pearls

- Paget disease is a rare form of breast cancer, characterized by the presence of intraepidermal tumor cells, often involving the nipple.
- Appearance of the nipple includes pruritus and eczema.
- One to five percent of all breast cancers present as Paget disease.
- Paget disease is oftentimes associated with DCIS.
- DCIS is oftentimes high grade and comedo type.

Suggested Readings

Cardenosa, G. *Breast Imaging Companion*. 2nd ed. Philadelphia, PA: Lippincott Williams & Wilkins; 2001.

Dalberg K, Hellborn H, Waermberg F. Paget's disease of the nipple in a population based cohort. *Breast Cancer Res Treat*. 2008;111(2):313-319.

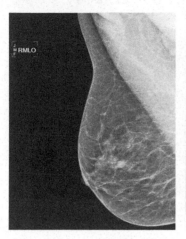
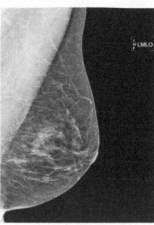
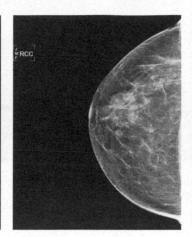
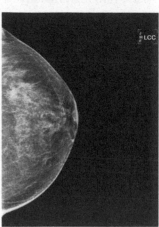

1. What is the pertinent finding?

2. What would be the next step in the workup of a spiculated mass seen on additional diagnostic mammogram?

3. What would be the next step in the workup of a questionable mass on screening mammogram?

4. What is the appropriate BI-RADS classification of the screening exam?

5. What would change if patient had nipple discharge?

Case ranking/difficulty:

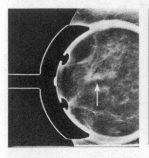

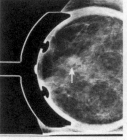

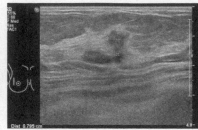

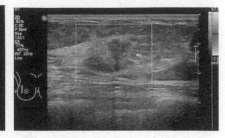

Diagnostic mammogram, right MLO view demonstrating mass with "irregular" shape right 11:00 close to the nipple.

Diagnostic mammogram, right CC view confirming the presence of mass with "irregular" shape close to the nipple at 11:00.

Ultrasound of right breast confirming the presence of an "irregular and angulated" mass.

Ultrasound of right breast with duplex confirming the presence of a spiculated, angulated anechoic mass with some flow in the periphery on duplex.

Answers

1. Noted is a "questionable mass" in the right retroareolar breast, middle depth. This would be an appropriate description on a screening mammogram report because diagnostic views need to confirm if the suspected mass is real. Mass can then be further described on spot compression views.

2. Ultrasound is in general the next step because ultrasound-guided biopsy is preferred over stereotactic biopsy.

3. Next step is to call the patient back for additional SC views and if the spiculated mass persists, then additional ultrasound targeted to the area of concern.

4. This is typical situation for an indeterminate finding on screening mammogram, which requires further workup with diagnostic mammogram and therefore it should be called BI-RADS 0 ("incomplete").

5. If patient had nipple discharge, study should be diagnostic mammogram and not a screening mammogram. Otherwise, workup would still include spot compression views and ultrasound. Since there is an abnormality that can explain discharge, no need for ductogram.

Pearls

- Ultrasound is always indicated if new "mass" or "asymmetry" is seen on mammogram.
- Any biopsy performed on ultrasound is in general easier to perform and more convenient than biopsy performed on the stereotactic biopsy table or upright stereotactic system.
- If ultrasound fails to show corresponding finding, stereotactic biopsy should be performed.

Suggested Readings

Meyer JE, Kopans DB, Stomper PC, Lindfors KK. Occult breast abnormalities: percutaneous preoperative needle localization. *Radiology*. 1984;150(2):335-337.

Sickles EA. Mammographic features of "early" breast cancer. *AJR Am J Roentgenol*. 1984;143(3):461-464.

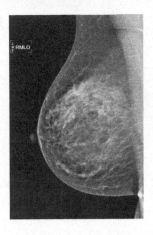
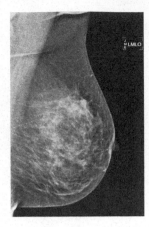
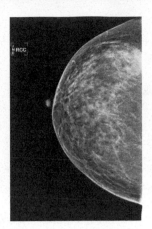
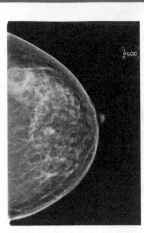

1. What is the BI-RADS category for this screening exam?

2. Where in the breast do you think the lesion lies?

3. What are the appropriate tests during diagnostic workup in this patient?

4. How would you describe the calcifications, shown?

5. What is the likely pathology in this patient?

Case ranking/difficulty:

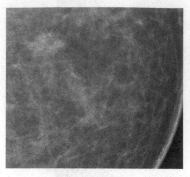

Left CC spot magnification shows ill-defined mass, and a cluster of amorphous calcifications anterior to the index lesion.

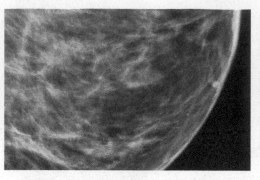

Left ML close-up view shows that the mass lies in the lower half of the breast, and not in the upper breast as we first thought. This was confirmed with MRI, which showed only the single index cancer at 6 o'clock.

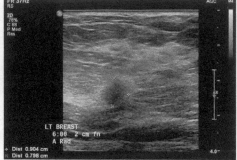

Targeted ultrasound to the mammographic finding shows an "ill-defined mass" deep in the breast disc with a "wide zone of transition" (bright halo).

Answers

1. This is an abnormal screening exam, so a BI-RADS 0 for further workup is indicated.

2. Based on the images at screening, we thought the lesion was going to be in the 12 o'clock position in the left breast. It was only when we did the diagnostic views that the subtle appearances of a mass were seen in the lower half, and the upper half asymmetry was confirmed to be superimposition only.

3. Many views may be appropriate, especially when you suspect something strongly and the follow-up films do not assist in the diagnosis or to target the lesion with ultrasound. In this patient, spot magnification views showed no abnormality in the upper half of the left breast. In these cases, MRI is useful to ensure that there is only a single lesion, and also to establish its position in the breast. You can then use second look ultrasound to identify the lesion and target biopsy. That is the approach we took with this patient. Some centers use "screening" ultrasound to determine position, rather than using targeted ultrasound. This is easier with automated breast ultrasound.

4. The calcific particles are difficult to characterize in this patient. They have no specific form, and are therefore "amorphous." "Punctate calcifications" are fine pin-prick-like calcifications with well-defined smooth outlines. They should be less than 0.5 mm in size. Stereotactic core biopsy showed microcystic change with benign microcalcifications.

5. Although fat necrosis can mimic malignancy (even giving BI-RADS 5 appearances), there is no history of trauma to support this, or hematoma. This lesion is likely to be a standard invasive ductal adenocarcinoma.

Pearls

- Localizing a lesion in a quadrant is important when you want to perform targeted ultrasound.
- Tomosynthesis should assign the, problem of the one view asymmetry, to the history books.

Suggested Reading

Venkatesan A, Chu P, Kerlikowske K, Sickles EA, Smith-Bindman R. Positive predictive value of specific mammographic findings according to reader and patient variables. *Radiology*. 2009;250(3):648-657.

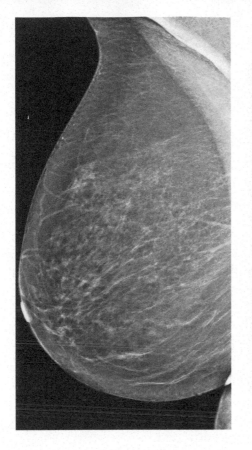 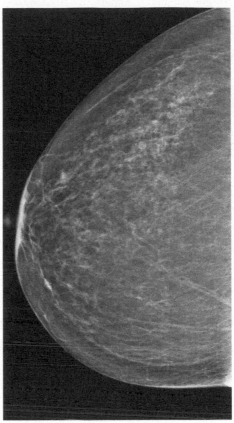

1. What is the abnormality?

2. What is the next step if there is a group of "pleomorphic" calcifications on magnification views?

3. What histological diagnosis would be concordant with the imaging?

4. Why is it important to try to differentiate between low- and high-grade DCIS?

5. What do descriptors imply?

Case ranking/difficulty:

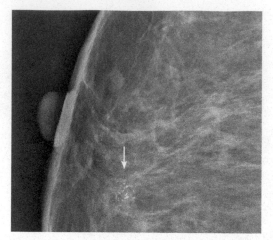

Diagnostic mammogram, right magnification ML view demonstrating group of "pleomorphic" calcifications.

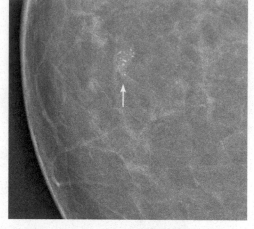

Diagnostic mammogram, right magnification CC view demonstrating group of "pleomorphic" calcifications.

Answers

1. Group of calcifications in the retroareolar breast, inferior and medial. Based on a screening mammogram, findings should not be further characterized but called "indeterminate" and more detailed characterization and assessment should be based on the further workup with diagnostic mammogram including magnification views.

2. Stereotactic biopsy is the next step to get a histological diagnosis. After the result is obtained, a decision has to be made if the results are concordant with the imaging finding.

3. DCIS is the most likely corresponding diagnosis—it could be low grade, but in this case it is more likely higher grade given the "pleomorphic" appearance of the calcifications. An invasive component could also be part of the process.

4. High-grade DCIS is a serious condition, which will progress rapidly and oftentimes come with an associated soft-tissue abnormality (mass) that can be detected by additional ultrasound. Low-grade DCIS is a very slow progressive change, which, only in some cases, might eventually progress into higher grade malignancy.

5. BI-RADS descriptors such as "round and oval" and "amorphous and indistinct" correlate to the Tabar descriptors such as "pearl like" and "powdery," which are more likely found in low-grade DCIS. BI-RADS

descriptors such as "coarse and heterogeneous," "pleomorphic," and "linear and branching" correlate to the Tabar descriptors such as "coarse granular," "crushed stone," and "casting," which are more likely found in high- and intermediate-grade DCIS.

Pearls

- DCIS can be divided into high- and low-grade DCIS, which have different clinical behavior and significance.
- Shapes such as "pleomorphe" and "fine and linear" (BI-RADS) and also "casting" or "crushed stone" (Tabar) are more likely to represent high-grade DCIS.
- Shapes such as "round and oval," "amorphous or indistinct" (BI-RADS), and "fine granular" or "powdery" (Tabar) are more likely to represent low-grade DCIS.

Suggested Readings

Bird RE. Critical pathways in analyzing breast calcifications. *Radiographics*. 1995;15(4):928-934.

D'Orsi CJ, Bassett LW, Berg WA, et al. *Breast Imaging Reporting and Data System: ACR BI-RADS–Mammography*. 4th ed. Reston, VA: American College of Radiology; 2003.

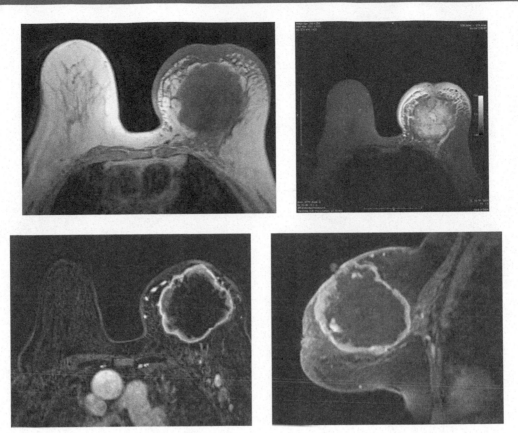

1. What are the typical findings of an abscess?

2. What would be included in the management of an abscess.

3. What is idiopathic granulomatous mastitis?

4. Why was MRI performed as first test?

5. What would be the likely differential diagnosis?

Case ranking/difficulty:

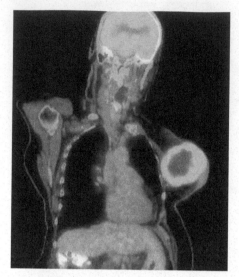

Coronal PET CT demonstrating large mass in the left breast taking up FDG.

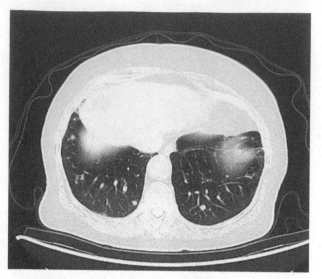

CT demonstrating nodules in both lung bases consistent with metastasis.

Answers

1. Unfortunately, some symptoms are not very specific, such as lymphadenopathy and thickening of the skin. More specific in favor of an abscess in comparison with tumor are the presence of fever and more sudden development of the mass.

2. Depending on the size, the first choice will be to treat the patient with antibiotics. If this does not yield any improvement, the thought should include malignancy and biopsy should be performed (in general ultrasound guided). In general, surgeons prefer surgical excision of an abscess over drainage. Steroids are not a preferred choice and would make the situation worse.

3. This is a rare entity, which can be found oftentimes in middle eastern countries and oftentimes in younger patients. It is in general a diagnosis of exclusion based on the lack of improvement of a presumed inflammation with antibiotics and subsequent biopsy showing granulomas. Treatment usually includes local excision and steroids.

4. In general, the first choice would be mammogram and then ultrasound. In this particular case, the pain of the patient was so strong that she did not tolerate mammogram.

5. The differential diagnosis to abscess it poorly differentiated carcinoma.

Pearls

- This case illustrates the need for a good clinical correlation with the imaging findings to determine the correct diagnosis.
- Most often, skin erythema, tenderness, and fever as seen in abscess are not present with breast cancer.
- However, inflammatory breast carcinoma and lymphoma can present with similar symptoms and imaging appearance as an abscess.
- Any failure of traditional management to resolve symptoms of an abscess or infection should prompt tissue diagnosis to exclude malignancy.

Suggested Readings

Bani-Hani KE, Yaghan RJ, Matalka II, et al. Idiopathic granulomatous mastitis: time to avoid unnecessary mastectomies. *Breast J*. 2004;10(4):318-322.

Bland KI, Copeland EM et al. *The Breast 4th Ed*. Saunders Elsevier; 2009:145-149.

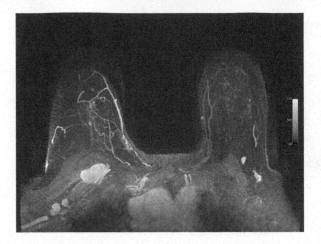

1. In which plane is this mass sited?

2. What is the likely underlying pathology?

3. What type of enhancement do you expect on a delayed scan?

4. What signal do you expect this mass to show on T2 images?

5. What biopsy technique would you recommend to get a diagnosis?

Case ranking/difficulty:

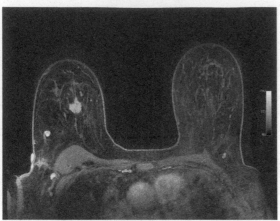

MRI breast with contrast. This slice is below the level of the Rotter node and shows the primary breast cancer as well as a metastatic intramammary lymph node.

Answers

1. This is a "Rotter node," which lies in the plane between the pectoralis major and minor.

2. This is a metastatic Rotter node. This is not normally excised if the patient is having axillary clearance. MRI is the best method for detecting this type of nodal metastasis. If not treated by excision, potentially it is a source of recurrent disease.

3. This is a lymph node and therefore washes out rapidly. It has a suspicious kinetic curve.

4. Nodes are typically T2 bright.

5. These nodes are usually visualized on ultrasound, and either FNA cytology or core biopsy under ultrasound guidance is suitable for tissue sampling. Usually, the node is noticed on MRI, and the ultrasound is a second look, as with axillary staging, these are not within our examination field.

Pearls

- Rotter nodes are a rare finding.
- They are not usually found on ultrasound.
- They are usually found on MRI scans for proven cancer.

Suggested Readings

Bembenek A, Schlag PM. Lymph-node dissection in breast cancer. *Langenbecks Arch Surg.* 2000;385(4):236-245.

Chandawarkar RY, Shinde SR. Interpectoral nodes in carcinoma of the breast: requiem or resurrection. *J Surg Oncol.* 1996;62(3):158-161.

Cody HS, Egeli RA, Urban JA. Rotter's node metastases. Therapeutic and prognostic considerations in early breast carcinoma. *Ann Surg.* 1984;199(3):266-270.

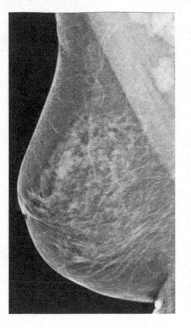
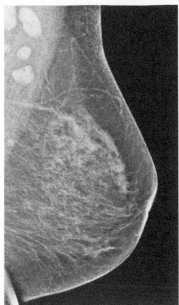

1. What is the significance of abnormal lymph
   nodes seen on mammogram?

2. What is the next step in evaluation
   of the lymph nodes?

3. What are the typical ultrasound features
   for malignancy of lymph node?

4. If lymphoma is suspected, what tests
   are preferred?

5. What could be the etiology for calcifications
   within axillary lymph nodes?

Case ranking/difficulty:

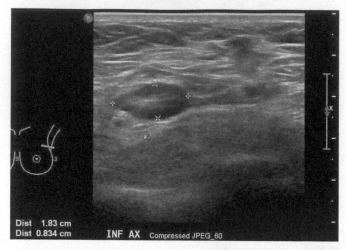

Dist 1.83 cm
Dist 0.834 cm
INF AX Compressed JPEG_60

Ultrasound of left axilla demonstrates eccentric thickening of the cortex of the lymph nodes (more than 3 mm).

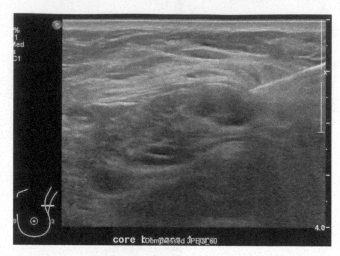

core Compressed JPEG_60

Ultrasound-guided needle biopsy with 14-gauge device.

Answers

1. Although there are studies suggesting 3.3 cm length for a non–fat-containing lymph node as threshold for possible malignancy, ultrasound is superior to mammography in evaluating lymph nodes. In a clinically asymptomatic patient, even smaller nodes can be suspicious in the appropriate setting, as seen in this case. It was in particular concerning, since lymph node had developed since last mammogram.

2. Most helpful is further evaluation with ultrasound. Morphological features such as thickening of the cortex of lymph node (more than 3 mm), penetrating cortical vessels, are seen only on ultrasound and help to decide if biopsy is necessary.

3. Suspicious features are irregular eccentric thickening of the cortex of the lymph node more than 3 mm in diameter and the presence of penetrating vessels outside the hilum at the cortex of the lymph node.

4. Primary lymphoma of the breast is extremely rare— about 2.5% of all extranodal forms of lymphoma. Core biopsy is preferred to obtain enough material for immunohistochemistry. However, if core biopsy cannot be performed due to the location of the node, fine needle aspiration is an alternative.

5. Metastatic breast carcinoma is the most common etiology for axillary lymph node calcifications as seen in about 3% of breast malignancies. In rare cases, axillary lymph nodes with calcifications could be related to

metastases from extramammary primary carcinoma, in particular with metastatic ovarian carcinoma. Axillary lymph nodes calcifications can also be seen in association with benign processes such as granulomatous disease, for example, rheumatoid arthritis.

Pearls

- Evaluation of lymph nodes on mammography is limited and changes over time, and size of the nodes is an important feature for possible concern.
- According to the study of Walsh et al. (1997), the length of non-fatty lymph node of more than 33 mm had specificity for malignancy of 97%.
- In general, core biopsy of lymph nodes is feasible. If technically not possible, fine needle aspiration can be performed.

Suggested Readings

Abe H, Schmidt RA, Kulkarni K, Sennett CA, Mueller JS, Newstead GM. Axillary lymph nodes suspicious for breast cancer metastasis: sampling with US-guided 14-gauge core-needle biopsy—clinical experience in 100 patients. *Radiology*. 2009;250(1):41-49.

Walsh R, Kornguth PJ, Soo MS, Bentley R, DeLong DM. Axillary lymph nodes: mammographic, pathologic, and clinical correlation. *AJR Am J Roentgenol*. 1997;168(1):33-38.

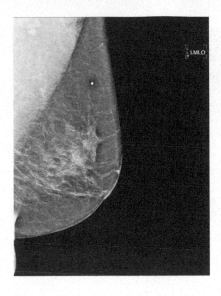
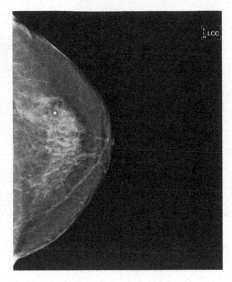
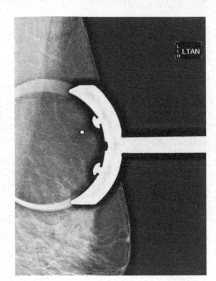

1. What is the finding on mammogram?

2. Why is this not a fibroadenoma?

3. What would be the reason to perform biopsy?

4. Why is follow-up not needed, despite the fact that it is palpable?

5. What is the difference between lipoma and adenolipoma?

Case ranking/difficulty:

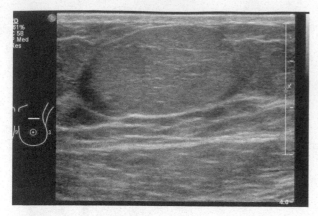

Ultrasound directed to the area of lump demonstrating "oval mass" with "circumscribed margins," "hyperechoic" in comparison with the surrounding fat.

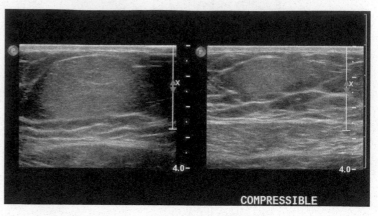

Ultrasound with compression demonstrates deformity of the mass with pressure.

Answers

1. The area marked with BB demonstrates fatty tissue best seen on the MLO projection and no focal abnormality.

2. Although fibroadenomas are more common in young patients, they can also be seen in older patients. This is especially the case in the presence of hormone replacement therapy. In this particular case, the mass is not seen at all on mammogram and is very soft under compression. This is typical for the presence of lipoma.

3. In general, palpable findings are suspicious because we can assume that they did grow—since they were not palpable previously—and therefore biopsy should be considered. This also applies in general to relatively benign-looking lesions such as masses most consistent with fibroadenomas or "complicated cysts" or "complex masses" with cystic components. However, if a palpable finding demonstrates typical morphology of fibroadenoma, many mammographers tend to follow the lesion over 2 years and call it probably benign. If there are multiple scattered similar benign-appearing lesions, the level of suspicion will be lower and follow-up might be considered of multiple benign-appearing palpable findings. In case of a simple lipoma, in general, no follow-up is required.

4. There are no case reports of malignant transformation of a lipoma into malignancy in the literature. There is only one report of transformation of a adenolipoma (hamartoma) of the breast with the presence of lobular carcinoma in situ. Therefore, in general, BI-RADS 2 is adequate and concern is less in comparison with a fibroadenoma that contains fibroglandular tissue and has therefore a higher potential for malignant transformation. If the lesion remains growing in size, excision, however, could be considered.

Remember, even the more complex fat-containing lesions (hamartomas) are called benign (BI-RADS 2).

5. If the lesion contains only fat, it is called lipoma—if there is more complex on imaging, it is called, in general, fibroadenolipoma or hamartoma. This implies that it contains fat, glandular, and fibrous tissue. Bottom line—as soon as a lesion contains fat on mammogram and has no features suggesting malignancy, it is benign (BI-RADS 2). This includes the more complex of the three entities, hamartoma.

Pearls

- In young patients, the most common mass is fibroadenoma.
- In older patients, the most common mass is cyst.
- In postmenopausal females, it is unusual to see development of fibroadenoma, which requires, in general, stimulation by estrogens.
- If mass is benign in appearance on ultrasound and there is no mass seen on corresponding fatty-replaced mammogram, finding is lipoma and benign.

Suggested Readings

Mendiola H, Henrik-Nielsen R, Dyreborg U, et al. Lobular carcinoma in situ occurring in adenolipoma of the breast. Report of a case. *Acta Radiol Diagn (Stockh)*. 1982;23(5):503-505.

Stavros TA. *Breast Ultrasound*. 1st ed. Philadelphia, PA: Lippincott Williams & Wilkins; 2004.

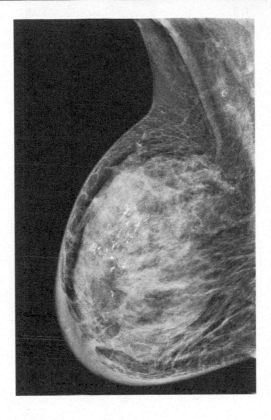 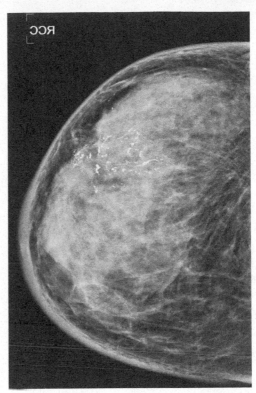

1. What BI-RADS classification should be used here?

2. What BI-RADS descriptors would you use for this calcifications?

3. Calcifications are seen in the lymph nodes. What is the differential diagnosis?

4. What is the likely pathology in this case?

5. What is the most likely type of tumor that the patient had conservation for?

Case ranking/difficulty:

Category: Diagnostic

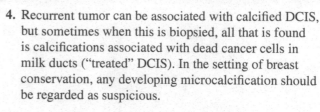

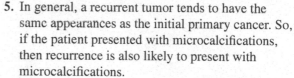

Right CC spot magnification view shows "segmental" distribution of "fine pleomorphic" microcalcifications: "casting type" (Tabar classification indicating calcification within ducts and not terminal ductal lobular units (TLDUs)).

4. Recurrent tumor can be associated with calcified DCIS, but sometimes when this is biopsied, all that is found is calcifications associated with dead cancer cells in milk ducts ("treated" DCIS). In the setting of breast conservation, any developing microcalcification should be regarded as suspicious.

5. In general, a recurrent tumor tends to have the same appearances as the initial primary cancer. So, if the patient presented with microcalcifications, then recurrence is also likely to present with microcalcifications.

Pearls

- Larger areas of DCIS preop are more likely to recur, even after full radiation therapy.
- Usually between years 2 and 4 posttreatment.
- Easy to spot, as developing calcifications in treated breast.

Answers

1. Classic "linear" and branching "pleomorphic microcalcifications" consistent with high-grade DCIS, in a background of residual postradiation change. BI-RADS 5: highly suspicious for malignancy.

2. This is a great example of "fine pleomorphic" calcifications. Many of the individual calcific particles have irregular borders with both a "crushed stone" and "casting" appearance (Tabar classification indicating site within TLDU and ducts). Secretory calcifications are "linear" and "branching" and are a BI-RADS special case, and look different to these calcifications. "Dystrophic" calcifications: the calcifications of DCIS are a type of dystrophic calcifications from dead cancer cells, but dystrophic calcifications postradiation are usually related to fat necrosis.

3. This patient did not have concomitant lymphoma, although it is a cause of calcified nodes. Sarcoid is the most common cause of nodal calcifications. Tattoo ink uses heavy metal pigments, and this may travel up the lymphatics into the nodes and present as calcified nodes. Extravasated silicone may also end up as densities within the lymph nodes.

Suggested Readings

Kane RL, Virnig BA, Shamliyan T, Wang SY, Tuttle TM, Wilt TJ. The impact of surgery, radiation, and systemic treatment on outcomes in patients with ductal carcinoma in situ. *J Natl Cancer Inst Monogr.* 2010;2010(41):130-133.

Lewis-Jones HG, Whitehouse GH, Leinster SJ. The role of magnetic resonance imaging in the assessment of local recurrent breast carcinoma. *Clin Radiol.* 1991;43(3):197-204.

Ralleigh G, Walker AE, Hall-Craggs MA, Lakhani SR, Saunders C. MR imaging of the skin and nipple of the breast: differentiation between tumour recurrence and post-treatment change. *Eur Radiol.* 2001;11(9): 1651-1658.

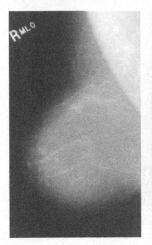 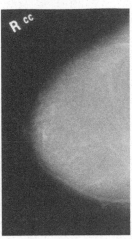 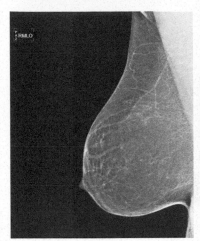 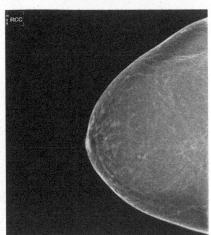

1. What is the subtle finding comparing the new images with the old screening mammogram?

2. What would be the first step of the workup of the patient?

3. What is the next step of the workup?

4. What is your final assessment and how would you choose your next step?

5. What are the next steps after the ultrasound-guided biopsy?

Case ranking/difficulty:

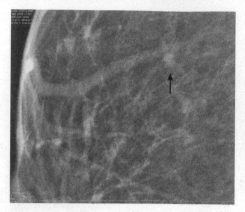

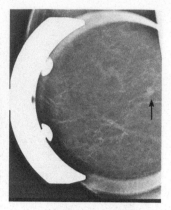

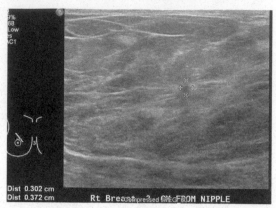

Mammogram right spot compression MLO view confirming the presence of small mass in the right breast at 12:00 orientation. The mass demonstrates "irregular" shape and "indistinct" margins.

Mammogram right spot compression CC view confirming the presence of small mass in the right breast at 12:00 orientation. The mass demonstrates "irregular" shape.

Ultrasound confirms small mass in the right breast at 12:00 orientation: "taller-than-wide" (Stavros) and "angular" shape.

Answers

1. Noted is a new small "focal asymmetry" in the right superior breast. The term 'nodular density' should not be used as it is not a BI-RADS descriptor.

2. The appropriate workup would include a spot compression MLO and CC views and a full-field ML view to better localize the lesion. The purpose is to confirm that the lesion is real and that this is not due to projection of normal fibroglandular tissue. Additional views will also assess the lesion further to determine the final assessment and level of concern. At this point, biopsy is feasible if the mammogram workup confirms the presence of the abnormality.

3. Next step would be to see if ultrasound is able to visualize the small lesion. If yes, this can further assess the level of concern and also will be able to be used as guidance for biopsy. If the lesion is not seen on ultrasound—based on the mammogram finding alone—biopsy is required. In case of negative ultrasound, stereotactic biopsy would be warranted.

4. This is based on BI-RADS descriptors: "mass," "irregular shape," "indistinct margin" (on mammogram), and "antiparallel" or "taller than wide" (Stavros) on ultrasound and therefore suspicious in nature and should be classified as BI-RADS 4—you could argue it might be even BI-RADS 5. Difference would be that if pathology demonstrates no malignancy, and classification as BI-RADS 5, pathology cannot be trusted and excisional biopsy is required. In this case, however, focal fibrosis—

maybe after a trauma—could be an outcome that could explain the finding and therefore BI-RADS 4 was chosen.

5. It is crucial to leave a clip to mark the area of biopsy and also to confirm that the clip is in the correct position by repeating mammogram of the right breast. This will allow you to find the area for subsequent needle localization and surgery.

Pearls

- Any developing "focal density" or new "mass" is worrisome for malignancy.
- "Nodule" is not a BI-RADS term.
- Ultrasound is able to show 3-mm suspicious mass, even in fatty-replaced breast.
- If ultrasound fails to demonstrate corresponding finding, stereotactic biopsy is recommended.
- After ultrasound-guided biopsy, it is important to leave a clip to mark the area.

Suggested Readings

D'Orsi CJ, Bassett LW, Berg WA, et al. *Breast Imaging Reporting and Data System: ACR BI-RADS–Mammography.* 4th ed. Reston, VA: American College of Radiology; 2003.

Stavros AT, Thickman D, Rapp CL, Dennis MA, Parker SH, Sisney GA. Solid breast nodules: use of sonography to distinguish between benign and malignant lesions. *Radiology.* 1995;196(1):123-134.

50-year-old woman with screening exam (the two figures on the extreme right) and prior exam (the two figures on the extreme left)

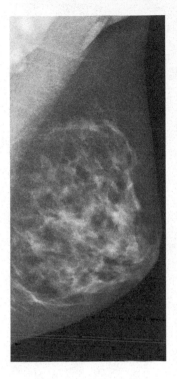 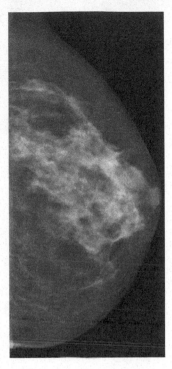 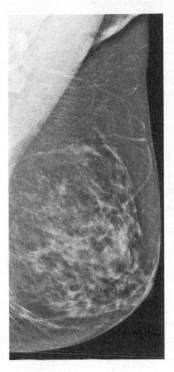 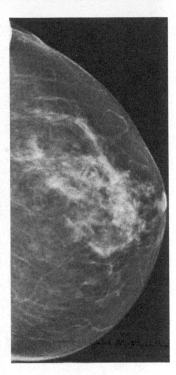

1. What is the epidemiology of invasive lobular carcinoma (ILC)?

2. What are the typical features of ILC in mammography and ultrasound?

3. What are the typical features of ILC on MRI?

4. Why is the ILC a difficult tumor to detect by a radiologist?

5. Why is breast MRI important, in particular, for ILC?

Case ranking/difficulty: 🌸🌸

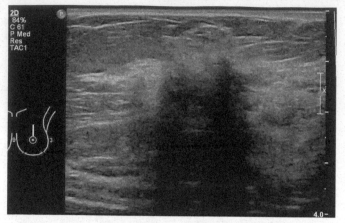

Ultrasound demonstrates large 2-cm "irregular mass" with "posterior acoustic shadowing" in the left retroareolar breast.

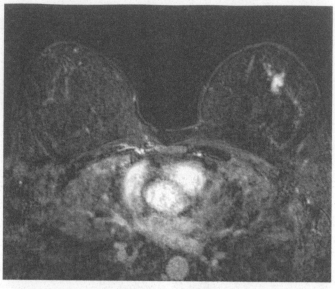

MRI, T1-weighted images after IV contrast demonstrating area of increased enhancement in the left superior breast.

Answers

1. ILC has increased in incidence from 9.5% in 1987 to 15.6% in 1999. It accounts for approximately 10% to 15% of all invasive breast cancers.

2. Because of lack of desmoplastic reaction, the density of ILC on mammography is less than other breast cancers, and the growth pattern is oftentimes diffuse. Mammography oftentimes shows a spiculated mass with "architectural distortion" or "focal asymmetry." ILC is oftentimes better seen on CC than on the MLO view. Ultrasound demonstrates, in general, an "irregular" mass with "posterior acoustic shadowing." However, sometimes ILC appears with more subtle findings on ultrasound, such as thickening of the cooper ligaments and diffuse septal hypoechoic thickening.

3. MRI demonstrates the same characteristics as on the other imaging such as "spiculated, irregular" mass. The enhancement pattern is not very specific and shows a variety of possible kinetics. Oftentimes, however, there is increasing contrast enhancement over time. Washout enhancement is not very often seen. On T2-weighted sequences, the signal is usually decreased and there might be perifocal edema identified.

4. Because of lack of desmoplastic reaction, there are less likely secondary signs such as nipple retraction. The false-negative rate from mammography is high and sensitivity is only between 57% and 81%.

5. MRI does help to show additional findings, since in 32% there is additional ipsilateral disease and about 7% additional contralateral disease. This is oftentimes missed with mammography and ultrasound.

Pearls

- Detection of ILC with mammography is limited and ILC is oftentimes difficult to see in dense breast tissue.
- Any patient with palpable abnormality needs additional ultrasound.
- Breast MRI is, in particular, important for preoperative assessment of ILC, since the extent of the tumor can be better delineated on MRI.
- Comparison with old mammograms is crucial, in particular in case of lobular carcinoma and in general for all screening mammograms.

Suggested Readings

Lopez J, Bassett L. Invasive lobular carcinoma of the breast: spectrum of mammographic, US, and MRI imaging findings. *Radiographics*. 2009;29:165-176.

Veltman J, Boetes C, Van Die L, et al. Mammographic detection and staging of invasive lobular carcinoma. *Clin Imaging*. 2006;30(2):94-98.

CT for suspected pulmonary embolus

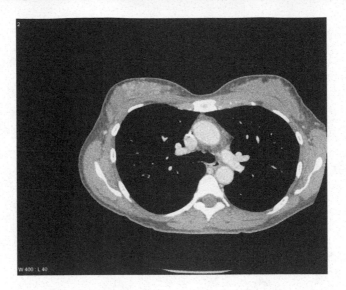

1. What are the causes of enhancing breast tissue on CT?

2. What BI-RADS classification should be used here?

3. What is the most likely cause for these appearances?

4. What is the next best imaging test?

5. What lesions on CT are ill defined?

Case ranking/difficulty:

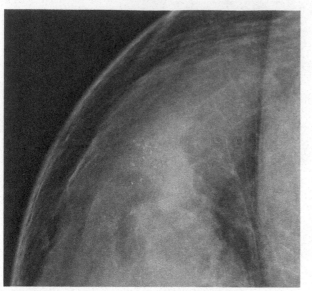

Right CC spot magnification view showing the extensive suspicious pleomorphic segmental microcalcification, consistent with high-grade DCIS.

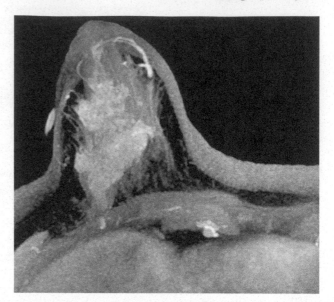

MIP reconstruction to show extensive non–mass-like enhancement in the right breast (of a different patient).

Answers

1. All of the above are potential causes of enhancing breast tissue. Enhancing breast tissue is not common on CT, and if diffuse and unilateral, it may represent DCIS. If bilateral, think of hormonal change. Masses may enhance, but if smooth and circumscribed, more likely to be benign, and irregular masses are more likely to be malignant.

2. None. BI-RADS was not written to report findings on CT. The BI-RADS lexicon is used for reporting mammography, breast ultrasound, and breast MRI.

3. Although these appearances can occur unilaterally in only one breast in normal hormonal change, it is more usual to be bilateral and patchy. DCIS, which enhances, is usually high grade, analogous to clumped ductal enhancement on MRI. PASH does not usually enhance. Both invasive lobular carcinoma and invasive ductal carcinoma usually present as a mass on CT, which does not necessarily enhance.

4. Mammography should be performed to pick up any suspicious microcalcifications that may potentially represent DCIS. MRI is a good test in this situation, but judicious timing with the patient's cycle is important, as she is likely to have enhancing breast tissue given her CT appearances. Ultrasound can be used when an abnormality can be targeted. Screening ultrasound in this situation may give rise to a high false-positive rate. Both positron emission mammography (PEM) and breast

specific gamma imaging (BSGI) potentially could be used if conventional imaging is inconclusive.

5. Diffuse enhancement is usually benign or normal. More segmental change potentially could be DCIS. Fibroadenoma and phyllodes have similar benign-looking mass-like lesions on CT. Radial scar could potentially enhance with ill-defined margins if extensive proliferative change or DCIS is associated with the scar.

Pearls

- Segmental or regional enhancement of dense breast tissue warrants at least a breast imaging workup.
- In younger women, the DCIS may be noncalcified, and therefore unlikely to be seen on mammogram.
- Calcifications, if present, can usually be seen on the mammogram even in women with extremely dense breasts.
- MRI likely to be the best imaging test.

Suggested Readings

Lin WC, Hsu HH, Li CS, et al. Incidentally detected enhancing breast lesions on chest computed tomography. *Korean J Radiol.* 2011;12(1):44-51.

Taira N, Ohsumi S, Takabatake D, et al. Contrast-enhanced CT evaluation of clinically and mammographically occult multiple breast tumors in women with unilateral early breast cancer. *Jpn J Clin Oncol.* 2008;38(6):419-425.

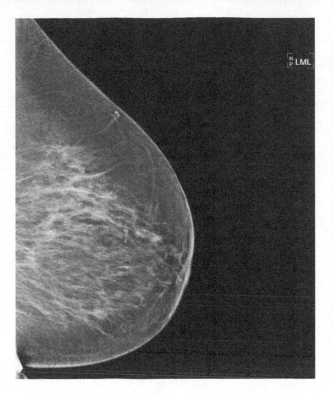
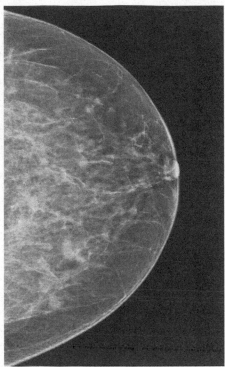

1. How often among breast cancers are mucinous carcinomas?

2. What is the characteristic appearance on ultrasound?

3. Why is it helpful to differentiate pure from mixed mucinous carcinomas?

4. What are the imaging features that favor the presence of pure form of mucinous carcinoma?

5. What is the difference between a mass and focal asymmetry according to BI-RADS?

Case ranking/difficulty:

Category: Diagnostic

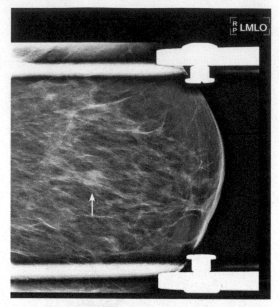

Diagnostic mammogram, left spot compression MLO view.

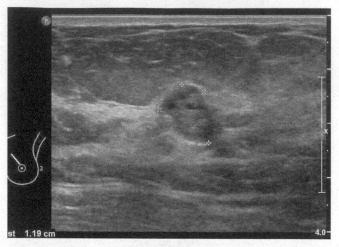

Ultrasound, B-mode demonstrates "mass" with "macrolobulated" with partially "irregular" shape (see *arrow*) but mostly "well circumscribed."

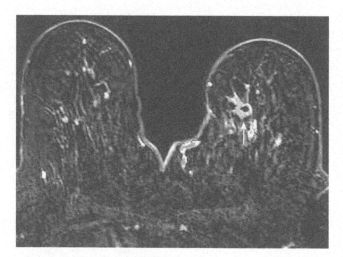

MRI T1-weighted sequence after IV contrast with mass in the left breast and clip in the center of the mass corresponding to the prior ultrasound-guided biopsy.

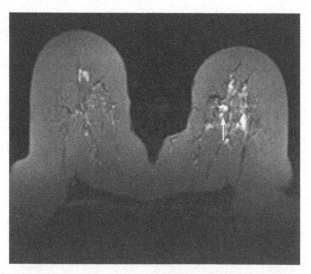

MRI T2-weighted sequence demonstrating corresponding high-signal mass.

Answers

1. Mucinous carcinoma makes up about 1% to 7% of all invasive mammary carcinomas. Prevalence is only 1% in women younger than 35 years.

2. Mucinous tumors are usually well circumscribed, round and oval, and isoechoic or hypoechoic to the subcutaneous fat. The pure form of mucinous carcinoma can show through transmission on ultrasound and sometimes can be very difficult to discern from surrounding fat. They might also present as heterogeneous complex masses with cystic elements (about 40%). Any diagnosis of a mucinous carcinoma of a mass with posterior acoustic shadowing will be highly suggestive of a more mixed and form of mucinous carcinoma or so-called intraductal carcinoma with colloid features.

3. The 10-year survival time among patient with pure mucinous tumors is 87% to 90.4% and that of among patients with mixed tumors is 54% to 66%. The likelihood of metastasis to the axilla is higher in mixed form.

4. Pure mucinous carcinomas more likely demonstrate well-circumscribed margins on imaging and appear to be more homogeneous, less likely demonstrate septations on MRI or heterogeneous echogenicity on ultrasound, and more likely demonstrate increasing enhancement over dynamic postcontrast images instead of washout enhancement.

5. The BI-RADS lexicon differentiates between "mass" and "asymmetry" in the way that an asymmetry does show up only on one projection. However, BI-RADS also describes the so-called "global asymmetry" and "focal asymmetry" as an area of increased density asymmetric to the other corresponding breast. "Focal density" is described as seen on two projections. Difference between "global asymmetry" and "focal asymmetry" is the size in relation to the size of the breast. Global asymmetries are most often consistent with normal fibroglandular tissue. However, special attention should be paid to any new or developing asymmetry.

Pearls

- As many as 21% of mucinous carcinomas might not be detected on mammogram.
- There are mucinous carcinomas with "pure" and "mixed" histology.
- The 10-year survival rate for "pure" form is 87% to 90% and for "mixed" form is 64% to 66%.
- MRI is the best modality to differentiate between both forms of mucinous carcinoma.

Suggested Readings

Lam WW, Chu WC, Tse MA, et al. Sonographic appearance of mucinous carcinoma of the breast. *AJR Am J Roentgenol.* 2004;182(4):1069-1074.

Monzawa S, Yokokawa M, Sakuma T, et al. Mucinous carcinoma of the breast: MRI features of pure and mixed forms with histopathologic correlation. *AJR Am J Roentgenol.* 2009;192:W125-W131.

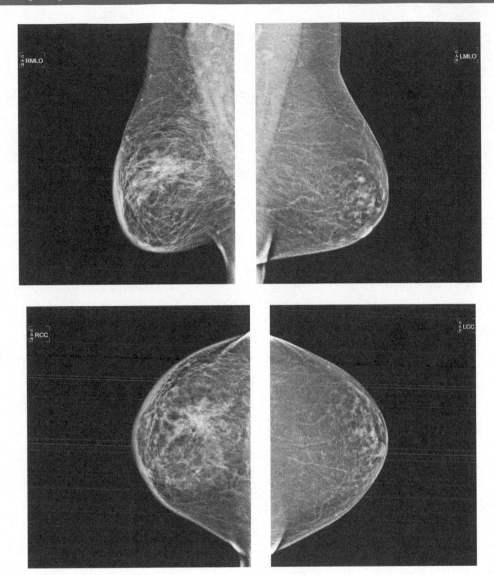

1. What are the pertinent findings in that symptomatic patient?

2. Does the MRI show any additional finding?

3. What is the appropriate description of the ultrasonography finding (image next page)?

4. What are the general reasons to perform mastectomy instead of lumpectomy?

5. What is the benefit of preoperative breast MRI?

Case ranking/difficulty:

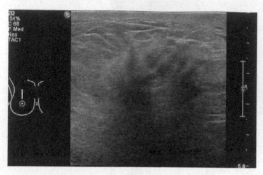

Gray-scale ultrasonography demonstrating large, highly suspicious mass in the right superior breast with "posterior acoustic shadowing" that corresponds to the mammogram finding.

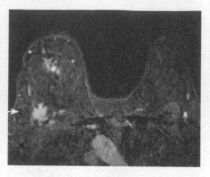

T1-weighted postcontrast sequence demonstrates the additional lesion near the chest wall.

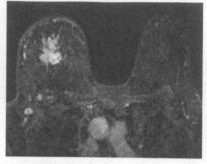

T1-weighted postcontrast sequence demonstrates the index lesion in the central right breast.

Answers

1. On the standard views (the spot compression views are not submitted), noted is a large area of "focal asymmetry" in the right superior breast with underlying "architectural distortion" and associated microcalcifications. Also noted is significant thickening of the right skin.

2. Noted on the MRI image is, in addition to the index lesion, additional 1.5-cm mass with strong enhancement in the lateral posterior right breast. This is better seen on the axial images. It is not well seen on the mammogram. It does show chest wall infiltration.

3. The index lesion as seen on mammogram demonstrates corresponding hypoechoic mass with strong posterior acoustic shadowing.

4. In general, the size of the lesion in comparison with the size of the breast will determine the need for mastectomy. In general, a mass or malignancy larger than 5 cm in an average-size breast likely requires mastectomy. Also the presence of skin or chest wall involvement and the presence of multicentric disease require mastectomy.

5. Based on a study by Fan et al looking at numbers of private community practice, surgical management is being changed after breast MRI in about 24%. Additional malignancies are being found in about 15% in the ipsilateral breast and in about 5% in the contralateral breast.

Pearls

- Adding breast MRI can show otherwise occult cancers in the ipsilateral and also in the contralateral breast.
- In a study performed in a community practice breast center, Fan et al found, in a population of 445 patients, 84 additional malignancies in 66 patients (14.8%) including 22 patients in contralateral breast (4.9%) and 48 patients with ipsilateral additional malignancies (10.8%).
- In 23.6% of these patients, MRI resulted in change of the surgical procedure.

Suggested Readings

Fan C, Nemoto T, Blatto K, et al. Impact of pre-surgical breast magnetic resonance imaging (MRI) on surgical planning—a retrospective analysis from a private radiology group. *Breast J*. 2013;19(2):134-141.

Gutierrez RL, DeMartini WB, Silbergeld JJ, et al. High cancer yield and positive predictive value: outcomes at a center routinely using preoperative breast MRI for staging. *AJR Am J Roentgenol*. 2011;196(1):W93-W99.

Schell AM, Rosenkranz K, Lewis PJ. Role of breast MRI in the preoperative evaluation of patients with newly diagnosed breast cancer. *AJR Am J Roentgenol*. 2009;192(5):1438-1444.

Patient with palpable abnormality in the left breast, history of type II diabetes—status post old benign biopsy in the left breast

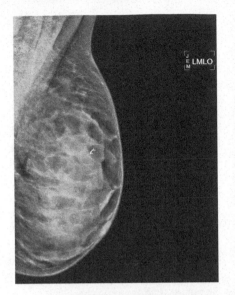

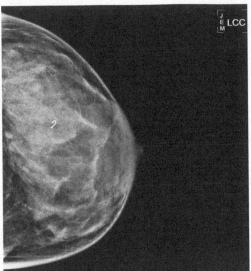

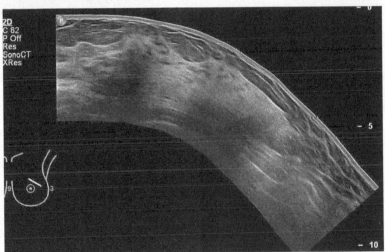

1. What are the findings on the mammogram?

2. What is the ultrasound finding corresponding to the palpable mass?

3. What is an appropriate next step?

4. What would be concordant pathology results of the previous left biopsy?

5. What is the consequence of the diagnosis of diabetic mastopathy?

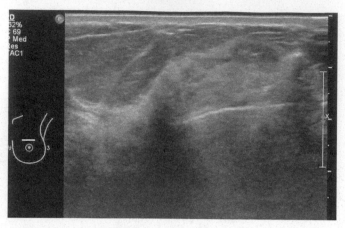

Ultrasound-guided biopsy of left breast.

Answers

1. This is a mammogram with extremely dense fibroglandular tissue. There is clip in the superior breast from prior biopsy.

2. Corresponding to the palpable abnormality is a large hypoechoic mass extending into all quadrants with "posterior acoustic shadowing." There was similar appearance of the right breast on ultrasound.

3. Ultrasound-guided core biopsy might be the first step. However, if patient had already prior biopsy, like in this case, which shows findings suggestive of diabetic mastopathy, and has a history of type I diabetes and if the finding on ultrasound is scattered throughout both breasts, it can be assumed that this is most likely a case of diabetic mastopathy and follow-up might be sufficient. There are reports that MRI might be helpful to distinguish malignancy from diabetic mastopathy.

4. All would be concordant, except the presence of benign fibroadenoma. The ultrasound finding could be malignant but would also be concordant with benign fibroproliferative changes including findings consistent with diabetic mastopathy. Diabetic mastopathy usually shows the presence of collagenous stromal fibrosis.

5. Diabetic mastopathy is a benign lesion and patient can return to screening mammography. Depending on the situation, further follow-up might be considered over a period of 2 years.

Pearls

- Diabetic fibrous mastopathy, a stromal proliferation, is found in patients with juvenile onset insulin-dependent diabetes (type I). Clinically, the most common manifestation is a firm-to-hard, nontender breast mass—there is no associated increase risk of breast cancer.
- Most of these lesions appear as masses at clinical or mammographic examination. On ultrasound, the lesions are mostly bilateral and can show suspicious appearance including the presence of "posterior acoustic shadowing."
- Fibroepithelial lesions are a combination of prominent stromal and glandular elements—fibroadenoma is the most common fibroepithelial lesion.
- Other benign fibroepithelial lesions include focal fibrosis, pseudoangiomatous stromal hyperplasia, and fibromatosis or desmoid tumor.

Suggested Readings

Gabriel HA, Feng C, Mendelson EB, Benjamin S. Breast MRI for cancer detection in a patient with diabetic mastopathy. *AJR Am J Roentgenol.* 2004;182(4):1081-1083.

Goel NB, Knight TE, Pandey S, Riddick-Young M, de Paredes ES, Trivedi A. Fibrous lesions of the breast: imaging-pathologic correlation. *Radiographics.* 2005;25(6): 1547-1559.

Sakuhara Y, Shinozaki T, Hozumi Y, Ogura S, Omoto K, Furuse M. MR imaging of diabetic mastopathy. *AJR Am J Roentgenol.* 2002;179(5):1201-1203.

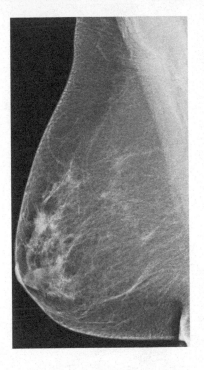
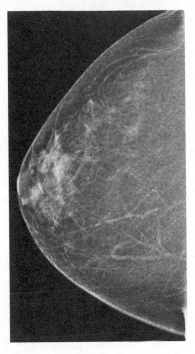
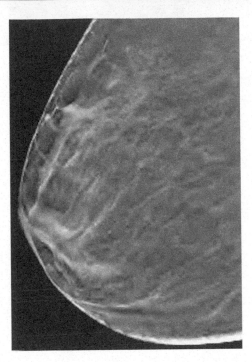

1. Is there any abnormality in the right upper outer quadrant?

2. What do you know about tomosynthesis?

3. How is tomosynthesis being used right now?

4. What do you know about primary lymphoma in the breast?

5. What is the appearance of lymphoma on imaging?

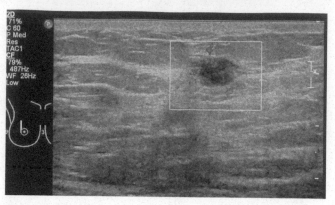

Ultrasound of right upper outer quadrant demonstrating mass at 11:00 close to the nipple. No increased flow on duplex.

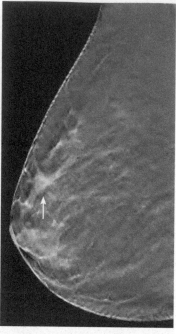

Tomosynthesis, right MLO, single 1-mm slice. Stack of slices replaces spot compression view.

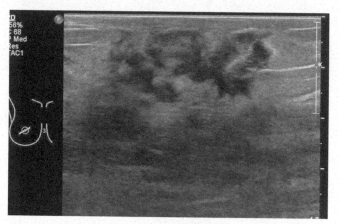

Ultrasound of retroareolar breast demonstrates the hypoechoic area, irregular in shape, which corresponds to the MRI.

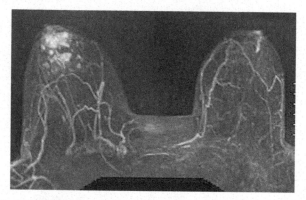

MRI maximum intensity projection (MIP) image after IV contrast demonstrates area of abnormal enhancement corresponding to the ultrasound finding.

Answers

1. This is a case where old pictures would be extremely important—a theme that cannot be repeated enough in breast imaging; thus: OLD IMAGES ARE THE KEY IN BREAST IMAGING. Yes there is a questionable mass in the right upper outer quadrant.

2. Tomosynthesis is a new mammographic technique that utilizes movement of the tube to create several slices of the breast. It is called 3D mammography and the machine looks the same and the patient does not realize any difference, but the radiologist receives multiple thin cuts in CC and MLO projection, which can be scrolled through on the workstation. The conventional current mammography machines can be referred to as 2D mammography in that context. One company got FDA approval in early 2011.

3. Tomosynthesis (3D mammography) was approved for diagnostic workup in 2011 but not to replace 2D mammography for screening. It is currently being used to replace spot compression views, since it creates multiple slices and has more information than a conventional compression view. It is more problematic in regard to calcifications. It is used in conjunction with 2D mammography as a combo (2D/3D mammography), especially for dense breasts. It is also FDA approved in conjunction with conventional mammography for screening.

4. Lymphomas contribute to about 0.15 of malignant mammary neoplasm. Less than 0.5% of all malignant mammary lymphomas involve the breast primarily. Primary breast lymphoma has an age peak at the 4th to 7th decade. The diagnosis of primary breast lymphoma is limited to patients with no evidence of systemic lymphoma or leukemia.

5. On mammogram, primary breast lymphoma, but lymphoma in general, presents often as mass, most frequently with "irregular" shape and "indistinct" margin. Other presentations include the presence of "focal asymmetry." Ultrasound demonstrates, in most cases, mass with "irregular" shape. Posterior to the mass, the echo can vary and could include "acoustic enhancement." Color Doppler imaging shows frequently hypervascularity. MRI demonstrates lobular mass, often hyperintense on T2-weighted images and heterogeneous enhancement with rapid uptake and washout. PET demonstrates vivid uptake of FDG.

Pearls

- This was a case where first invasive ductal carcinoma was the pathology result. However, after review it showed features of primary breast lymphoma.
- The treatment of primary breast lymphoma is controversial and lumpectomy is not the main focus; chemotherapy and radiation therapy are considered part of primary treatment. Approach depends on the extent of the disease, best assessed with PET CT.
- Tomosynthesis is an emerging technology, providing multiple 1-mm slices, FDA approved in 2011 for screening in conjunction with conventional mammography and for diagnostic workup as replacement for spot compression views.
- Tomosynthesis is particularly helpful to detect architectural distortion or subtle masses hidden in dense tissue and can help to eliminate need for additional spot compression views, and patient can go directly to ultrasound.
- Tomosynthesis is considered less helpful in workup of calcifications.

Suggested Readings

Hakim CM, Chough DM, Ganott MA, Sumkin JH, Zuley ML, Gur D. Digital breast tomosynthesis in the diagnostic environment: a subjective side-by-side review. *AJR Am J Roentgenol*. 2010;195(2):W172-W176.

Noroozian M, Hadjiiski L, Rahnama-Moghadam S, et al. Digital breast tomosynthesis is comparable to mammographic spot views for mass characterization. *Radiology*. 2012;262(1):61-68.

Yang WT, Lane DL, Le-Petross HT, Abruzzo LV, Macapinlac HA. Breast lymphoma: imaging findings of 32 tumors in 27 patients. *Radiology*. 2007;245(3):692-702.

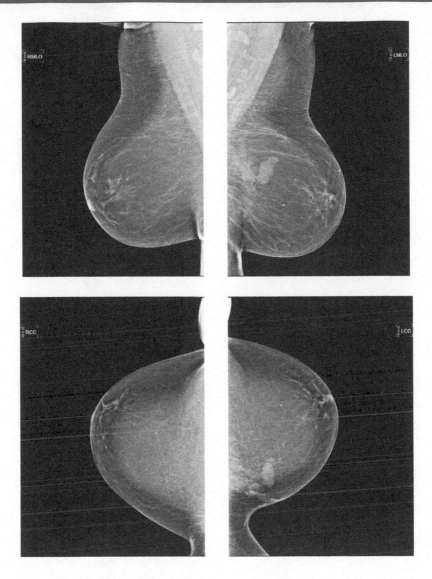

1. What BI-RADS classification should be used here?

2. What is the next imaging test?

3. What type of tumor does a chondrosarcoma arise from?

4. What determines whether a chondrosarcoma is primary breast or arising from another lesion?

5. What is the best way of treating a chondrosarcoma of the breast?

Case ranking/difficulty:

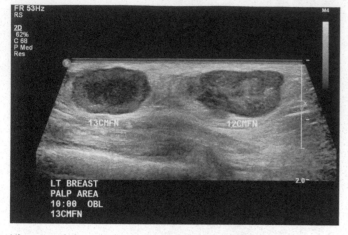

Ultrasound shows two circumscribed complex echogenicity masses. Note the acoustic enhancement behind the lesions. The mass on the left also shows a liquid necrotic center.

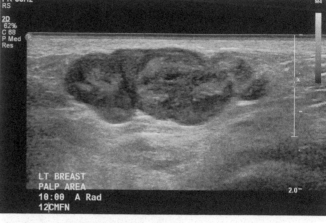

Ultrasound shows that although the mass is sharply marginated, the margins have a microlobulated appearance. There are some low echo slit-like areas raising the possibility of a phyllodes tumor.

Answers

1. Although these masses are not calcified and have circumscribed margins, their distribution is not normal. They are also palpable and feel hard, which does not fit with the normal presentation of fibroadenomas or tense simple cysts. A BI-RADS 4 assessment is the most suitable outcome.

2. Further evaluation with ultrasound is likely the best next investigation. You can perform further mammographic views if you think that the margins of the masses have not been demonstrated clearly. MRI is unlikely to give additional information to affect the management of the case.

3. Sarcomatous change has been reported in both phyllodes tumors and metaplastic carcinomas of the breast.

4. The presence of a primary sarcoma means that this is likely a secondary deposit. However, a chondrosarcoma can arise in a phyllodes tumor or a metaplastic carcinoma. Both of these lesions have an epithelial component, and so this should be excluded before calling a lesion a primary breast chondrosarcoma.

5. Treatment is primarily surgical. Chondrosarcoma of the breast is resistant to both chemotherapy and radiation therapy.

Pearls

- Multiple masses in a segmental distribution need further workup.
- Evaluate margins of lesion and then biopsy.
- With atypical pathology findings, think metaplastic carcinoma.
- Metaplastic carcinoma can cause a variety of tumor types.

Suggested Readings

Patterson JD, Wilson JE, Dim D, Talboy GE. Primary chondrosarcoma of the breast: report of a case and review of the literature [published online ahead of print]. *Breast Dis*. 2011.

Verfaillie G, Breucq C, Perdaens C, Bourgain C, Lamote J. Chondrosarcoma of the breast. *Breast J*. 2005;11(2):147-148.

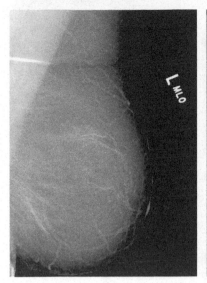 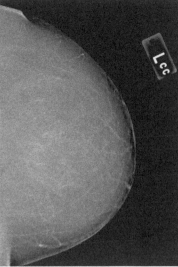 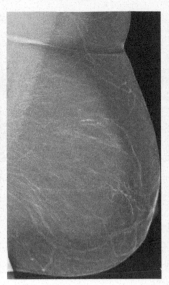 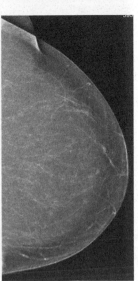

1. What is the finding on the screening mammogram?

2. Who qualifies for MRI screening?

3. What are the factors being considered for the risk calculator of the National Cancer Institute?

4. What is the average lifetime risk of women up to the age of 90?

5. What other exam would be available if patient does not qualify for MRI?

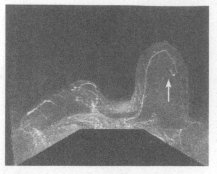

MRI of bilateral breast after IV contrast, maximum intensity projection (MIP) technique.

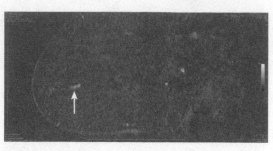

MRI, T1-weighted sequence after IV contrast, sagittal reformation.

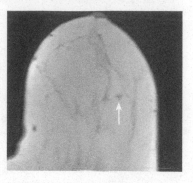

MRI of non–fat-suppressed T1-weighted sequence without contrast demonstrating small mass with "irregular" margin.

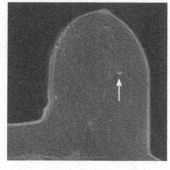

MRI of T1-weighted sequence after IV contrast demonstrates early enhancement of the small 4-mm mass.

Answers

1. This is a normal screening mammogram.

2. Patients with a lifetime risk of 20% to 25%, patient needs two first degree relatives with breast cancer, for example, mother and sister.

3. Factors that will put into the calculator are as follows:

   i. Personal history of breast cancer
   ii. Woman's age
   iii. Woman's age at the time of first menstrual period.
   iv. Woman's age at the time of her first live birth of a child
   v. Number of first-degree relatives with breast cancer
   vi. History of breast biopsies
   vii. Race/ethnicity

4. Lifetime risk depends on the age and ethnicity; for a 40-year-old white woman, it is about 12.4%, and for a 40-year-old African American, it is around 9.6%.

5. In case of not qualifying for breast MRI—and in particular if the patient has very dense breast tissue—the other exams that would be complementary to mammography and widely available would be breast ultrasound. Breast ultrasound in general is not accepted for screening but is being used by request of the referring physician. Tomosynthesis would also be a helpful adjunct to standard mammography to increase sensitivity.

Pearls

- Since 2007, most insurance companies in the United States pay for screening MRI for patients with 20% to 25% lifetime risk of breast cancer.
- There are several risk calculators available on the Internet, which help to calculate the lifetime risk based on several risk factors, for example, the National Cancer Institute webpage (www.cancer.gov/bcrisktool/).
- In general, patients with two close family members (mother and sister) will have a lifetime risk of about 25% and higher and therefore would qualify for screening breast MRI.
- This is an example where even in a fatty-replaced breast, a 5-mm-large invasive ductal carcinoma can be missed on mammogram.

Suggested Reading

Warner E, Messersmith H, Causer P, Eisen A, Shumak R, Plewes D. Systematic review: using magnetic resonance imaging to screen women at high risk for breast cancer. *Ann Intern Med.* 2008;148(9):671-679.

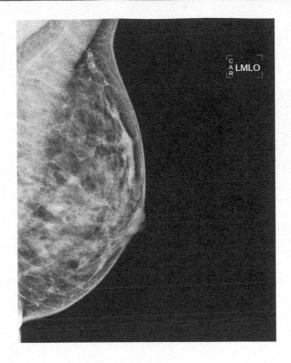
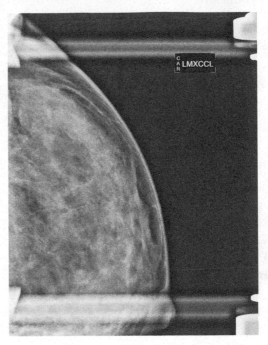

1. Would these calcifications require biopsy if they were there 2 years ago?

2. What would be the procedure if these calcifications cannot be biopsied with stereotactic approach?

3. What are two important quality-assuring steps for performing a stereotactic biopsy.

4. If the post-biopsy marker clip is displaced, what might be the consequence?

5. How can clip displacement be avoided?

Case ranking/difficulty: 🐾 🐾 🐾

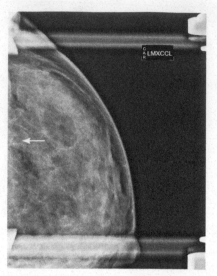

Diagnostic mammogram demonstrates group of suspicious calcifications in the left lateral, central, and posterior breast.

Diagnostic mammogram magnification XCCL view demonstrates group of suspicious calcifications in the left lateral breast.

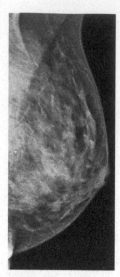

Mammogram of left breast MLO view after stereotactic biopsy demonstrates clip at the level of the nipple.

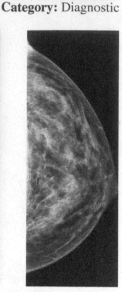

Left CC view after stereotactic biopsy after clip placement demonstrates 3-cm clip medial from the residual calcifications.

Answers

1. Calcifications—if they are suspicious based on morphological features—need to be biopsied, even if they are stable over several old mammograms. They could represent ductal carcinoma in situ (DCIS), which can progress slowly over time, in particular if it is low-grade DCIS.

2. If suspicious calcifications are seen on two projections, they can be approached with needle localization and surgical excision can be performed. Calcifications such as in this case are not accessible to stereotactic biopsy due to their location within the breast, for example, since they are located very posteriorly, patient needs to be send for needle localization and surgical excision.

3. It is important to get a specimen radiograph after stereotactic biopsy of suspicious calcifications to prove that a representative sample of the calcifications was obtained. It is not the goal to excise all calcifications. Also important is that the postbiopsy mammogram shows the clip in good position, which means that the clip is in the target zone where the specimen was collected from.

4. In most cases, it is sufficient to document the location of the misplaced clip in relation to the area that was biopsied. There are rare cases where it is helpful to place a second clip. This can be the case if the clip is short in correlation to the target and therefore the needle localization would be less accurate.

5. Clip displacement cannot be completely avoided. It is caused by the release of compression after a stereotactic biopsy.

Pearls

- Clip displacement is not uncommon, as seen on postbiopsy mammogram.
- Clip displacement is oftentimes due to traction during decompression on the stereotactic biopsy unit.
- Postbiopsy mammogram is crucial to confirm correct clip placement.
- Consequence of clip displacement can be placement of a new clip. If there are residual calcifications, or the clip is too deep, needle localization can be corrected accordingly. Important is to document the location of the clip in regard to the abnormality (target zone).

Suggested Reading

Esserman LE, Cura MA, DaCosta D. Recognizing pitfalls in early and late migration of clip markers after imaging-guided directional vacuum-assisted biopsy. *Radiographics*. 2004;24(1):147-156.

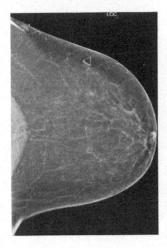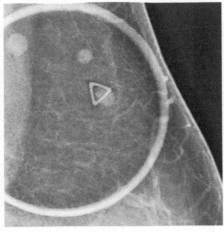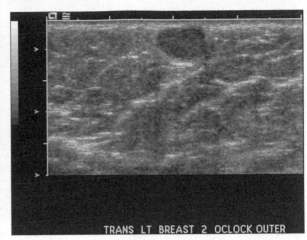

1. What BI-RADS classification should be used here?

2. What is the most likely pathology based on the imaging?

3. What is the next best imaging test?

4. What are the imaging features of a breast sarcoma?

5. What is the surgical treatment of breast sarcoma?

Case ranking/difficulty:

Category: Diagnostic

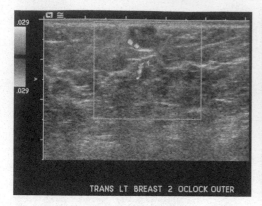

Left breast ultrasound with Doppler showing peripheral vessels—no surrounding vessels in subcutaneous tissues.

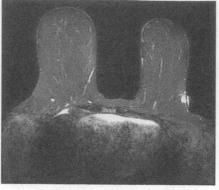

T2 axial MRI, shows homogeneous high signal circumscribed but superficial mass simulating fibroadenoma.

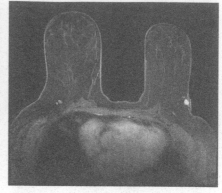

T1 fat sat axial 120 seconds following contrast injection.

Answers

1. BI-RADS 4—as the findings simulate fibroadenoma, there are some confounding features that allow you to recommend a biopsy.

2. Any of the first four answers can present as a circumscribed mass with peripheral vascularity. Interval change may help to differentiate a phyllodes tumor from a fibroadenoma. Metastases are common only when there is a known other cancer primary site setting. A simple cyst with proteinaceous debris should be belottable with gentle pressure on ultrasound. Seeing the internal echoes moving helps to distinguish form a solid mass.

3. The mass on mammography is circumscribed and similar to the nearby axillary lymph nodes. The initial ultrasound image shows that the mass is very superficial, unlike the normal position for a fibroadenoma, but could then be a node. Doppler ultrasound may show this mass to be highly vascular, including the surrounding breast tissue.

4. The characteristic features that make you suspect a sarcoma are the oval shape with indistinct margins, and marked vascularity on ultrasound. It is rare for a mass to be truly round unless it is a high tension simple cyst. Irregular margin to a mass is the suspicious finding arising from an invasive ductal carcinoma.

5. Lumpectomy with wide margins has been tried, but sarcomas when they recur are difficult to treat. The standard care has developed with mastectomy and no axillary procedure, as sarcoma rarely metastasizes to the locoregional lymph nodes. Mastectomy with reconstruction can be an option in sites with oncoplastic surgeons.

Pearls

- Rare sarcoma.
- Oval mass with indistinct margins, but can simulate a benign mass.
- MRI and ultrasound show similar features.
- Does not metastasize to the axillary nodes.
- Mastectomy without axillary dissection is standard care.

Suggested Readings

Babarović E, Zamolo G, Mustać E, Strčić M. High grade angiosarcoma arising in fibroadenoma. *Diagn Pathol.* 2011;6(1):125.

Cao Y, Panos L, Graham RL, Parker TH, Mennel R. Primary cutaneous angiosarcoma of the breast after breast trauma. *Proc (Bayl Univ Med Cent).* 2012;25(1):70-72.

Hui A, Henderson M, Speakman D, Skandarajah A. Angiosarcoma of the breast: a difficult surgical challenge. *Breast.* 2012;21(4):584-589.

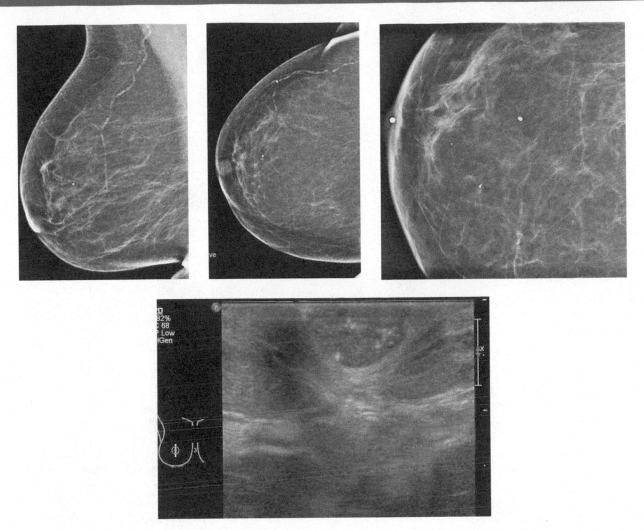

1. What is the abnormality?

2. What are typical features of Paget disease?

3. What is the differential diagnosis?

4. Patient has eczema of nipple but normal mammogram—what is the next step?

5. What is the best technique to assess retroareolar breast on ultrasound?

Case ranking/difficulty: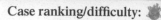

Category: Diagnostic

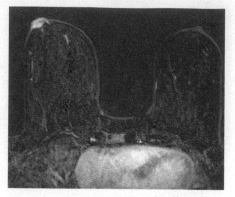

MRI T1-weighted sequence after IV contrast.

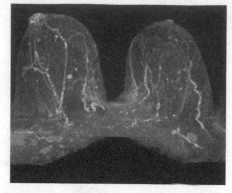

MRI T1-weighted sequence after IV contrast with CAD.

Answers

1. Noted is only minimal retraction of the nipple that was stable since prior studies (not submitted)—no other abnormality. Ultrasound does not demonstrate any abnormality neither.

2. Paget disease accounts for 2% to 3% of breast cancer. It is a clinical diagnosis with eczema of the nipple but has characteristic Paget cells within the dermis, which are consistent with adenocarcinoma. Mammograms are in most cases demonstrating findings related to high-grade ductal carcinoma in situ—however, mammograms can be normal as well.

3. Differential diagnosis could include scaring or eczema.

4. In general, ultrasound would be part of the workup to further exclude hidden abnormality in the retroareolar breast—especially in the presence of dense breast tissue. MRI can be helpful to evaluate for additional abnormalities or to further confirm abnormal nipple complex, but it is in general not required at this stage. Punch biopsy performed by breast surgeon is the crucial next step.

5. To assess the anterior retroareolar breast tissue on ultrasound and to avoid the posterior shadowing, it is helpful to compress the lateral aspect by hand and to elongate the tissue anteriorly and to approach the tissue with the transducer from the other lateral contour of the retroareolar breast. Any direct anterior approach at the level of the nipple will require large amount of gel to get rid of any air in between the transducer and the nipple.

Pearls

- Paget disease accounts for approximately 2% to 3% of breast cancers.
- Paget disease is a distinct entity, which includes erythema of the nipple areola complex that often has some underlying breast neoplasm—the characteristic histological finding is the presence of malignant Paget cells (adenocarcinoma) in the epidermis.
- Given the high incidence of underlying breast malignancy, as reported of up to 100%, it is believed that Paget cells arise in the secretory ducts and migrate into the skin of the nipple.
- Paget disease in general occurs in the age around 55 years.
- Mammography has been reported to be positive in only 40% to 50%—in most cases, it correlates to the presence of ductal carcinoma in situ.
- Early skin biopsy, called punch biopsy, is the important first step to get the diagnosis—any eczema of the breast for more than 2 weeks should be viewed with suspicion.
- Mastectomy is the standard treatment for Paget disease.
- In this particular case, however, the diagnosis was a surprise and pathology demonstrated findings consistent with solid papillary carcinoma, a relatively rare but pathologically distinct entity, which can be seen in the nipple region of elderly women.

Suggested Readings

Burke ET, Braeuning MP, McLelland R, Pisano ED, Cooper LL. Paget disease of the breast: a pictorial essay. *Radiographics*. 2000;18(6):1459-1464.

Haddad N, Ollivier L, Tardivon A, et al. Usefulness of magnetic resonance imaging in Paget disease of the breast. *J Radiol*. 2007;88(4):579-584.

Sundaram S, Prathiba D, Rao S, Rajkumar A, Rajendiran S. Solid variant of papillary carcinoma of nipple: an under recognized entity. *Indian J Pathol Microbiol*. 2011;53(3):537-540.

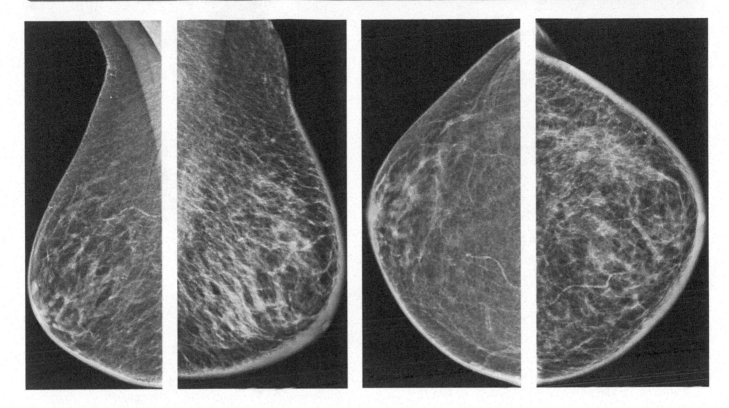

1. What is the pertinent finding on this diagnostic mammogram?

2. What is the next step of workup?

3. What are other important findings to exclude?

4. What could be the diagnosis?

5. What is the most likely diagnosis in the absence of skin alterations and the presence of edema in left leg?

Case ranking/difficulty: 🐞🐞🐞

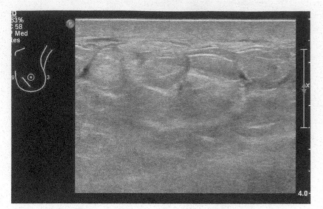

Ultrasound demonstrating interstitial edema.

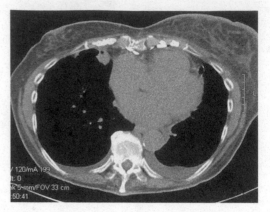

CT chest without contrast demonstrates the unilateral breast edema and pleural effusion after heart surgery.

Answers

1. Patient demonstrates uniform reticular edema of the left breast, swelling of the left breast, and uniform thickening of the skin.

2. The most important next step is the clinical evaluation. In this case, patient presented with unilateral edema including leg and arm after cardiac surgery. She also noticed the enlargement of the left breast.

3. In this particular case, it is important to exclude any focal abnormal morphology in the breast, such as masses, microcalcifications, and/or lymphadenopathy. This presentation of the left breast can be seen with inflammatory malignancy. However, inflammatory skin changes such as redness and swelling are usually seen in the presence of inflammatory malignancies of the breast.

4. Differential diagnosis could include infection, status postradiation, lymphoma, unilateral cardiac edema, and, most importantly, the presence of inflammatory carcinoma of the breast.

5. This is, given the corresponding chronicity after cardiac surgery and the presence of leg edema, likely due to a rare case of cardiac unilateral edema. If there is remaining clinical concern, punch biopsy can be performed to exclude diagnosis of inflammatory carcinoma.

Pearls

- In the absence of skin alteration, the presence of inflammatory breast cancer is extremely unlikely.
- This particular patient had recent cardiac surgery and left unilateral leg edema since surgery and was believed to represent a rare case of unilateral edema after cardiac surgery.
- However, since inflammatory cancer is a devastating malignancy, patient was send to breast surgeon for clinical evaluation—punch biopsy was not performed and patient was further followed clinically and with imaging.

Suggested Reading

Oraedu CO, Pinnapureddy P, Alrawi S, Acinapura AJ, Raju R. Congestive heart failure mimicking inflammatory breast carcinoma: a case report and review of the literature. *Breast J.* 2001;7(2):117-119.

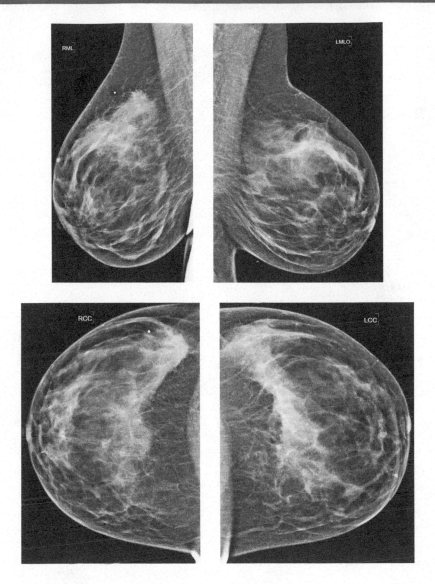

1. What BI-RADS classification should be used here?

2. What is the next imaging test?

3. What is the most likely pathological entity for these imaging appearances?

4. Dense breast tissue may have what effect on cancer detection?

5. According to BI-RADS, what are the mass margin descriptors?

Case ranking/difficulty:

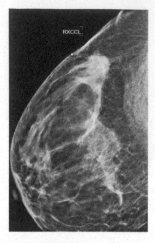

Right XCCL (exaggerated CC lateral)—this was performed rather than spot films. We do not have any images of the margins of the mass as a result. There are only scattered fibroglandular densities, but the breast tissue where the cancer is arising is dense enough to partially obscure the lesion.

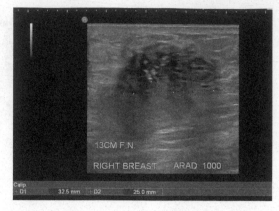

Ultrasound shows calcifications within the irregular mass.

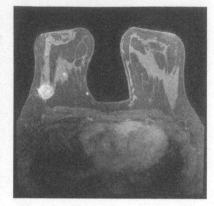

MRI was performed for extent of the lesion.

Answers

1. If this was a screening exam, then a BI-RADS 0 is appropriate. If the finding is palpable, then this would be a diagnostic exam and further images should be performed. We need to determine whether we can see the margins of the suspected mass, and perform an ultrasound scan.

2. The most appropriate examinations are as follows:

   i. Spot views to press out the normal tissue and reveal the underlying mass
   ii. Targeted ultrasound examination

   At this stage, MRI is not indicated, but if after a full workup you cannot determine the cause of the finding on imaging, and there is nothing to target for a biopsy, a troubleshooting MRI may help.

3. Pseudoangiomatous stromal hyperplasia can present as a suspicious mass, but tends to be less dense. Ductal carcinoma in situ (DCIS) typically presents with calcification. DCIS masses can occur, but are usually not calcified and may be circumscribed. Lobular cancer may be invisible, a mass (particularly on the CC view), or as distortion or a shrinking breast. Complex sclerosing lesions can occur as density with distortion, and may require excision to make the diagnosis.

4. Increased breast density is a personal risk factor for breast cancer. Dense breast tissue may obscure a cancer, even a large one. Significant calcification (DCIS) is rarely obscured by dense tissue.

5. "Oval" and "lobular" are descriptions of the shape of a mass (BI-RADS 4)—lobulated mass will be dropped from the 5th edition of BI-RADS. The mass margin descriptors include:

   i. "Circumscribed"
   ii. "Lobulated"
   iii. "Microlobulated"
   iv. "Angulated"
   v. "Spiculated"

Pearls

- Cancers can be difficult to see in dense breast tissue.
- Look for signs of displaced tissue or an asymmetry that does not follow normal tissue planes.
- Use spot/spot magnification views to further characterize the margins of a suspected mass.
- Tomosynthesis (if available) would likely help visualize the lesion in one examination.
- Do full mammographic workup prior to ultrasound.

Suggested Readings

Boyd NF, Melnichouk O, Martin LJ, et al. Mammographic density, response to hormones, and breast cancer risk. *J Clin Oncol.* 2011;29(22):2985-2992.

Checka CM, Chun JE, Schnabel FR, Lee J, Toth H. The relationship of mammographic density and age: implications for breast cancer screening. *AJR Am J Roentgenol.* 2012;198(3):W292-W295.

King V, Brooks JD, Bernstein JL, Reiner AS, Pike MC, Morris EA. Background parenchymal enhancement at breast MR imaging and breast cancer risk. *Radiology.* 2011;260(1):50-60.

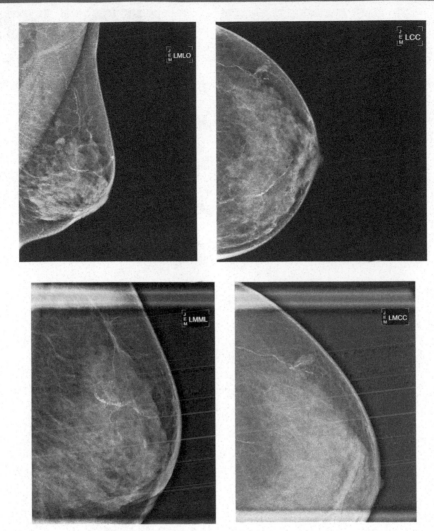

1. Why is it important to obtain postbiopsy mammogram?

2. What is the reason for clip displacement?

3. What can help in this situation after displacement of the clip?

4. How would you characterize the calcifications in the left breast?

5. What would be the next step to manage the situation?

Case ranking/difficulty:

Category: Diagnostic

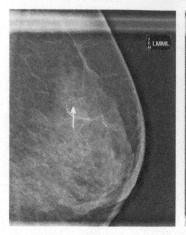 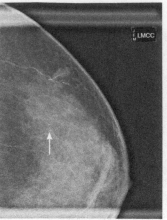 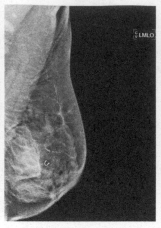 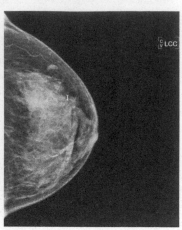

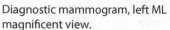

Diagnostic mammogram, left ML magnificent view.

Diagnostic mammogram, left CC magnificent view.

Mammogram, left MLO view, after clip placement.

Mammogram, left CC view, after clip placement.

Answers

1. Postbiopsy mammogram is absolutely necessary to determine if the clip is in good location, if the clip is in the same location at the calcifications sampled (see *arrows*).

2. The accordion effect explains the movement of a clip due to compression and release of compression during the stereotactic biopsy. Clip displacement can also be caused by bleeding or hematoma. All the other factors mentioned are not documented in the literature.

3. Any landmark or residual pathology can be helpful to improve accuracy doing the needle localization. If the pathology is completely removed, like in our case, it is tricky. If the clip is on the *z*-axis deeper than the biopsied target, it is reasonable to target the clip, given that the abnormality biopsied should be on the track of the wire. However, if the clip is short to the target zone, another modality might be helpful to see the scar from the biopsy and thus determine the actual target zone. MRI was performed, which demonstrated residual enhancement in the target zone and subsequently second clip was inserted with MRI guidance.

4. Noted are benign vascular calcifications and also a group of "irregular and pleomorphic" calcifications.

5. Next step would be stereotactic biopsy. Ultrasound could also be added to investigate if there is a solid component. However, just to do the stereotactic biopsy would also be not unreasonable.

Pearls

- If a small group of calcifications is completely removed by the vacuum-assisted core biopsy needle, it is crucial to prove that the clip is in the area biopsied by performing postbiopsy mammogram.

- In this particular case, post–core biopsy images (MLO and CC views) demonstrate that the clip is displaced about 4 cm inferior from the target zone and 1.5 cm anterior.

- Clip displacement has direct effect on the planning of the needle localization because the target zone cannot be directly targeted if there are no residual calcifications or other landmark that could be used for needle localization.

- Clip displacement can be deep or superficial to the target zone—the latter is the more complicated situation.

- Clip usually migrates along the *z*-axis (compression axis) at the time of compression release due to the fact that clip might not be anchored to the wall of the biopsy cavity but to the adjacent tissue and that the distance is minimal during compression but can extend after decompression ("accordion effect").

Suggested Reading

Esserman LE, Cura MA, DaCosta D. Recognizing pitfalls in early and late migration of clip markers after imaging-guided directional vacuum-assisted biopsy. *Radiographics*. 2004;24(1):147-156.

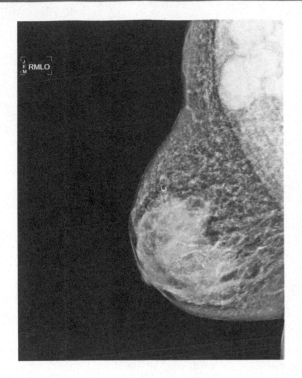 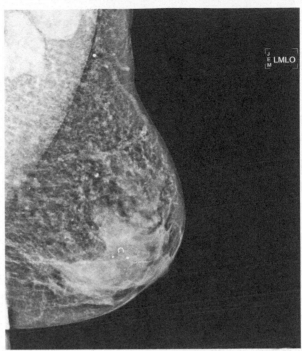

1. What are the findings seen on the screening mammogram?

2. What is part of differential diagnosis of bilateral axillary lymphadenopathy?

3. What are typical findings related to amyloidosis in the breast?

4. What would be the appropriate workup of the lymph nodes in case of lack of old images?

5. What would be an appropriate approach to biopsy these lymph nodes?

Case ranking/difficulty:

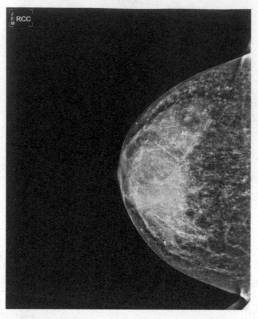

Screening mammogram, right CC view demonstrating scattered benign calcifications and clip from prior benign biopsy.

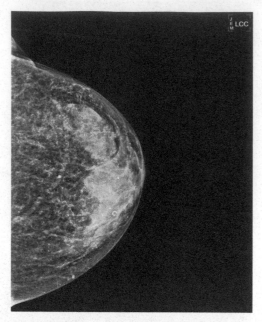

Screening mammogram, left CC view demonstrating benign scattered calcifications and clip from prior benign biopsy.

Answers

1. Noted is bilateral lymphadenopathy. Also noted are scattered benign-appearing calcifications bilaterally.

2. Differential diagnosis can include Rheumatoid Arthritis, Scleroderma, Sarcoidosis, Lymphoma, Leukemia, Lung cancer or melanoma.

3. Amyloidosis can result in the presence of masses; they can appear suspicious and oftentimes, biopsy is necessary. Also possible in the presence of calcifications—they are more likely scattered and more coarse.

4. The patient history is the key. In this case, the presence of systemic disease, such as rheumatoid arthritis, explains the situation. If any remaining concern, ultrasound should be performed and possible biopsy.

5. Ultrasound-guided core biopsy is the best choice. Alternative could be ultrasound-guided fine needle aspiration.

Pearls

- Amyloidosis is characterized by protein deposition within extracellular tissue. It involves primarily the heart, kidneys, skin, musculoskeletal system, and lungs.
- It can be a primary systemic disease or secondary to inflammatory systemic conditions, such as autoimmune disease.
- Presentation of amyloidosis on mammogram is rare. It can present as an incidental or palpable mass but also as clustered microcalcifications.

Suggested Readings

Cao MM, Hoyt AC, Bassett LW. Mammographic signs of systemic disease. *Radiographics*. 2011;31(4):1085-1100.

Munson-Bernardi BD, DePersia LA. Amyloidosis of the breast coexisting with ductal carcinoma in situ. *AJR Am J Roentgenol*. 2006;186(1):54-55.

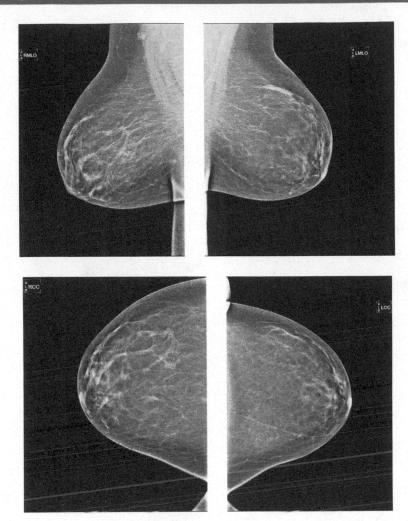

1. What is the BI-RADS category for this screening exam?

2. What was the abnormality you saw that prompted recall from screening?

3. What is the best description for the distribution of calcifications?

4. What is the likely final pathology in this patient?

5. What should be the next radiological investigation to determine the extent of this disease?

Case ranking/difficulty:

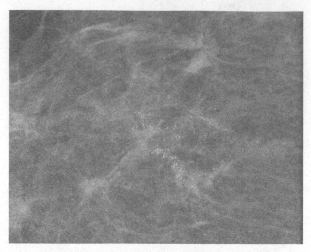

Spot compression with magnification. This shows the small "indistinct" masses with calcifications in a "segmental" distribution between the masses.

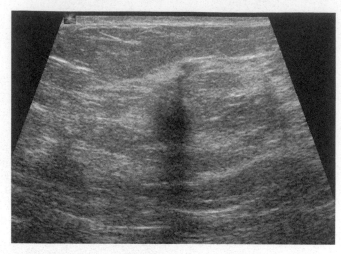

Ultrasound shows a "non-parallel" irregular mass with "acoustic shadowing," consistent with malignancy.

Answers

1. This is a screening exam; therefore, only BI-RADS 0, 1, and 2 are allowed. Further imaging required. Recommend inclusion of spot magnification views to further characterize the calcification particles.

2. Some readers find it easier to perceive cancers when they are associated with calcifications, especially in dense breasts. In this case, there is at least one spiculated mass and several clusters and segmental calcifications, associated with focal asymmetries, suggesting multifocal or even multicentric disease.

3. The calcifications reflect a segment of the milk ducts (a suspicious feature). Multiple clusters of calcifications could be used, but clustered calcification is a nonspecific descriptor. If you feel the calcifications are likely suspicious, and they conform to a segment, then segmental calcifications can be used to indicate your suspicion.

4. The radiological features of the calcifications are highly suspicious of DCIS. The individual calcific particles are pleomorphic and have sharp irregular margins. According to the Tabar classification, these are a crushed rock appearance. The distribution is composed of clusters arranged in a segmental pattern, with some of the calcium rearranging themselves into a more linear pattern.

5. Ultrasound is routinely performed but may not show the extent of the disease. Multiple areas of shadowing may be observed, which may not necessarily be due to further disease. PEM has been advocated particularly in women

with dense breasts, where the technique may pick up additional foci not visualized on the mammogram. MRI would be the best next radiological exam to determine the extent of disease and to stage the disease, lymph nodes, and contralateral breast.

Pearls

- Multifocal disease is within the same anatomic segment of breast tissue.
- Multicentric disease affects multiple areas of the breast with discontinuous disease, and there could be occult disease that has not yet been detected.
- DCIS may be seen in continuity between the tumor masses.

Suggested Readings

Ustaalioglu BO, Bilici A, Kefeli U, et al. The importance of multifocal/multicentric tumor on the disease-free survival of breast cancer patients: single center experience. *Am J Clin Oncol.* 2011;35(6):580-586.

White J, Achuthan R, Turton P, Lansdown M. Breast conservation surgery: state of the art. *Int J Breast Cancer.* 2011;(2011):107981.

Yerushalmi R, Tyldesley S, Woods R, Kennecke HF, Speers C, Gelmon KA. Is breast-conserving therapy a safe option for patients with tumor multicentricity and multifocality? *Ann Oncol.* 2012;23(4):876-881.

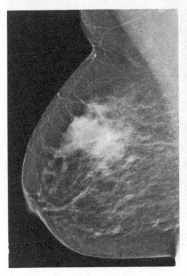 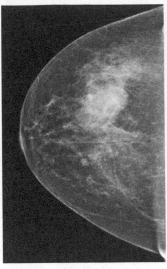 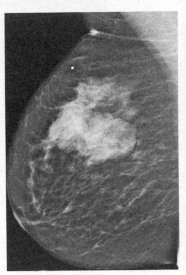 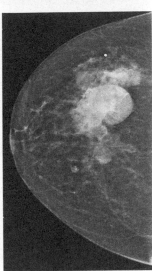

1. Is there any pertinent abnormality seen?

2. What could be the pitfalls in this particular case?

3. Why was an MRI performed in that case?

4. Is it important to work up the masses each time patient comes to screening?

5. What would be the appropriate management of screening mammogram of an asymptomatic patient with known fibrocystic changes?

Case ranking/difficulty:

Category: Diagnostic

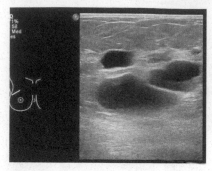

Ultrasound directed to the area of concern demonstrates multiple simple cysts.

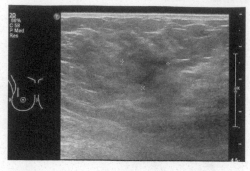

Ultrasound directed to the area of concern demonstrates an area of low echogenicity located close to the fibrocystic changes. It is "irregular" in shape and about 1.3 cm in maximum diameter.

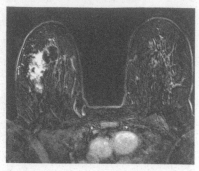

MRI postcontrast demonstrating large area of non–mass-like enhancement.

Answers

1. Patient has history of fibrocystic changes as described on prior ultrasound exams. Again noted are multiple benign-appearing masses, which have fluctuated over time. There is a questionable new "focal asymmetry" on right superior MLO view.

2. Any palpable abnormality requires first diagnostic workup with additional spot compression views and BB marker on the area of concern (not submitted in this particular case—but performed)—then ultrasound should be performed in any circumstance to better characterize the abnormality.

3. Breast MRI in this case is helpful to better address the extent of the lesion and subsequently the appropriate surgical approach. It is also helpful to address the situation in the contralateral breast and to address possible lymphadenopathy.

4. If a screening exam shows multiple bilateral scattered benign-appearing masses and in the past patient has had ultrasound demonstrating benign cysts, there is no need to work up the cysts each time. This is true even if the mammographically benign-appearing masses fluctuate slightly in size. However, if there are new suspicious morphological features, such as "architectural distortion," new "focal asymmetry," or calcifications, patient needs to be called back for additional workup.

5. If a patient has multiple bilateral scattered benign-appearing masses on mammogram, which have been shown in the past on ultrasound to represent benign cysts, even if they fluctuate in size, there is no need to perform a diagnostic workup. Cysts can fluctuate in size (see Leung and Sickles, 2000). Assessment can be BI-RADS 2.

Pearls

- Despite history of benign fibrocystic changes and mammogram showing corresponding waxing and waning masses, consistent with cysts as seen on prior ultrasound, any new palpable mass raises concern and could be due to additional malignancy that can be obscured by the surrounding benign cysts.
- Most mucinous carcinomas present as mass on ultrasound, oftentimes with microlobulation. However, if the tumor is not pure mucinous in nature, ultrasound can also represent irregular shaped hypoechoic mass, like in this case.
- MRI was also performed and demonstrated large area of abnormal non–mass-like enhancement that was significantly larger than it appeared on the ultrasound.

Suggested Readings

Lam WW, Chu WC, Tse GM, Ma TK. Sonographic appearance of mucinous carcinoma of the breast. *AJR Am J Roentgenol.* 2004;182(4):1069-1074.

Leung JW, Sickles EA. Multiple bilateral masses detected on screening mammography: assessment of need for recall imaging. *AJR Am J Roentgenol.* 2000;175(1):23-29.

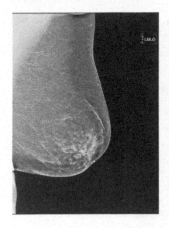 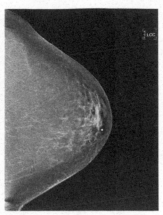 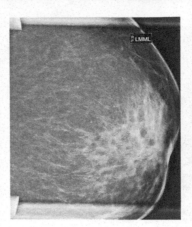 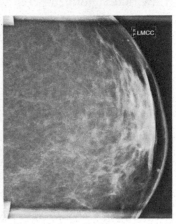

1. What is the next step after a normal mammogram when patient has palpable lump?

2. If ultrasound is normal as well, what is the next step?

3. Is an additional MRI standard of care to evaluate palpable breast abnormality after normal mammogram and ultrasound?

4. What is the significance of an ultrasound (image next page) finding?

5. What is the reason to add an MRI preoperatively?

Case ranking/difficulty:

Category: Diagnostic

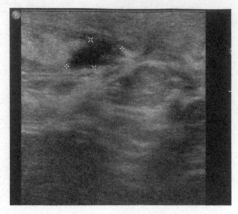

Ultrasound demonstrates hypoechoic solid area in the medial left breast in the area of palpable abnormality.

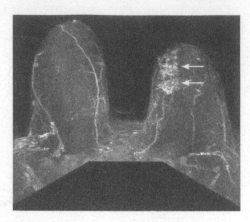

MRI does confirm a larger than expected area of "non–mass-like enhancement."

Answers

1. Standard of care is to perform diagnostic mammogram including spot compression views and ultrasound for a palpable abnormality.

2. If mammogram and ultrasound are unremarkable, the exam can be called BI-RADS 1 ("negative"). However, it is helpful to add a statement that "despite normal imaging further evaluation of the palpable abnormality should be based on clinical grounds." That can include biopsy of the palpable abnormality by a breast surgeon if the palpable abnormality is suspicious enough.

3. After normal mammogram and ultrasound in a patient of palpable abnormality, it is not standard of care to add MRI. However, in selected cases, MRI could be helpful as additional test to evaluate palpable abnormality. This is in particular the case if the breast tissue is very dense on mammogram and if the palpable abnormality is highly suspicious based on the clinical evaluation or in the setting of very strong family history.

4. Ultrasound finding is consistent with hypoechoic nodule—it does not show posterior enhancement and does not fulfill all the criteria of simple cyst. Therefore, and in particular since the finding was palpable, ultrasound-guided biopsy was performed and demonstrates findings consistent with lobular invasive carcinoma.

5. MRI is helpful to assess the extent of the disease and to look for additional malignancy, to exclude multifocal (same quadrant) or multicentric (different quadrants) disease.

Pearls

- In case of palpable abnormality, despite a normal diagnostic mammogram, ultrasound is crucial for further evaluation.
- The most common ultrasound presentation of an infiltrative lobular carcinoma is an irregular or "angular" mass with "ill-defined" or "spiculated" margins. However, there are also other ultrasound presentations of ILC, which includes even the presence of a "well-circumscribed" mass as in this case.
- In general, the false-negative rate of mammograms for ILC is much higher than for invasive ductal carcinoma due to the diffuse growth pattern of lobular carcinomas ("Indian file pattern of growth" as described by the pathologists).

Suggested Reading

Lopez JK, Bassett LW. Invasive lobular carcinoma of the breast: spectrum of mammographic, US, and MR imaging findings. *Radiographics*. 2009;29(1):165-176.

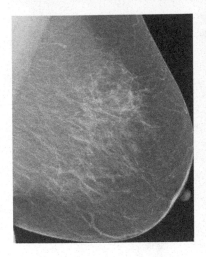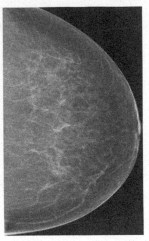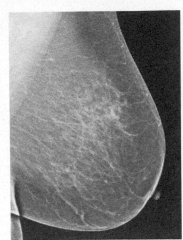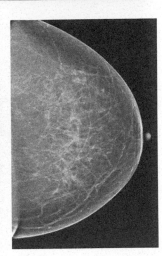

1. If you suspect subtle "architectural distortion," what is the next step?

2. What can be the etiology for "architectural distortion"?

3. If there is architectural distortion and no abnormality on ultrasound, what is the next step?

4. Why is it challenging to see subtle "architectural distortion"?

5. Why is the history of the patient important?

Case ranking/difficulty: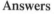

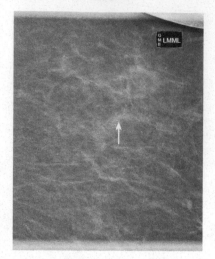

Diagnostic mammogram, left spot compression ML view demonstrating very subtle "architectural distortion."

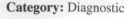
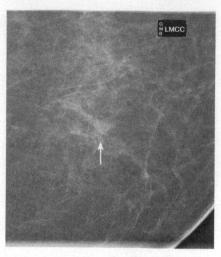

Diagnostic mammogram, left spot compression CC view demonstrating subtle "architectural distortion."

Answers

1. Next step is diagnostic mammogram with spot compression views.

2. "Architectural distortion" can be caused by variety of different etiologies, including prior biopsy or surgery and atypical ductal hyperplasia.

3. If there is no abnormality on ultrasound, stereotactic biopsy is the next step.

4. To find subtle "architectural distortion" is the most challenging topic in mammography and yet very important, since oftentimes "architectural distortion" is related to the presence of invasive ductal carcinoma.

5. Excisional biopsy or lumpectomy would cause architectural distortion—all other procedures as mentioned above in general do not result in the presence of distortion, although in rare cases can cause some distortion as well.

Pearls

- If there is presence of architectural distortion on mammogram, as confirmed on spot compression views, despite normal ultrasound, stereotactic biopsy is recommended.

- Since it is documented that between 4% and 54% of lesions reported on core biopsies as atypical ductal hyperplasia are upgraded on further surgical excision to invasive carcinoma, surgical intervention is recommended.

Suggested Readings

Deshaies I, Provencher L, Jacob S, et al. Factors associated with upgrading to malignancy at surgery of atypical ductal hyperplasia diagnosed on core biopsy. *Breast*. 2011;20(1):50-55.

Samardar P, de Paredes ES, Grimes MM, Wilson JD. Focal asymmetric densities seen at mammography: US and pathologic correlation. *Radiographics*. 2002;22(1):19-33.

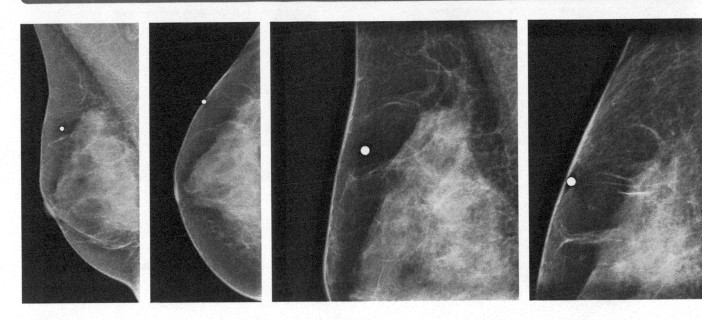

1. What do you do if palpable mass does not show up on diagnostic mammogram?

2. What do you do if mammogram and ultrasound are normal in the area of palpable abnormality?

3. What characterizes an adenoid cystic carcinoma?

4. What are the typical imaging features of adenoid cystic carcinoma?

5. What is the most likely treatment?

Case ranking/difficulty: 🪲🪲🪲

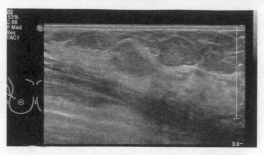

Ultrasound of the right breast, area of concern. Mass with "angular" margin.

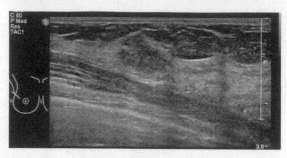

Ultrasound of the right breast, area of concern with harmonic imaging that helps to increase contrast between mass and fat nodules.

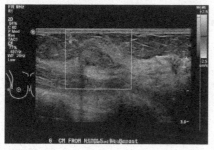

Ultrasound of the right breast, area of concern with duplex confirming flow in the mass.

Answers

1. This is a good example where ultrasound does show the abnormality. Thus, it is critical not to stop after a normal mammogram workup but to perform ultrasound.

2. A mass felt by the patient is always an important issue and critical for the radiologist to take seriously. If mammogram including diagnostic workup with spot compression views is normal and ultrasound is normal, the likelihood that patient has any malignancy is low, but there are cases where despite normal imaging there is a malignancy. The likelihood is higher in dense breast tissue. Thus, in general, the decision whether palpation-based biopsy (not imaging-based biopsy) should be performed by a breast surgeon will depend on the clinical situation and the level of concern based on the palpation. Since the breast exam in the ultrasound is in general not done by the radiologist, a statement like "further management should be based on clinical grounds" is appropriate.

3. It is a subgroup of adenocarcinoma with low rate of lymph node metastasis but not infrequent presence of distant metastasis, in general, to the lungs.

4. It usually presents as an asymmetry or indistinct mass on mammogram, without calcifications. On ultrasound,

it usually demonstrates an angular and microlobulated mass with mixed echogenicity. It might not show up at all on ultrasound and mammogram.

5. In most cases, tumor is treated with surgical resection and radiation therapy, which will lower the rate of possible recurrence.

Pearls

- Adenoid cystic carcinoma of the breast is a rare tumor accounting for less than 0.1% of all breast cancers. It is a variant of an adenocarcinoma with relative good prognosis. Distant metastasis, most likely to the lung, can occur, with axillary metastasis being rare.
- Mammography demonstrates in general "lobular"-shaped mass with "microlobulated" or "indistinct" margin. Calcifications were not reported.
- On sonography, adenoid cystic carcinoma of the breast shows "irregular"-shaped mass with hypoechoic or heterogeneous echotexture. Margins are often "angular" or "indistinct."

Suggested Readings

Glazebrook KN, Reynolds C, Smith RL, et al. Adenoid cystic carcinoma of the breast. *AJR Am J Roentgenol*. 2010;194(5):139-126.

Stavros T. *Breast Ultrasound*. 1st ed. Lippincott Williams & Wilkins. Philadelphia, PA; 2004.

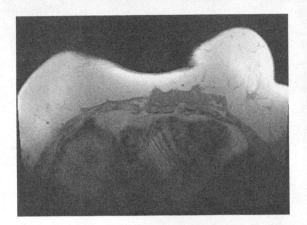
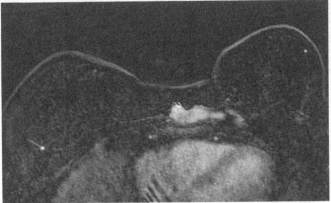

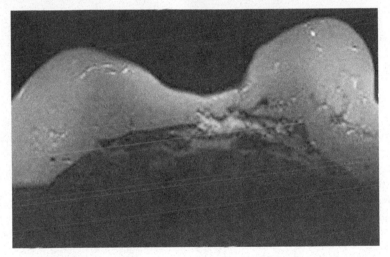

1. What are the findings on the MRI?

2. Based on the MRI what is the situation in regard to the chest wall?

3. What is the practical consequence of these images?

4. What is a desmoid of the breast?

5. What is the treatment for desmoid of the breast?

Case ranking/difficulty:

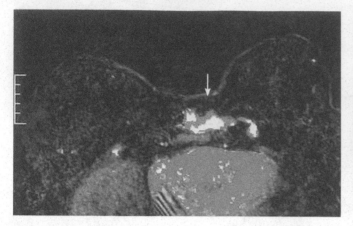

MRI T1-weighted sequence after IV contrast, with subtraction and CAD color coding demonstrating mass in the medial left breast near chest wall with mixed enhancement kinetics.

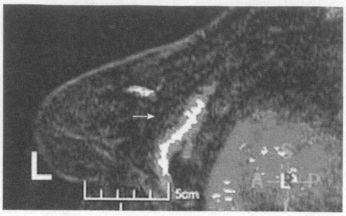

MRI T1-weighted sequence after IV contrast, with subtraction and CAD with mass in the posterior breast near chest wall.

Answers

1. Noted is strongly enhancing mass near the chest wall in the left medial breast. It does enhance strongly after IV contrast and is suspicious for malignancy.

2. Chest wall involvement can be assessed on MRI. There is no fat plane remaining and enhancement of the chest wall—therefore, this is consistent with chest wall infiltration.

3. Because of the very posterior location of the lesion, correlation with ultrasound is crucial, since ultrasound-guided biopsy is easier than MRI or stereotactic biopsy. Mammogram is always indicated as the base of all breast imaging.

4. Mammary fibromatosis or desmoid is a rare form of breast mass, which consists of benign proliferative stromal tissue. It has a high rate of recurrence.

5. First line of treatment is surgical resection. Radiation therapy might be added to obtain local control in recurrent fibromatosis. Hormonal agents might be added, since some desmoids show estrogen receptor or progesterone receptor activity. Low-dose chemotherapy also has been shown to be effective in some cases.

Pearls

- Mammary fibromatosis presents usually as palpable mass that is clinically suspicious for malignancy.
- Mammary fibromatosis may occur spontaneously or can occur after trauma or surgical procedure, such as breast reduction.
- The best imaging technique to evaluate the extent of the tumor is breast MRI. Signal on T1-weighted sequences is in general isointense to muscle. T2-weighted images show a variety of signal intensities. Enhancement patterns are usually more dominated by benign-progressive enhancement instead of washout enhancement.
- Differential diagnosis includes metaplastic carcinoma, spindle cell type, low-grade fibrosarcoma, nodular fasciitis, and scar after surgery.
- Treatment includes complete surgical resection. Radiation therapy has been used to obtain local control in recurrent fibromatosis.

Suggested Reading

Glazebrook KN, Reynolds CA. Mammary fibromatosis. *AJR Am J Roentgenol.* 2009;193(3):856-860.

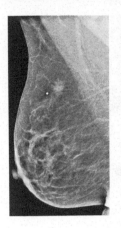
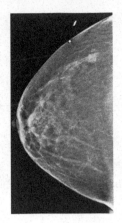
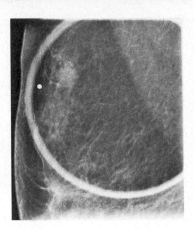
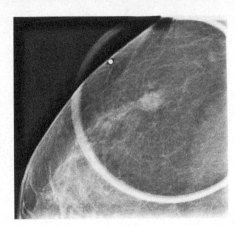

1. What is the next step given this mammogram with "focal asymmetry" and palpable lump?

2. What ultrasound finding could explain the mammogram finding?

3. What are typical features of spindle cell tumor of the breast?

4. What is the prognosis of spindle cell tumor?

5. What are the characteristic features of squamous cell carcinoma of the breast?

Case ranking/difficulty: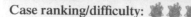

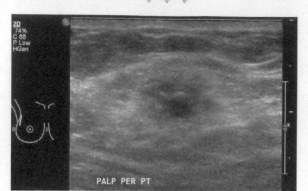

Ultrasound demonstrates "complex mass" with hypoechoic center and thick hyperechoic halo.

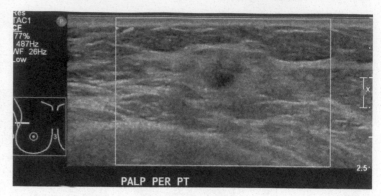

Duplex demonstrates no increased flow.

Answers

1. Any palpable abnormality has to raise high alert and biopsy has to be considered. This is especially the case if there is any morphological abnormality that correlates to the finding. All BI-RADS 3 ("probably benign") findings are in general not palpable, such as benign-appearing "round and oval" mass, "focal asymmetry" without ultrasound finding, and "round and oval" group of calcifications as seen on first screening mammogram.

2. If there was an appropriate history of trauma or surgery, fat necrosis or hematoma could have the same appearance. Also, invasive ductal carcinoma or even a phyllodes tumor with cystic changes could appear similar.

3. It is a very rare entity that consists of spindle cells with island of squamous cells. It can contain, in addition, in situ or invasive lobular or ductal carcinoma. But it is believed to derive from epithelial elements. There is no typical or specific morphological feature.

4. Spindle cell tumor has in general a good prognosis despite lack of estrogen receptors but due to the fact that it does not in general metastasize.

5. Very rare tumor with bad prognosis due to frequent distant metastasis. Tumor derives from epithelial cyst, either from the skin or from deep dermoid cysts.

Pearls

- Spindle cell carcinoma is a very rare type of breast cancer and appears as well-circumscribed tumor containing cystic areas.
- It has also been described as squamous carcinoma with spindle metaplasia due to histology showing sheets of spindle-shaped cells with islands of cells with squamous cell differentiation.
- Other names for the same entity are pseudocarcinoma and sarcomatoid carcinoma.
- Spindle cell carcinomas are low in estrogen receptors, but they are considered less likely to metastasize and have overall good prognosis.
- Spindle cell carcinoma should not be confused with squamous cell carcinoma of the breast, which is more aggressive and has higher rate of metastasis and which is related to epidermis cells, for example, from a deep-seated dermoid cyst.

Suggested Reading

Maemura M, Iino Y, Oyama T, et al. Spindle cell carcinoma of the breast. *Jpn J Clin Oncol.* 1997;27(1):46-50.

68-year-old woman with history of left lumpectomy—new malignancy in the right breast: patient currently on neoadjuvant chemotherapy. Two lesions in the left breast: lesion 1 (top left image) and lesion 2 (top right image). Repeat MRI 10 days later. MRI (bottom left) and second look ultrasound (bottom right)

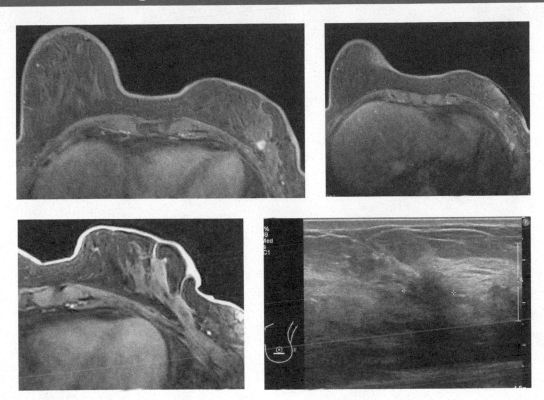

1. What can be a reason for fluctuating enhancement seen on MRI at different timing of the same patient?

2. Why is it helpful to perform second look ultrasound?

3. What is the key to perform ultrasound-guided biopsy?

4. In this case, despite disappearing lesion 1 ultrasound demonstrates abnormality—what is the next step?

5. What is the influence of chemotherapy on contrast enhancement on MRI?

Fluctuating enhancement after chemotherapy: lesion 1 with loss of enhancement (atypical ductal hyperplasia) and lesion 2 (the middle figure, the figure on the extreme right (top) and the bottom figure) with stable enhancement (fibrosis)

311

Case ranking/difficulty: **Category:** Diagnostic

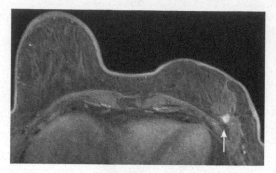

MRI, T1-weighted sequence after IV contrast demonstrating mass no. 1 in the left breast.

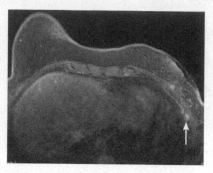

MR, T1-weighted sequence after IV contrast demonstrating mass no. 2 near chest wall.

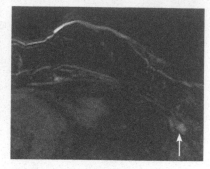

MRI, T1-weighted sequence after IV contrast, 10 days later still demonstrates mass no. 2 near chest wall.

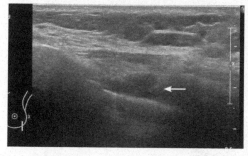

Second look ultrasound for lesion 2, left breast, demonstrates corresponding small "mass." Ultrasound-guided biopsy was performed and demonstrated hyalinized fibrosis.

Answers

1. Enhancement can be fluctuating due to compression by the coil—different timing in regard to the cycle due to hormonal stimulation—and, if there is no appropriate injection. This can be determined by looking at the enhancement of the heart. Also enhancement can fluctuate due to application of chemotherapy.

2. Second look ultrasound can be helpful to see a lesion since ultrasound-guided biopsy is easier to perform. In some cases, MRI-guided biopsy is technically impossible and ultrasound has to be performed to find the abnormality. Ultrasound is not more specific than MRI.

3. Important is close correlation of the ultrasound with the MRI in regard to location of the suspicious lesion. This can be done by a physician or a technologist under the guidance of a physician. Subtle findings on ultrasound can be meaningful if it correlates in size and location to the MRI finding.

4. In general, any lesion with suspicious morphology such as the ultrasound finding—despite normal second MRI—

requires biopsy. It demonstrated atypical hyperplasia in this case and was subsequently excised.

5. Chemotherapy does decrease the uptake of contrast and can even completely eliminate contrast enhancement.

Pearls

- Fluctuating enhancement on MRI between two different exams of the same patient after short time period can be explained in a premenopausal woman with different timing of the exam in relationship to her menstrual cycle.
- MRI of the breast should be performed between days 6 and 12 of the cycle to minimize influence of hormonal simulation.
- In this postmenopausal woman, fluctuating enhancement can be due to prior chemotherapy, changing vascularization of the tumor.
- Second look ultrasound is an important next step for lesions that are seen on MRI but not accessible for core biopsy due to their location.

Suggested Readings

Abe H, Schmidt RA, Shah RN, et al. MR-directed ("Second-Look") ultrasound examination for breast lesions detected initially on MRI: MR and sonographic findings. *AJR Am J Roentgenol.* 2010;194(2):370-377.

Partridge SC, Gibbs JE, Lu Y, Esserman LJ, Sudilovsky D, Hylton NM. Accuracy of MR imaging for revealing residual breast cancer in patients who have undergone neoadjuvant chemotherapy. *AJR Am J Roentgenol.* 2002;179(5):1193-1199.

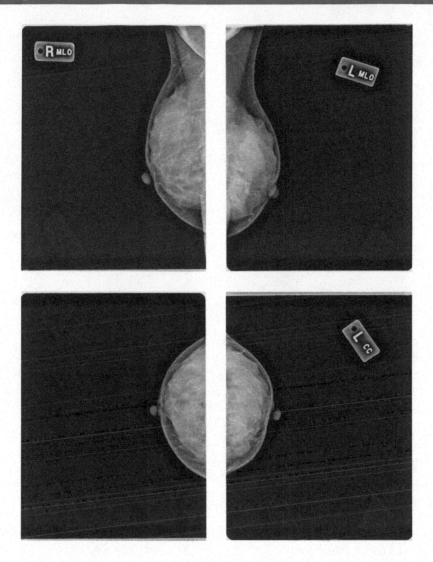

1. What is the BI-RADS category for this diagnostic exam?

2. What pathologies typically present as distortion only?

3. If the biopsy shows a radial scar, what is the likelihood of associated malignancy?

4. What is the breast density in this patient?

5. What should be the next radiological investigation to determine the extent of this disease?

Case ranking/difficulty:

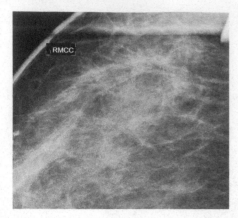

Another case with vague "architectural distortion" only. Difficult to see, even though you know the patient has pathologically enlarged nodes.

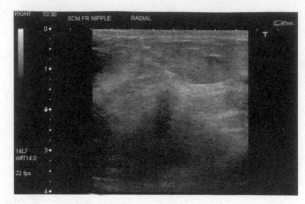

Targeted ultrasound of this second case shows a vague mass deep in the breast.

Answers

1. This is a diagnostic exam; therefore, BI-RADS 0 is not allowed. Findings of distortion in the left lower inner quadrant. With the presence of an obvious cancer on physical exam (if you have examined the patient), you could equally give this a BI-RADS 5.

2. Virtually all of the above can present as distortion. Even a rapidly growing fibroadenoma can present as distortion but would occur with an obvious mass.

3. Radial scars (or complex sclerosing lesions) are frequently associated with low-grade DCIS or may be the "benign" part of a tubular carcinoma with long spicules. Accurately sampling a radial scar may allow these lesions to be followed rather than excised, but there are two schools of thought on this. One says *all* radial scars should be excised, and the other says that sampling all parts of the periphery is enough if no malignancy is found.

4. These breasts are extremely dense, and a lobular cancer, which can be difficult to spot at the best of times, can be harder in dense breasts. Look for progressive distortion or shrinking of a breast on subsequent mammograms. Often may need a prior from at least 5 years earlier to appreciate the changes in the breast.

5. While many of the above tests have been used, MRI is the only test of proven benefit to study the extent of disease and screen the contralateral breast.

Pearls

- ILC may present in atypical ways.
- Distortion and asymmetry are found in place of a mass in around 25% of cases, but a mass may still be found.

Suggested Readings

Albayrak ZK, Onay HK, Karataǧ GY, Karataǧ O. Invasive lobular carcinoma of the breast: mammographic and sonographic evaluation. *Diagn Interv Radiol*. 2011;17(3):232-238.

Evans WP, Warren Burhenne LJ, Laurie L, O'Shaughnessy KF, Castellino RA. Invasive lobular carcinoma of the breast: mammographic characteristics and computer-aided detection. *Radiology*. 2002;225(1):182-189.

Michael M, Garzoli E, Reiner CS. Mammography, sonography and MRI for detection and characterization of invasive lobular carcinoma of the breast. *Breast Dis*. 2008;30(30):21-30.

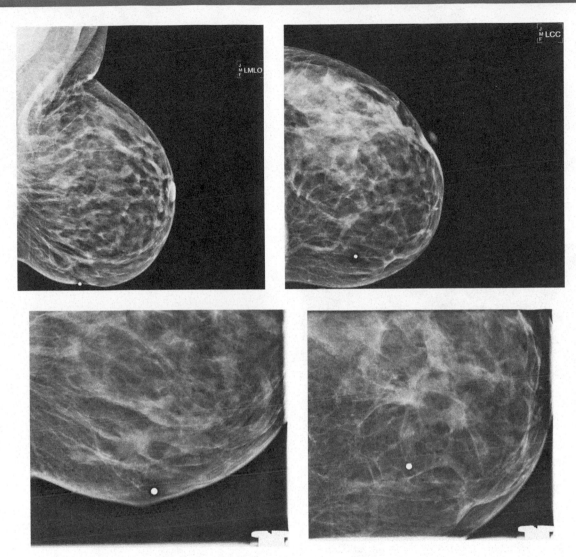

1. What is the initial reason for additional images?

2. What is the pertinent finding best seen on the spot compression views?

3. What is the next step?

4. What is the next step if ultrasound is normal?

5. What can cause the presence of architectural distortion on mammogram?

Case ranking/difficulty: **Category:** Diagnostic

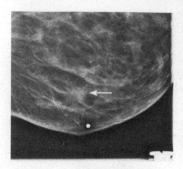

Left spot compression MLO view demonstrating subtle architectural distortion.

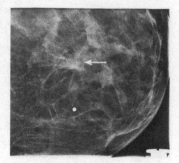

Left spot compression CC view demonstrating subtle architectural distortion.

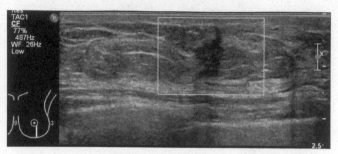

Ultrasound demonstrates "mass" with "posterior shadowing" corresponding to palpable abnormality.

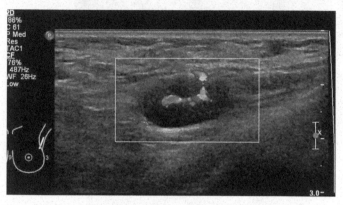

Ultrasound with duplex of axilla demonstrating suspicious penetrating cortical vessel.

Pearls

- Ultrasound is superior to mammography in assessing morphology of lymph node and to determine if lymph node is pathological.
- If lymph node presents on ultrasound with cortex of more than 3-mm thickness, in particular, if the thickening is eccentric and if there is the presence of penetrating cortical vessels, there is concern for malignancy.
- If there is concern, based on morphology, fine needle aspiration or core biopsy can be performed.

Answers

1. Patient felt lump in the left breast.

2. At the area of palpable abnormality, noted is subtle distortion, as best seen on the spot compression views.

3. Next step is ultrasound in further evaluation of the palpable abnormality.

4. If ultrasound is normal, there remains the issue of palpable abnormality and the presence of architectural distortion seen on mammogram. Subsequently, stereotactic biopsy should be attempted.

5. The etiology of architectural distortion can include underlying malignancy, proliferative changes like radial scar, old biopsy. In rare cases, even prior infection or bruise could cause architectural distortion.

Suggested Readings

Jung J, Park H, Park J, Kim H. Accuracy of preoperative ultrasound and ultrasound-guided fine needle aspiration cytology for axillary staging in breast cancer. *ANZ J Surg.* 2010;80(4):271-275.

Mainiero MB, Cinelli CM, Koelliker SL, Graves TA, Chung MA. Axillary ultrasound and fine-needle aspiration in the preoperative evaluation of the breast cancer patient: an algorithm based on tumor size and lymph node appearance. *AJR Am J Roentgenol.* 2010;195(5): 1261-1267.

Walsh R, Kornguth PJ, Soo MS, Bentley R, DeLong DM. Axillary lymph nodes: mammographic, pathologic, and clinical correlation. *AJR Am J Roentgenol.* 1997;168(1):33-38.

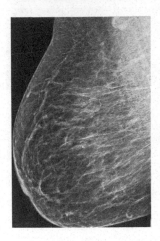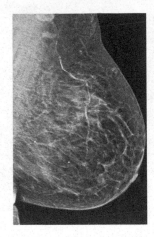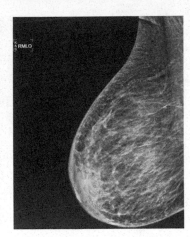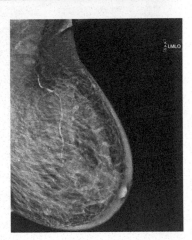

1. What are the findings seen on that mammogram?

2. What would be the differential diagnosis if that finding was only seen in one breast?

3. What are the characteristics of inflammatory breast cancer?

4. What are the symptoms that differentiate mastitis from inflammatory carcinoma?

5. How can inflammatory breast cancer be diagnosed?

Case ranking/difficulty: 🔨 🔨 🔨

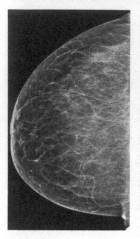

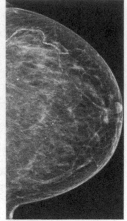

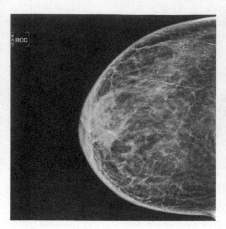

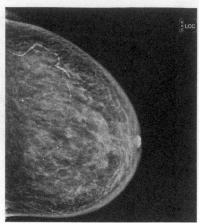

Screening mammogram, right CC view 2007.

Screening mammogram, left CC view 2007.

Screening mammogram, right CC view 2009 demonstrates reticular markings and skin thickening.

Screening mammogram, left CC view 2009 demonstrating reticular markings and skin thickening.

Answers

1. This is a typical case of bilateral, symmetric thickening of the skin and trabecular/parenchymal thickening due to congestive heart failure.

2. In case of this finding being present only in one breast, the differential diagnosis includes radiation-induced edema, inflammatory breast cancer, and mastitis. Most important is not to miss an inflammatory breast cancer. Even CHF in rare cases can affect only one side.

3. Inflammatory breast cancer is the most aggressive and fatal form with a 5-year survival period of around 5% being treated with surgery or radiation therapy. It can manifest with redness of the skin and could present like a mastitis. It is generally unilateral. Inflammatory breast cancer usually affects rather younger females.

4. Inflammatory breast cancer is most frequently unilateral, but can be bilateral in rare circumstances. It demonstrates thickening of the skin with orange peel appearance of the skin due to swelling of the follicles pits. There are, in general, no sings of infection such as leukocytosis, fever, and so on. Mastitis is more common in lactating females.

5. While all methods above can help to describe the findings and raise concern for underlying breast cancer. The best choice to diagnose inflammatory breast cancer is punch biopsy of the skin, which can demonstrate the pathognomonic feature of presence of numerous dermal tumor emboli in the papillary and reticular dermis. Punch biopsy is usually performed by a breast surgeon.

Pearls

- Reticular pattern within the breast and skin thickening can be due to cardiac heart failure (CHF). This is most likely bilateral but can be present unilateral in rare cases.
- If these findings are seen unilateral, differential diagnosis includes inflammatory breast cancer and radiation-induced edema.
- It is crucial not to miss an inflammatory breast cancer, since they are rapidly progressive with 5-year survival rate of less than 5%.
- Inflammatory breast cancer accounts for only 2.5% of all breast cancers.
- Skin punch biopsy, performed by breast surgeon, can confirm diagnosis of inflammatory breast cancer if skin is involved.

Suggested Readings

Ezeugwu C, Gidwani U, Oropello J, Benjamin E. Unilateral breast enlargement in association with congestive heart failure. *N J Med*. 1995;92(6):391-392.

Kamal RM, Hamed ST, Salem DS. Classification of inflammatory breast disorders and step by step diagnosis. *Breast J*. 2010;15(4):367-380.

Oraedu CO, Pinnapureddy P, Alrawi S, Acinapura AJ, Raju R. Congestive heart failure mimicking inflammatory breast carcinoma: a case report and review of the literature. *Breast J*. 2001;7(2):117-119.

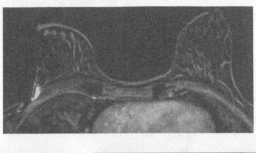
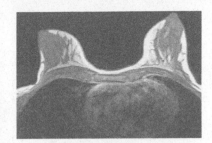

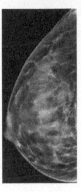
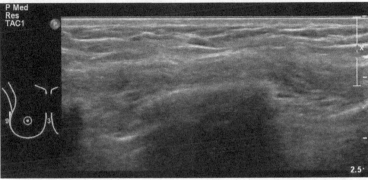

1. What artifacts can sometimes be seen on breast MRI?

2. What could be the solution for positioning related artifact?

3. How can malpositioning cause increased enhancement?

4. What could be the other reason why you might get motion artifact?

5. What is the remedy to misregistration artifact?

Case ranking/difficulty:

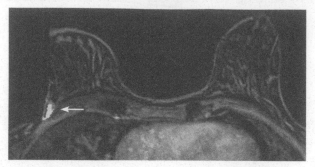

MRI after IV contrast and subtraction demonstrating area of "increased enhancement" in the right lateral breast near chest wall.

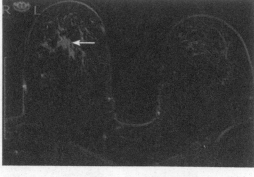

MRI postcontrast with subtraction demonstrating area of "washout enhancement" in the right central breast.

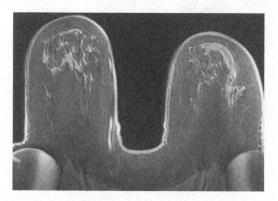

Corresponding source images, T1 postcontrast after IV contrast does not demonstrate focal suspicious abnormality or enhancement.

Answers

1. Misregistration artifacts can be seen at subtraction images due to motion and causing mass-like structures oftentimes overlaying fat parenchyma interfaces. Susceptibility artifacts are seen as drop out of signal and tissue distortion and are more common on gradient echo sequence due to lack of 180-degree pulses. Inhomogeneous fat suppression can be due to altered magnetic field such as due to metallic objects, or air in the chest. The remedy is to improve the tuning of the shim.

2. The patient could be called back and the MRI can be repeated. Ultrasound and mammogram might be helpful for correlation. Physical exam is helpful but is not sufficient without additional or repeat imaging to exclude malignancy.

3. Blood flow can be changed due to compression. An example can be the nipple that might be compressed against the coil and cause increased enhancement.

This can also result in increased enhancement due to mechanical compression elsewhere in the breast parenchyma.

4. Open door could cause interference with the signal causing "zipper artifact" through interference with outside RF impulse. All other factors on the list can cause movement artifacts.

5. The remedy is not to rely on the color-coded images, provided by the CAD workstation, but to use the source images (nonsubtracted images) to see if the enhancement is real.

Pearls

- MRI artifacts can be a reason to repeat the MRI scan.
- Enhancement caused by positioning can be confused with possible malignancy.
- Ghost artifacts are often motion induced and more prominent in phase-encoding direction.
- Misregistration on subtracted images is due to motion and can result in artifacts on the color-coded images on the workstation.
- Always look at the source images and do not entirely rely on the color-coded images on the workstation.

Suggested Reading

Ojeda-Fournier H, Choe KA, Mahoney MC. Recognizing and interpreting artifacts and pitfalls in MR imaging of the breast. *Radiographics*. 2007;27(Suppl 1):S147-S164.

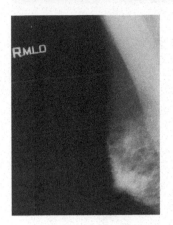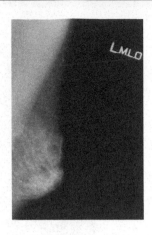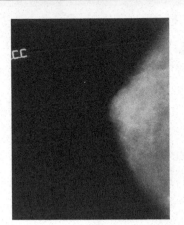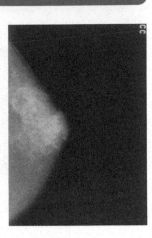

1. What is the BI-RADS category for this screening exam?

2. What is the differential diagnosis of an asymmetry in this position?

3. What is the next best imaging test?

4. What type of biopsy should be performed?

5. It is a solid lesion. Core biopsy shows fibrosis and apocrine metaplasia. Is the finding concordant?

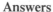
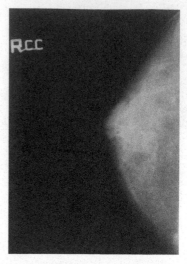

Medially turned CC—the mass is still at the medial edge of the film.

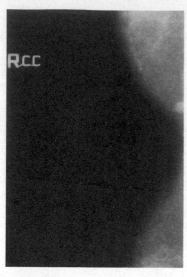

Cleavage view again shows the mass. Often this view is the most helpful in very medially placed tumors.

Answers

1. This is not a normal variant based on just this one image. Although it could be a sternalis muscle, further workup is required. If the features were characteristic of a sternalis muscle, then you can either describe the finding and give it a BI-RADS 2, or not describe it at all and give it a BI-RADS 1.

2. Most of the above can give rise to an "asymmetry" in the medial aspect of the breast. Sebaceous cysts often occur in the bra-line, and are difficult to tell apart from a malignancy, unless the tech has placed a skin marker on the lesion prior to the mammogram. The sternalis muscle is a common variant, normally seen on the right CC, which can look triangular or mass like. Ectopic breast tissue can occur in the lower medial breast, often with a nipple, although the most common presentation of this is accessory breast tissue in the axilla.

3. Tomosynthesis may not be helpful for lesions traditionally found at the edge of the film, due to the positioning. Currently, there are no data on this. Specialized diagnostic views to include cleavage views and medially exaggerated CC views may assist. Once localized, then ultrasound scanning should enable you to characterize the mass.

4. While any of the answers could be correct in differing situations, the best fit is that if the mass is seen to be solid, a biopsy should be recommended. A developing lesion this medial is much more likely to be malignant. Surgical excision is not warranted, unless the patient is extremely needle phobic, or there is another good reason not to perform a needle biopsy. MRI for a small mass should not necessarily be required, as it would be low

yield for a finding that would alter patient management A sebaceous cyst in the skin does not need excision unless it has gotten infected, and then you need to wait until the infection has settled. Simple cysts do not require drainage. If they are palpable or painful, you may be requested by a patient to aspirate it.

5. The findings are concordant. Routine follow-up would be the norm. However, if the patient is uncomfortable with leaving it in place, then you can offer vacuum-assisted diagnostic excision or surgical excision. There is no risk of the lesion being upgraded, and there is an absence of pathological evidence of atypia.

Pearls

- Case of malignancy at the margin of the film.
- One danger area to be aware of on any exam, especially if you have not yet seen an abnormality on the exam.

Suggested Readings

Leung JW, Sickles EA. Developing asymmetry identified on mammography: correlation with imaging outcome and pathologic findings. *AJR Am J Roentgenol.* 2007;188(3):667-675.

Sickles EA. The spectrum of breast asymmetries: imaging features, work-up, management. *Radiol Clin North Am.* 2007;45(5):765-771, v.

Venkatesan A, Chu P, Kerlikowske K, Sickles EA, Smith-Bindman R. Positive predictive value of specific mammographic findings according to reader and patient variables. *Radiology.* 2009;250(3):648-657.

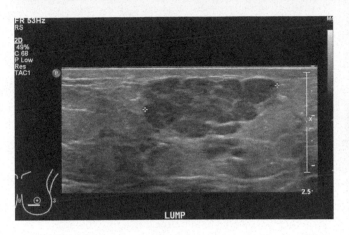

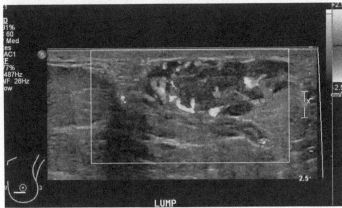

1. What is a lactating adenoma?

2. What is the connection of lactating adenoma to breast cancer?

3. What is the sonographic feature of lactating adenoma?

4. What is the management of palpable abnormality in pregnancy?

5. What is the management of a palpable breast mass during pregnancy?

Case ranking/difficulty: 🦷🦷🦷

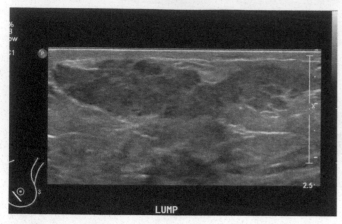

Mass on gray-scale ultrasound is heterogeneous in echogenicity, and extends "parallel to the chest wall" and is located in the anterior portion of the breast tissue.

Answers

1. Lactating adenoma is a benign condition and the most prevalent breast lesion in pregnant women and during puerperium. It occurs most likely in the third trimester of pregnancy. High concentrations of estrogen, progesterone, and prolactin promote the growth of ducts and formation of tubulo-alveolar structures. It consists of benign stromal alterations, although the etiology remains unclear.

2. The risk of associated breast cancer is not negligible, although the presence of lactating adenoma does not carry an increased risk of breast carcinoma. Lactating adenomas have been shown to express high amount of prolactin receptors, whose stimulation in a fully primed breast, as a result of lactation, could promote rapid growth of existing foci of breast cancer cells. Breast cancer is the second most common malignancy in pregnancy (1:1000).

3. Lactating adenomas are generally located in the anterior breast and are nontender on physical exam but firm and mobile. Sonographically, it had been described as oval, sharply circumscribed, solid hypoechoic mass, often with prominent central tubular structures presumed to be a dilatated duct. Occasionally, a lobulated contour or an ill-defined margin can be present. Most are orientated parallel to the chest wall. The mass mostly demonstrates posterior acoustic enhancement and rarely posterior acoustic shadowing.

4. Imaging of the pregnant or lactating patient is, in general, necessary for the evaluation of a palpable mass, bloody nipple discharge, suspicious findings for infection or abscess, pagetoid alterations of the nipple, or persistent axillary adenopathy. Ultrasound is the first choice due to lack of radiation and also due to the fact that the value of mammography is limited during pregnancy up to the 4th to 5th months after stopping lactation due to proliferation of breast tissue resulting in increased density. If ultrasound does not show the abnormality or if further imaging is necessary to assess additional lesions or microcalcifications, mammography can be performed.

5. In general, ultrasound-guided biopsy is the management of choice. If the lesion demonstrates only benign features, and the time of discovery is close to delivery, the lesion might be followed (BI-RADS 3).

Pearls

- Imaging of the symptomatic pregnant woman is necessary and can be performed with ultrasound and as second choice mammography.
- Standard 4 image mammogram results in dose of 0.4 rad, which is of no clinical concern. Dose of 10 rad or greater is considered to cause fetal malformations.
- Indication for core biopsy is same as for nonpregnant women.
- MRI should be avoided in pregnancy, since impact of gadolinium on fetus is under investigation and unclear at this point.
- Most breast masses in pregnancy are benign. However, breast cancer is the second most common malignancy in pregnancy (1:1000 pregnancies).

Suggested Readings

Behrndt VS, Barbakoff D, Askin FB, Brem RF. Infarcted lactating adenoma presenting as a rapidly enlarging breast mass. *AJR Am J Roentgenol.* 1999;173(4):933-935.

Magno S, Terribile D, Franceschini G, et al. Early onset lactating adenoma and the role of breast MRI: a case report. *J Med Case Rep.* 2009;3(3):43.

Sumkin JH, Perrone AM, Harris KM, Nath ME, Amortegui AJ, Weinstein BJ. Lactating adenoma: US features and literature review. *Radiology.* 1998;206(1):271-274.

Subject Index

Difficulty Level Index

Easy Cases

1626, 730, 1572, 1642, 1753, 1298, 583, 306, 1728, 394, 1646, 1307, 582, 586, 1864, 737, 602, 379, 1870, 610, 305, 1610, 1796, 340, 1574, 169, 680, 678, 1863, 615, 343, 616, 1741, 581, 167, 309, 165, 1765, 307, 1311, 1738, 1302, 1312, 607, 378, 1303, 1842, 734, 595, 324, 1843, 1862, 1749, 673, 596, 1583, 675, 1589, 622, 696, 617, 620, 599, 381, 609, 318, 601, 588, 377, 591, 613, 1744, 589, 677, 1573, 1641, 1643, 623, 585, 592, 580, 587, 119, 608, 731, 618

Moderately Difficult Cases

1865, 1308, 1797, 1868, 1310, 1838, 1762, 1309, 1761, 1304, 1754, 1306, 1745, 1742, 733, 1580, 321, 1578, 1625, 762, 761, 1612, 1627, 1000, 1611, 1001, 1628, 763, 688, 998, 729, 687, 758, 686, 683, 291, 674, 117, 614, 387, 413, 398, 397, 676, 395, 612, 390, 341, 611, 320, 593, 319, 317, 597, 314, 313, 594, 312, 310, 579, 292, 290, 1577, 264, 590, 263, 262, 584, 259, 606, 258, 684, 203, 202, 672, 201, 200, 681, 168, 164, 619, 163, 162, 1795, 141, 139, 224, 137

Most Difficult Cases

1305, 999, 764, 600, 393, 322, 1581, 759, 1299, 1740, 997, 755, 603, 732, 389, 353, 352, 351, 323, 311, 605, 257, 256, 204, 679, 69

Author Index